Sleep Disorders in Neurology

Sleep Disorders in Neurology

A Practical Approach

Edited by Sebastiaan Overeem and Paul Reading

Second Edition

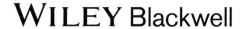

Registered Office(s)
John Wiley & Sons, Inc., 111 River Street, Hoboken, NJ 07030, USA
John Wiley & Sons Ltd, The Atrium, Southern Gate, Chichester, West Sussex, PO19 8SQ, UK

Editorial Office
9600 Garsington Road, Oxford, OX4 2DQ, UK

For details of our global editorial offices, customer services, and more information about Wiley products visit us at www.wiley.com.

Wiley also publishes its books in a variety of electronic formats and by print-on-demand. Some content that appears in standard print versions of this book may not be available in other formats.

Library of Congress Cataloging-in-Publication Data

Names: Overeem, Sebastiaan, editor. | Reading, Paul, editor.
Title: Sleep disorders in neurology : a practical approach / edited by Sebastiaan Overeem,
    Paul Reading.
Other titles: Sleep disorders in neurology (Overeem)
Description: Second edition. | Hoboken, NJ : Wiley, 2017. | Includes bibliographical references
    and index. |
Identifiers: LCCN 2018007682 (print) | LCCN 2018008043 (ebook) | ISBN 9781118777244 (pdf) |
    ISBN 9781118777220 (epub) | ISBN 9781118777268 (cloth)
Subjects: | MESH: Sleep Wake Disorders–complications | Nervous System Diseases–complications
Classification: LCC RC547 (ebook) | LCC RC547 (print) | NLM WL 108 | DDC 616.8/498–dc23
LC record available at https://lccn.loc.gov/2018007682

Cover Design: Wiley
Cover Image: © Marjot/iStock

Set in 10/12pt Warnock by SPi Global, Pondicherry, India
Printed in Singapore by C.O.S. Printers Pte Ltd

10 9 8 7 6 5 4 3 2 1

Contents

List of Contributors

Kirstie N. Anderson
Regional Sleep Service
Newcastle upon Tyne Hospital NHS
Foundation Trust
Newcastle upon Tyne
UK

Isabelle Arnulf
Sleep Disorders Unit
Pitié-Salpêtrière Hospital (APHP),
Sorbonne University
Paris
France

Claudio L. Bassetti
Department of Neurology
Bern University Hospital
Bern
Switzerland

Christian R. Baumann
Department of Neurology
University Hospital Zurich
Zurich
Switzerland

Sushanth Bhat
JFK Neuroscience Institute
Hackensack Meridian Health-JFK
Medical Center
Edison
USA

Valérie Cochen De Cock
Department of Neurology and Sleep
Disorders
Clinique Beau Soleil
Montpellier
France

Chris Derry
Department of Clinical Neurosciences
Western General Hospital
Edinburgh
UK

J. Gert van Dijk
Department of Neurology and Clinical
Neurophysiology
Leiden University Medical Centre
Leiden
The Netherlands

Jeroen J.J. van Eijk
Department of Neurology
Jeroen Bosch Hospital
Den Bosch
The Netherlands

Luigi Ferini-Strambi
Sleep Disorders Center
University Vita-Salute San Raffaele
Milan
Italy

Joop van Gerven
Centre for Human Drug Research
Leiden
The Netherlands

Francesc Graus
Neurology Service
Hospital Clínic de Barcelona
Barcelona
Spain
and
Institut d'Investigació Biomèdiques
August Pi i Sunyer (IDIBAPS)
Barcelona
Spain

Dirk M. Hermann
Department of Neurology
University Hospital Essen
Essen
Germany

Alex Iranzo
Neurology Service
Hospital Clínic de Barcelona
Barcelona
Spain
and
Institut d'Investigació Biomèdiques
August Pi i Sunyer (IDIBAPS)
Barcelona
Spain
and
Centro de Investigación Biomédica
en Red sobre Enfermedades
Neurodegenerativas (CIBERNED)
Barcelona
Spain

Brigit A. de Jong
Department of Neurology
VU University Medical Center
Amsterdam
The Netherlands

Gert Jan Lammers
Department of Neurology and Clinical
Neurophysiology
Leiden University Medical Centre
Leiden
The Netherlands
and
Sleep Wake Centre SEIN Heemstede
Heemstede
The Netherlands

José Enrique Martínez-Rodríguez
Neurology Service
Hospital del Mar
IMAS
IMIM
Barcelona
Spain

Geert Mayer
Sleep Disorders Unit
Hephata Klinik
Schwalmstadt-Treysa
Germany

Christine Norra
LWL Hospital Paderborn and
Department of Psychiatry, Psychotherapy
and Preventive Medicine
Ruhr University Bochum
Bochum
Germany

Sebastiaan Overeem
Centre for Sleep Medicine
'Kempenhaeghe'
Heeze
The Netherlands
and
Eindhoven University of Technology
Eindhoven
The Netherlands

Dirk Pevernagie
Centre for Sleep Medicine
'Kempenhaeghe'
Heeze
The Netherlands

Angelique Pijpers
Centre for Sleep Medicine
'Kempenhaeghe'
Heeze
The Netherlands

J. Steven Poceta
Scripps Clinic Sleep Center
Division of Neurology
Scripps Clinic
La Jolla
USA

Timothy G. Quinnell
Respiratory Support and Sleep Centre
Royal Papworth Hospital
Cambridgeshire
UK

Jeanetta C. Rains
Center for Sleep Evaluation at Elliot
Hospital
Manchester
USA

Paul Reading
Department of Neurology
James Cook University Hospital
Middlesbrough
UK

Gé S.F. Ruigt
Clinical Consultancy for Neuroscience
Drug Development
Oss
The Netherlands

Mojca van Schie
Department of Neurology and Clinical
Neurophysiology
Leiden University Medical Centre
Leiden
The Netherlands

Markus H. Schmidt
Department of Neurology
Bern University Hospital
Bern
Switzerland

Pieter Jan Simons
Centre for Sleep Medicine
'Kempenhaeghe'
Heeze
The Netherlands

Bart Willem Smits
Department of Neurology
Maasstadziekenhuis
Rotterdam
The Netherlands

Karel Šonka
Department of Neurology
1st Medical Faculty
Charles University and General Teaching
Hospital
Prague
Czech Republic

Thom P.J. Timmerhuis
Department of Neurology
Jeroen Bosch Hospital
Den Bosch
The Netherlands

Ingrid Verbeek
Centre for Sleep Medicine
'Kempenhaeghe'
Heeze
The Netherlands

Johan Verbraecken
Department of Pulmonary Medicine and
Multidisciplinary Sleep Disorders Centre
Antwerp University Hospital and
University of Antwerp
Antwerp
Belgium

Marie Vidailhet
Movement Disorders Unit
Pitié-Salpêtrière Hospital (APHP),
CRICM UMR 975, and Paris 6 University
Paris
France

Thomas C. Wetter
Department of Psychiatry and
Psychotherapy
University of Regensburg
Regensburg
Germany

Sue J. Wilson
Psychopharmacology Unit
Dorothy Hodgkin Building
University of Bristol
Bristol
UK

Preface

An increasingly held perception is that medical textbooks have become the extinct 'dinosaurs' of information transfer and education. Indeed, the global availability of knowledge and thirst for brand new data, the inevitable delays in producing written multi-authored texts, the expense of books together with the demise of traditional libraries would all appear to support this contention. In a rapidly changing environment, therefore, books, like dinosaurs, need to evolve in parallel and certainly be clearer in their aims than previously. Edited by a sleep physician and a general neurologist with a subspecialist interest in sleep, this book was conceived as a counterpoint to the established large encyclopaedic reference volumes currently available. The intentions were to cover areas not always addressed by standard sleep medicine or, indeed, neurology textbooks, at least from a practical perspective. The book is specifically aimed at clinicians and health care professionals not specifically trained or experienced in sleep medicine who nevertheless need to manage neurologically damaged patients with increasingly recognised sleep–wake disturbances. As such, we envisage the book will serve as an easily digested and practical handy companion, rather than as an exhaustive and fully referenced factual tome.

Largely for historical reasons, most neurologists receive little formal training in academic and clinical aspects of sleep medicine. Most sleep units are run solely by physicians primarily interested in breathing-related sleep disorders and patients under their care may have little access to neurological expertise. This may seem paradoxical given conditions such as narcolepsy that are clearly 'neurological' with recently defined specific neuropathology and neurochemistry. The lack of exposure to sleep medicine naturally tends to produce neurologists with an unconfident, at best, or nihilistic, at worst, approach to sleep-related symptoms in the clinic. By necessity, the situation is changing, especially given the increasingly recognised relevance of poor sleep or impaired wakefulness to quality of life issues in chronic neurological patients. Furthermore, it is clear to most clinicians that deterioration in sleep often coincides with or even causes worsening control of many chronic neurological conditions such as epilepsy.

Most neurologists would not expect to be referred cases of primary insomnia or obvious obstructive sleep apnoea although may well encounter them incidentally. Despite their high prevalence, there is relatively little emphasis on these common sleep disorders in this book and the focus is on those specific symptoms commonly experienced by neurological patients, assuming they are asked about them.

When sleep 'goes wrong' it impacts highly on all aspects of a subject's well-being and often their carer's. As a result, increasing attention to patient choice has appropriately led to a higher expectation that such symptoms should be taken seriously. However, many neurologists with traditional approaches might feel that sleep problems are not disabling enough to warrant detailed attention. We would counter-argue that 'sleep is for the brain' and without enough of it, the brain suffers. It is perhaps worthwhile recalling somewhat distasteful experiments from the late nineteenth century demonstrating that puppies could survive longer without water than without sleep.

The reputation that neurology is a discipline in which successful therapeutic options play second fiddle to diagnostic acumen is only partly true. Perhaps counter-intuitively, treating sleep symptoms in neurology is often particularly rewarding, patients and carers appreciating even partial improvements in controlling their sleep–wake cycle. A recurrent theme in the book is that drugs to improve sleep are often selected using 'medicine-based' evidence and personal experience than the gold standard of evidence-based medicine. Despite this, together with the relative limited armamentarium of drugs available to the sleep physician, we believe that the majority of patients can be helped with a flexible and pragmatic approach. When drugs are mentioned, their proposed use is often 'off licence' and any prescriber will need to take responsibility for monitoring and progress. Similarly, doses of drugs are often approximate recommendations and it is not intended to provide strict or didactic guidelines. In many of the sleep-disordered populations covered in the book, it is appropriate to suggest long-term therapy on the assumption spontaneous improvement is unlikely. This often needs to be emphasised to primary care physicians who are more accustomed to providing short-term prescriptions for sleep-related problems.

The point or threshold at which a general neurologist should engage the help of a sleep specialist clearly depends on a number of factors. However, an exchange of views and expertise in a multidisciplinary setting, if possible at an early stage, would seem to be the best approach if facilities allow. We would encourage neurologists to forge stronger links with physicians more dedicated to sleep medicine in the firm belief any 'cross fertilisation' will benefit both sides.

By necessity, there is some overlap in the topics covered by some of the chapters. However, given the personal and practical approach we have espoused throughout the book, we hope different perspectives will improve rather than hinder understanding and effective symptom management in sleep-disordered neurological patients.

In the Second Edition

The second edition of our handbook incorporates the changes outlined in the third International Classification of Sleep Disorders (ICSD-3), published in 2014. The organisation of the book has also changed such that three parts now cover 'General Sleep Medicine'; 'Primary Sleep Disorders'; and 'Sleep in Neurological Disorders'. It is hoped that the book will be a useful tool for those planning to gain a formal 'somnologist' qualification, given the increasing availability of a certification process in Europe, for example. Indeed, one encouraging development in many countries is the realisation that sleep medicine should be recognised as an important subspeciality with a formalised curriculum and specific assessment process. Inevitably, this will encourage and incentivise those fascinated by sleep and facilitate career pathways.

Eindhoven, The Netherlands
and Middlesborough, UK, January 2018

Sebastiaan Overeem
Paul Reading

Part One

General Sleep Medicine

Part One

General Sleep Problems

1

The Sleep History

Paul Reading[1] and Sebastiaan Overeem[2,3]

[1] Department of Neurology, James Cook University Hospital, Middlesbrough, UK
[2] Centre for Sleep Medicine 'Kempenhaeghe', Heeze, The Netherlands
[3] Eindhoven University of Technology, Eindhoven, The Netherlands

Introduction

It is a commonly held misperception that practitioners of sleep medicine are highly dependent on sophisticated investigative techniques to diagnose and treat sleep-disordered patients. However, it is relatively rare for detailed tests to add indispensable diagnostic information, provided a detailed, credible and accurate 24-hour sleep–wake history is available. In fact, there can be few areas of medicine where a good, directed history is of more diagnostic importance. In some situations, this can be extremely complex due to interacting social, environmental, medical and psychological factors. Furthermore, obtaining an accurate sleep history often requires collateral or corroborative information from bed partners or close relatives, especially in the assessment of parasomnias.

In sleep medicine, neurological patients can present particular diagnostic challenges. It can often be difficult to determine whether a given sleep–wake symptom arises from the underlying neurological disorder and perhaps its treatment or whether an additional primary sleep disorder is the main contributor. The problem is compounded by the relative lack of formal training in sleep medicine received by the majority of neurology trainees that often results in reduced confidence when faced with sleep-related symptoms. However, it is difficult to underestimate the potential importance of disordered sleep in many chronic and diverse neurological conditions such as epilepsy, migraine, multiple sclerosis and parkinsonism.

The following framework is a personal view on how to approach sleep–wake complaints from a neurological perspective. Although the focus is on individual or particular symptoms, it should be realised that several conditions can produce a variety of symptoms across the full 24-hour sleep–wake period. In Chapters 2 and 3, the various ways in which sleep and sleepiness can be recorded are discussed. Then, in Chapter 4, an 'integrative' approach to diagnosis is outlined, illustrated by case examples.

Sleep Disorders in Neurology: A Practical Approach, Second Edition.
Edited by Sebastiaan Overeem and Paul Reading.
© 2018 John Wiley & Sons Ltd. Published 2018 by John Wiley & Sons Ltd.

Excessive Daytime Sleepiness

Excessive daytime sleepiness (EDS) is an increasingly recognised symptom that is deemed worthy of assessment. It is relatively prevalent and disabling both in general and neurological populations [1]. Many excessively sleepy patients may present to the medical profession indirectly, most often due to adverse indirect effects on cognition, motivation or mood. Indeed, the inability to focus or maintain concentration is often the most disabling aspect of conditions causing EDS, described as 'brain fog' or even masquerading as dementia. A not uncommon question posed to general neurologists is whether a sleepy patient might have narcolepsy or a similar primary, presumed 'central' sleep disorder. Furthermore, 'secondary' or 'symptomatic' narcolepsy is evolving as a valid concept given recent major advances in unravelling the neurobiology of sleep regulation. In particular, a variety of pathologies predominantly affecting the hypothalamus can mimic elements of idiopathic (primary) narcolepsy [2].

It is widely perceived that EDS is a normal phenomenon associated with the ageing process. In fact, objective measures of sleepiness suggest that healthy elderly subjects are actually less prone to falling asleep when unoccupied during the day compared with their younger counterparts. Although afternoon planned naps are probably a normal phenomenon with many elderly people in all cultures, evidence for EDS beyond this level should be taken seriously in all age groups.

In the initial assessment of EDS, it is essential to gain an impression of the severity of symptoms and how they are impacting on an individual subject. It is also crucial to confirm that the complaint is that of true excessive somnolence rather than simple fatigue or lethargy. Although sleepiness questionnaires are widely used and can act as an effective screening tool in this respect (Chapter 4), they rarely help with actual diagnosis. Directly asking a subject about particularly unusual, unplanned or inappropriate sleep episodes can therefore provide valuable insight. Habitual mid-afternoon or late evening naps when unoccupied could be considered normal phenomena whereas regularly dropping to sleep mid-morning or in public places usually indicates a problem. A history of invariably napping as a car passenger for journeys of over an hour may suggest pathological levels of sleepiness as may a complete inability to watch any film all the way through. In narcolepsy, the subject may describe sleep onset even whilst engaged in physical activities such as writing or standing. Furthermore, in severe EDS, the subject may report awakening from naps unaware of any prior imperative to sleep. So-called 'sleep attacks' are recognised in narcolepsy and have been widely reported in sleepy parkinsonian patients. Regarding the latter population, recent evidence suggests that they may be particularly poor at monitoring their levels of subjective sleepiness, making the history from relatives particularly important [3].

The commonest causes of mild and severe EDS are probably insufficient sleep and poor quality overnight sleep, respectively. A directed history, perhaps backed by a sleep diary, usually helps in diagnosing the former and can indicate causes of the latter. If a subject regularly and reliably reports at least seven or eight hours of continuous sleep, yet remains significantly somnolent during the day, it is most likely that there is a disturbance of sleep architecture and, usually, that insufficient deep or restorative sleep is being obtained. An overabundance of light (stage N2) sleep compared with deep non-rapid eye movement (REM) sleep (stage N3) is frequently seen in sleep-related breathing disorders and periodic limb movement disorder. These diagnoses can easily be missed from the history if the subject is not a typical phenotype for the former or if they sleep alone. However, leading questions such as 'do you invariably awake with a dry mouth?' or 'are the bed clothes usually disrupted on waking?' can provide diagnostic pointers. Morning headaches or general sensations of 'heaviness' are traditionally associated with obstructive sleep apnoea although are equally common in a variety of sleep disorders.

A drug history including alcohol habit is also clearly relevant in assessing EDS as numerous agents given before bed may appear to induce drowsiness and aid sleep onset but actually worsen nocturnal sleep quality overall. Tricyclic preparations and benzodiazepines are frequently associated with unrefreshing sleep yet are frequently given primarily as hypnotic agents. It is worth noting that most antidepressants will potentially worsen restless legs syndrome or periodic limb movement disorder (Chapter 13).

Less recognised causes of disturbed nocturnal sleep may be picked up by a focused history. Nocturnal pain, frequent nocturia, persistent wheeze and acid reflux are usually fairly obvious 'toxins' to sleep and are generally readily reported. However, more subtle phenomena such as teeth grinding (bruxism) may not be recognised by the subject and only suspected if direct questions are asked about teeth wear, temporomandibular joint dysfunction or jaw pain, especially on waking.

A number of primary neurological disorders, including narcolepsy, disrupt the continuity of nocturnal sleep, most likely as a result of pathology in various brain regions intimately involved in sleep–wake control. A new symptom of sleep fragmentation and daytime somnolence in a patient with inflammatory brain disease such as multiple sclerosis, for example, might sometimes suggest inflammatory pathology in the pontomedullary area [4] or around the hypothalamus [5]. Idiopathic Parkinson's disease is strongly associated with EDS, especially in the advanced stages. Although there are many potential causes, including dopaminergic medication, primary Lewy body brainstem pathology itself is a likely substrate for most of the sleep–wake dysregulation, especially with regards to REM sleep [6]. If a neurological patient complains of significant EDS and no obvious cause such as Parkinson's disease is determined after a detailed history and subsequent sleep investigations, magnetic resonance brain imaging can be justified to exclude unexpected inflammatory or even structural pathology. This may particularly apply to sleepy, overweight children, for example [7].

There are usually sufficient clues from a patient's history to suggest a specific diagnosis of narcolepsy, the quintessential primary disorder of sleep–wake dysregulation (Chapter 8). Typically, narcolepsy causes symptoms from early adolescence and profound delays in receiving a diagnosis are still commonplace. A detailed history, therefore, exploring issues of excessive sleepiness around schooling can be illuminating. Apart from its severity, the nature of sleepiness is not particularly exceptional or unique in narcolepsy. However, even short naps, planned or unplanned, tend to be restorative, allowing a 'refractory' wakeful period of 3–4 hours. Given that REM sleep is particularly dysregulated in narcolepsy, it is also useful to enquire about the presence of dreams, dream-like experiences or sleep paralysis during short naps. Even when alert, the majority of narcoleptics will be prone to automatic behaviours and reduced powers of concentration or vigilance, potentially reflecting brief 'micro-sleeps'. These can be explored from a full history. Losing objects around the house or placing inappropriate objects such as mobile phones in the fridge are particularly common examples of this phenomenon.

Cataplexy is present in two-thirds of narcoleptics and is very rarely seen in other situations. It is therefore an extremely specific phenomenon and important to recognise with confidence. Full-blown episodes of temporary paralysis triggered by positive emotions or their anticipation are generally easy to pick up from the history. Subtle or atypical variants may be missed, however, especially since 'going weak at the knees' with laughter or other strong emotions is probably a normal phenomenon. Typically, cataplexy occurs in a relaxed or intimate environment in the company of friends or family. It is usually manifested by descending paralysis in a rostro-caudal direction over two or three seconds, preceded by head bobbing or facial twitching. Subjects often learn to anticipate the situations in which they are at risk of attacks and may even develop social phobias as a result. Common precipitants include positive emotions such as surprise at meeting an old acquaintance or watching comedy on television. Some report that the anticipation of a positive emotion, perhaps as a punchline is approaching, acts as the most potent stimulus. Negative emotions such as frustration, particularly that induced by children or pets, can also induce episodes in many. Partial attacks can be missed or hidden. Indeed, minor facial twitching, head bobbing, mild neck weakness or a stuttering dysarthria when telling a joke may reflect the only observable manifestations of cataplexy. On the other hand, cataplexy is a doubtful explanation if episodes are very sudden or prolonged. Similarly, if conscious levels are significantly impaired or if injuries frequently incurred during attacks, alternative diagnoses need consideration.

Nocturnal symptoms in narcolepsy are extremely varied but frequently significant. Often to the surprise of physicians inexperienced with narcolepsy, restless sleep with impaired sleep maintenance and even sleep onset insomnia is common, as are excessive limb movements during sleep. The latter may reflect simple restlessness or periodic limb movements. Many narcoleptics also exhibit dream enactment during REM sleep although it generally appears as a more benign phenomenon to that commonly seen in neurodegenerative disease [8]. In particular, the movements tend to be less explosive or violent in narcolepsy and there is not the striking male predominance as observed in Parkinson's disease, for example.

Unpleasant dreams that are particularly vivid and difficult to distinguish from reality are commonplace in narcolepsy. Indeed, narcoleptic children often become fearful of sleep as a result, so-called 'clinophobia'. Frank hallucinatory experiences in a variety of modalities including tactile may not be mentioned spontaneously through fear of being labelled mentally ill. These experiences are commonest around the sleep–wake transition periods or in states of drowsiness. A common example is the unpleasant sensation of a stranger in the bedroom in the absence of a frank hallucinatory vision or auditory perception. A full history should therefore actively explore such dream-like experiences in detail.

A less common sleep disorder, idiopathic hypersomnolence (IH), can often mimic narcolepsy although certain historical pointers may help with the differential diagnosis [9]. IH in its classical form is characterised by long yet unrefreshing overnight sleep with prolonged napping during the day and continuous perception of reduced alertness. Difficulty with morning waking or prolonged confusion on forced waking are typical symptoms as are frequent acts of automatic behaviour during the day. Important negative historical features might include the lack of prominent REM sleep-related phenomena. Overnight sleep is also usually undisturbed by arousals or excessive movement. It is recognised that mood disorders may be particularly common in IH although it is likely they are simply a consequence of the sleep disorder [10].

Although not a symptom routinely presented to neurologists, difficulty with morning waking is not uncommon and can lead to significant problems either with education or maintaining employment. If the sleep history indicates that the most likely cause is an abnormally late time of nocturnal sleep onset, the possibility of delayed sleep phase syndrome should be considered. This primarily affects adolescents and is often assumed simply to reflect socio-behavioural factors. However, although bad habits may worsen the situation, it is often a defined disorder of circadian timing such that subjects are 'hard wired' to sleep and rise later than average, acting as extreme 'night owls' [11]. The diagnosis, if suspected, can be deduced from the history and subsequently supported by investigations.

Insomnia

Chronic insomnia either at sleep onset or through the night is undoubtedly common and most often reflects a combination of psychological and poorly defined constitutional factors. Although a patient's history might indicate severe symptoms, it should be noted that a minority will have so-called 'paradoxical insomnia' and will actually sleep fairly well when objectively investigated.

Many chronic insomniacs are able to identify a significant event or lifestyle change that seemed to trigger their sleep disturbance. Despite seemingly severe symptoms of poor nocturnal sleep and reported lethargy, most primary insomniacs are unable to nap during the day. The diagnosis of primary insomnia should therefore be questioned, and secondary causes sought in the presence of significant daytime somnolence. This is particularly relevant to neurological populations as insomnia symptoms are common and frequently adversely affect long-term conditions such as epilepsy.

One of the commonest and most under-recognised contributors to delayed sleep onset, sleep fragmentation and, indeed, daytime somnolence is restless legs syndrome (RLS) and associated periodic limb movement disorder (Chapter 13). RLS is defined solely from a positive history [12]. There should be frank restlessness, usually, but not always, in the lower limbs, most often associated with ill-defined sensory symptoms that worsen in the late evening. Symptoms are triggered by rest or immobility and eased, at least temporarily, by movement or rubbing the affected limb or limbs. Associated involuntary jerks can be significant and intrude during wakefulness or light sleep, often adversely affecting sleep quality and causing daytime somnolence. The condition may not be suspected if the upper limbs are predominantly involved or if the symptoms are mistakenly attributed to arthritis or poor circulation, for example. In patients with underlying neuropathies, radiculopathies or demyelinating disease, RLS may be secondary to the primary diagnosis and should not be overlooked. Particularly in younger patients, a positive family history is common and should be actively sought from the history.

Discrete or identifiable brain pathology rarely leads to insomnia as an isolated phenomenon. However, it is relatively common both in neurodegenerative diseases and inflammatory disorders such as multiple sclerosis in the context of more obvious physical neurodisability [13]. Furthermore, insomnia can also be an apparent direct consequence

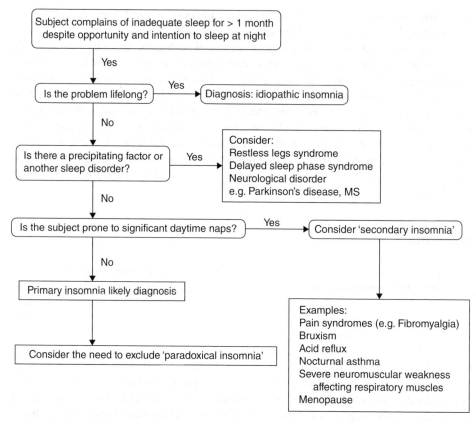

Figure 1.1 Algorithm outlining a diagnostic approach to some of the common causes of primary and secondary insomnia that might present to neurologists.

of head injuries or strokes, particularly those producing subcortical pathology and potentially involving the paramedian thalamic region [14]. Insomnia and severely disturbed sleep are also increasingly recognised accompanying features of limbic encephalitis, a rare disorder in which fluctuating confusion, seizures and autonomic symptomology usually predominate [15]. Finally, delayed sleep phase syndrome sometimes presents as insomnia although, unlike the typical case of primary insomnia, by definition, there are also major problems in waking at a conventional hour.

A simple algorithm to assess insomnia presenting to a neurologist is shown in Figure 1.1.

Nocturnal Disturbances

Neurologists are frequently asked to assess patients with abnormal nocturnal behaviours or experiences, often to exclude epilepsy as a potential explanation. Distinguishing parasomnias from epileptic or psychiatric phenomena can clearly be difficult, especially given the practical issues of investigating nocturnal symptoms that are invariably intermittent (Chapter 12). However, a full history supported by spouses and family members together with a detailed background knowledge of parasomnias and their spectrum usually allow for a confident diagnosis.

Sleep–wake transition disorders are poorly studied but often alarming phenomena that may require reassurance if not treatment. They are relatively easy to recognise from the history. Most people are familiar with an occasional and slightly unpleasant sensation of sudden falling through space at the point of sleep onset. In sleep–wake transition disorders this phenomenon is amplified, more frequent and often accompanied by a variety of unusual and disturbing sensory or experiential symptoms such as loud auditory or intense visual stimuli. At the more severe end of the spectrum, the so-called 'exploding head syndrome' has been described [16]. If frequent or recurrent, significant insomnia at sleep onset and through the night may result.

Parasomnias arising from non-REM sleep are not rare in young adults and probably affect at least 1%. They usually reflect incomplete and abnormal arousals from deep non-REM or slow wave sleep that can lead to a variety of complex and occasionally disturbing nocturnal behaviours. The events themselves usually have relatively little impact on daytime functioning or levels of sleepiness. For a confident diagnosis, it is important to ask about sleep-related phenomena in early childhood as the majority will have a positive history for night terrors, confusional arousals, sleep walking, or all three. Given the likely genetic component to non-REM parasomnias, a family history of nocturnal disturbances, including sleep talking, can also be insightful. In adults, a frequency of one or two events a month is typical, often with identifiable precipitants. These include sleep deprivation, alcohol intake before bed or sleeping in an unfamiliar or uncomfortable environment. Coinciding with the first period of deep non-REM sleep, the nocturnal disturbance will generally occur within an hour or two of sleep onset and will rarely recur through the night. Subsequent recollection of the event by the subject is at best hazy although agitated events may produce vague memories of non-specific threats or frightening situations. Detailed or bizarre dream narratives are rare. Events can be prolonged and the subject may appear superficially awake, responding in a limited way to questions and commands. Relatively complex motor tasks such as eating, performing housework and driving are certainly possible.

Distinguishing adult non-REM parasomnias from nocturnal complex partial seizures can be difficult as both may produce complicated behaviours and confusion (Chapter 12). Epileptic episodes are often of frontal lobe origin and can occur several or many times a night from any sleep stage, except REM sleep. If detailed descriptions or, ideally, video clips of several events demonstrate strictly stereotyped episodes, especially with fixed or dystonic limb posturing, a diagnosis of epilepsy is likely. Alternatively, if episodes are long-lasting with an indistinct termination or if they appear to wax and wane, a parasomnia is favoured. Strongly expressed emotions or leaving the bed are not particularly discriminatory features.

In a neurological setting, it is commoner to see parasomnias arising from REM sleep, particularly in the context of parkinsonian neurodegenerative disease. In particular, REM sleep behaviour disorder (RBD) typically affects men in late middle-age, often many years in advance of any motor or, indeed, cognitive symptomology [17]. The nocturnal disturbances are usually of more concern to the bed partner who may incur injuries from violent dream enactment. The episodes themselves are generally more frequent and prolonged at the end of the night when REM sleep is more prevalent. Movements are often associated with vocalisation and tend to be defensive, brief and undirected, typically involving the upper limbs with eyes generally closed. The subject is usually fairly easy to arouse to full wakefulness and will often recall a vivid dream, perhaps involving previous acquaintances or occupations. In certain conditions such as multiple system atrophy and narcolepsy, RBD seems to affect females equally [18]. Moreover, in narcolepsy, the dreams and movements may be relatively banal and probably reflect differing underlying pathogenetic mechanisms to those seen in parkinsonism.

The causes of generally restless sleep can be difficult to diagnose from history alone even if detailed witnessed accounts and videos are available. Periodic limb movement disorder can exist in the absence of RLS and is relatively common. Persistent rocking or stereotyped rolling movements involving virtually any body part may reflect a so-called rhythmic movement disorder. This often evolves from childhood 'head banging' at sleep onset although can occur in any sleep stage, even REM sleep, in adults [19]. As with many parasomnias, the bed partner is usually the main complainant.

Conclusions

As within many areas of neurology, a detailed and directed history is paramount when trying to diagnose sleep disorders. The need for a full 24-hour sleep–wake history should be emphasised, corroborated where possible by observers or family members. At the very least, a good history usually provides a credible differential diagnosis which investigations may subsequently further refine. However, if significant diagnostic doubt remains after obtaining a full sleep history, it is relatively rare for sleep investigations to fully elucidate the problem. Furthermore, given the expense and patchy distribution of specialist sleep centres, the sleep history assumes particular diagnostic importance.

Disordered sleep is undoubtedly prevalent in neurological disease and may exacerbate underlying conditions such as migraine and epilepsy. Aside from their direct deleterious effects on daily and nightly functioning, there is therefore ample justification for taking sleep-related symptoms seriously in a neurological setting.

Key Points

- The patient history is the single most important diagnostic tool in neurological sleep medicine.
- In neurological patients, it can sometimes be difficult to determine whether a sleep–wake symptom is due to an underlying neurological disorder, its treatment or a coexisting primary sleep disorder.
- Excessive daytime sleepiness is not uncommon, and may easily be missed or mistaken for fatigue, cognitive impairment or mood disorder.
- Additional symptoms not directly related to the sleep–wake cycle may be crucial for the diagnosis (e.g. cataplexy in the case of narcolepsy).
- Sleep onset or sleep maintainance insomnia can reflect an idiopathic or primary phenomenon but is more often secondary to a variety of disorders, including other primary sleep disorders (e.g. RLS), psychiatric (e.g. depression) or neurological disease (e.g. multiple sclerosis, neurodegenerative diseases or stroke).
- A knowledge of the typical pattern and spectrum of the various parasomnias normally allows a confident history from history alone and helps exclude epilepsy as a diagnosis.

References

1 Bixler EO, Kales A, Soldatos CR, et al. Prevalence of sleep disorders in the Los Angeles metropolitan area. *Am J Psychiatry* 1979; 136(10):1257–1262.
2 Nishino S, Kanbayashi T. Symptomatic narcolepsy, cataplexy and hypersomnia, and their implications in the hypothalamic hypocretin/orexin system. *Sleep Med Rev* 2005; 9(4):269–310.
3 Merino-Andreu M, Arnulf I, Konofal E, et al. Unawareness of naps in Parkinson's disease and in disorders with excessive daytime sleepiness. *Neurology* 2003; 60(9):1553–1554.
4 Mathis J, Hess CW, Bassetti C. Isolated mediotegmental lesion causing narcolepsy and rapid eye movement sleep behaviour disorder: a case evidencing a common pathway in narcolepsy and rapid eye movement sleep behaviour disorder. *J Neurol Neurosurg Psychiatry* 2007; 78(4):427–429.
5 Oka Y, Kanbayashi T, Mezaki T, et al. Low CSF hypocretin-1/orexin-A associated with hypersomnia secondary to hypothalamic lesion in a case of multiple sclerosis. *J Neurol* 2004; 251(7):885–886.
6 Arnulf I, Konofal E, Merino-Andreu M, et al. Parkinson's disease and sleepiness: an integral part of PD. *Neurology* 2002; 58(7):1019–1024.
7 Marcus CL, Trescher WH, Halbower AC, Lutz J. Secondary narcolepsy in children with brain tumors. *Sleep* 2002; 25(4):435–439.
8 Nightingale S, Orgill JC, Ebrahim IO, et al. The association between narcolepsy and REM behavior disorder (RBD). *Sleep Med* 2005; 6(3):253–258.
9 Anderson KN, Pilsworth S, Sharples LD, et al. Idiopathic hypersomnia: a study of 77 cases. *Sleep* 2007; 30(10):1274–1281.
10 Bassetti C, Aldrich MS. Idiopathic hypersomnia. A series of 42 patients. *Brain* 1997; 120(Pt 8):1423–1435.
11 Archer SN, Robilliard DL, Skene DJ, et al. A length polymorphism in the circadian clock gene Per3 is linked to delayed sleep phase syndrome and extreme diurnal preference. *Sleep* 2003; 26(4):413–415.
12 Benes H, Walters AS, Allen RP, et al. Definition of restless legs syndrome, how to diagnose it, and how to differentiate it from RLS mimics. *Mov Disord* 2007; 22(Suppl. 18):S401–S408.
13 Tachibana N, Howard RS, Hirsch NP, et al. Sleep problems in multiple sclerosis. *Eur Neurol* 1994; 34(6):320–323.
14 Bassetti CL. Sleep and stroke. *Semin Neurol* 2005; 25(1):19–32.
15 Vincent A, Buckley C, Schott JM, et al. Potassium channel antibody-associated encephalopathy: a potentially immunotherapy-responsive form of limbic encephalitis. *Brain* 2004; 127(Pt 3):701–712.
16 Sachs C, Svanborg E. The exploding head syndrome: polysomnographic recordings and therapeutic suggestions. *Sleep* 1991; 14(3):263–266.
17 Schenck CH, Bundlie SR, Ettinger MG, Mahowald MW. Chronic behavioral disorders of human REM sleep: a new category of parasomnia. 1986 [classical article]. *Sleep* 2002; 25(2):293–308.
18 Iranzo A, Santamaria J, Rye DB, et al. Characteristics of idiopathic REM sleep behavior disorder and that associated with MSA and PD. *Neurology* 2005; 65(2):247–252.
19 Stepanova I, Nevsimalova S, Hanusova J. Rhythmic movement disorder in sleep persisting into childhood and adulthood. *Sleep* 2005; 28(7):851–857.

2

Polysomnography

Recording, Analysis and Interpretation

Pieter Jan Simons[1] and Sebastiaan Overeem[1,2]

[1] Centre for Sleep Medicine 'Kempenhaeghe', Heeze, The Netherlands
[2] Eindhoven University of Technology, Eindhoven, The Netherlands

Introduction

The field of sleep medicine is an area that has particularly benefited from Hans Berger's invention of electroencephalography (EEG). Soon after its introduction, EEG was being used to investigate sleeping subjects and by the 1930s distinct sleep stages were first described by Loomis. Phenomena including K-complexes as reactions to external stimuli during sleep were recognised and rapid eye movement (REM) sleep was described in the early 1950s.

In the 1970s, the term polysomnography (PSG) was coined for the combination of EEG sleep recordings with additional physiological parameters such as respiratory movements, airflow, oxygen saturation, body position and electrocardiography (ECG). Over time, the type and number of signals that can be recorded simultaneously has expanded considerably such that multichannel electromyography, full montage EEG, respiratory effort through oesophageal pressure sensors and transcutaneous or end-tidal capnography can now all be measured. Finally, in the digital age, long term time-synchronized video recordings have become an indispensable addition, allowing the detailed visual assessment of the behavioural or motor aspects of sleep.

Following a consensus meeting with sleep experts in 1968, Rechtschaffen and Kales described a set of standard criteria to divide sleep into different stages in a standardized manner [1]. Since then, the basic principles of staging sleep in 30-second epochs has not fundamentally changed in clinical practice. The current most widely accepted criteria for the recording, scoring and interpretation of sleep studies is documented in the *American Academy of Sleep Medicine (AASM) Manual for the Scoring of Sleep and Associated Events* [2]. This is a continuously updated document which details the finer aspects of sleep staging as well as providing more precise criteria for transitions between sleep stages. It also advises on the standardised recording and scoring of all the additional polygraphic signals.

This chapter outlines the basics of polysomnography as used in daily practice. It addresses the clinical application of (video)-PSG, its merits and limitations, and aims to provide insight in the 'art' of PSG interpretation and reporting. The text deals only with

Sleep Disorders in Neurology: A Practical Approach, Second Edition.
Edited by Sebastiaan Overeem and Paul Reading.
© 2018 John Wiley & Sons Ltd. Published 2018 by John Wiley & Sons Ltd.

PSG in adults, highlighting the most important elements and finishing with additional pointers and pitfalls. The subtly different PSG scoring rules for children are not discussed but can be found in the AASM manual.

The Use of Polysomnography: Considerations and Indications

Given the importance of a comfortable sleeping environment and the fact that many sleep disorders show significant night-to-night variability, one may question the value of performing one night of PSG with the associated discomfort and unfamiliar surroundings of the hospital. This highlights the importance of knowing the limitations of PSG and, most importantly, the need for a clear clinical question and/or diagnostic hypothesis before performing a study.

In specific clinical situations such as likely significant sleep-disordered breathing, it is appropriate to consider a limited recording setup with only cardiorespiratory polygraphic measurement. However, when resources allow, performing full PSG confers important advantages that include the recording of synchronised video and monitoring by a sleep technologist during the night, primarily to allow correction of technical issues. It also allows proper safeguarding of patients with possible parasomnias and may be crucial for concomitant interventions such as continuous positive airway pressure (CPAP) titration. Increasingly, many advocate to perform sleep recordings with ambulatory equipment, so the patient can sleep in his or her own home environment. Although this may well improve the quality of any sleep observed and may appear to reduce costs, the advantages of home studies need to be weighed against the disadvantages, including technical faults and limits on the information gained.

In general, PSG can be used to increase diagnostic confidence of a specific sleep disorder, initially deduced from the patient's history and clinical examination. However, often it is also important to check for the presence of additional 'co-morbid' disorders such as sleep-related breathing disorders that may trigger or worsen a parasomnia, for example.

Several consensus papers describe the indications for PSG in detail, separately for adults and children [3–5]. Specific indications for PSG in the adult population include the diagnosis of entities such as sleep-related breathing disorders, sleep-related disorders in neuromuscular diseases, hypersomnias, complex and/or violent behaviours with a differential diagnosis of epilepsy and parasomnias, and periodic limb movement disorder. In addition, PSG is indicated for the re-evaluation of a diagnosis, when a patient is not responding to first-line treatment strategies. Finally, PSG may be used in the evaluation of a therapy of a primary sleep disorder, most often in the case of sleep-related breathing disorders. Due to the fact that children do not always present in 'textbook' fashion, the threshold for performing PSG may be lower in paediatric practice although, again, available resources for this investigation are often the limiting factor.

Standardisation of Video-polysomnography

There are no accepted international standards for in-hospital PSG with respect to factors such as the dimensions of the room, furniture, lighting and sound proofing. Nevertheless, these are obviously important aspects to consider when interpreting PSG recordings. Another consideration relates to variations in patients' chronotype. Clearly, when a 'night owl' is asked to sleep at a relatively early bedtime because of the hospital routine, one should not diagnose sleep onset insomnia based on a long sleep latency. The level of monitoring during the night by staff is also not thoroughly defined although nursing and technical training and expertise should be available not only to provide patient care but at least to recognise and solve common technical issues including artifacts from badly attached electrodes. When analysing a sleep study, it is often productive to let the patient fill out a small sleep diary in the morning, allowing comparisons of a night in the sleep laboratory to a typical night at home.

The AASM manual provides detailed standards on the technical aspects of the sleep recording, analysis and reporting. Parameters and settings necessary for routine sleep studies are marked as 'recommended', while the use of several 'optional' ones will depend on the clinical indication. The manual provides minimal criteria with respect to recording hardware, such as type of sensors, sampling rates and filter settings. The software criteria such as viewing features, montages and aspects of automatic analyses implicitly assume that digital recording and analysis is the gold standard.

General parameters to be recorded and recommended by the AASM are: frontal, central and occipital EEG leads (one-sided, with the other side as backup); electrooculogram (EOG); submental electromyogram (EMG); airflow signals; respiratory effort signals; oxygen saturation; body position; ECG and tibialis anterior EMG. Video recording is not listed as an absolute requirement but technical specifications are provided. In the hospital setting there is no reason to omit audio-visual registrations given the state of present day technology. When a sensor is not available or fails during recording, in some cases other physical sensors can take over or be substituted by derivations from other signals. An example is the scoring of likely hypopneas by summing the respiratory inductance signals.

In selected cases, it is useful to add capnography, for example when nocturnal hypoventilation is suspected. While oesophageal pressure sensing is the gold standard for respiratory effort measurement, its invasive nature precludes its routine use in many instances.

Table 2.1 lists some details on the recommended signals according to the AASM manual.

Recorded signals are presented as continuous data. Once recorded, recordings are scored off-line and 'event' data are generated by a sleep technologist, sometimes aided by automatic analysis. The discrete assessment of sleep stages results in the hypnogram as a graphical depiction of sleep structure through the night. The combined assessment of respiratory signals enables the definition of 'breathing events' such as obstructive apnoeas. These events can then be expressed in indices or other numerical indicators, such as the apnoea–hypopnoea index (AHI): the number of apnoeas plus hypopnoeas over the night divided by the total sleep time. Data that describe sleep structure and continuity include sleep latency, wake after sleep onset and sleep efficiency (total sleep time divided by the time in bed). Although these indices are widely used, they should always be interpreted with caution and in the clinical context. A detailed graphical representation of the whole night recording is indispensable.

Assessment that combines the hypnogram, scored cardiorespiratory and movement events in addition to whole-night raw signals is referred to as trend analysis. This allows the detection of clinically highly relevant patterns such as sleep-disordered breathing occurring in relation to specific body positions or sleep stages.

Table 2.1 Recommended signals to be obtained during polysomnogram recording, according to the AASM manual.

Parameter	Electrodes/Sensor	Primary Function in PSG	Additional remarks
EEG	F4-M1; C4-M1; O2-M1 Contralateral derivations as back-up	Sleep staging	Electrode position according to 10/20 system Epileptic activity can be detected but sensitivity and specificity is too low to use as a primary diagnostic instrument due to the limited montage
EOG	E1-M2; E2-M2 (Referencing to M1 if M2 fails)	Sleep staging	Frontal EEG activity is often mixed with the EOG signal
Chin EMG	Chin1 and Chin2 below and ChinZ above the inferior edge of the mandible. Use either Chin1-ChinZ or Chin2-ChinZ. Chin1-Chin2 may be used if ChinZ fails	Staging of REM sleep Arousal detection during REM sleep REM Sleep Behaviour Disorder	The signal consists of electrical activity of the M. mylohyoideus and M. digastricus Activity can also reveal e.g. bruxism, mouth-opening during snoring or talking
Leg EMG	Two electrodes on the m. tibialis anterior (bipolar derivation), bilateral	Detection of periodic limb movements	Other movement types, including ALMA, HFT, EFM defined according to the signal characteristics. Rhythmic activity (movement artifacts) can be seen during Rhythmic Movement Disorder
Airflow	Oronasal thermal airflow sensor (thermistor or thermocouple) (Δt in-/expiratory air)	Breathing pattern: detection of apnoeas	Cardio-ballistic artifact can be seen during central apnoea, in case of an open airway
	(Oro)nasal pressure transducer (Δp in-/expiration due to airflow)	Breathing pattern: detection of hypopneas and RERA	Turbulence during snoring can be seen as a high frequency signal on top of the low frequency breathing pattern
Respiratory effort	Thoraco-abdominal respiratory inductance plethysmography belts	Thoracic and abdominal volume changes during breathing; classification of obstructive versus central events	Phase shift between both signals with growing obstruction (phase angle 180° = [nearly] total obstruction) Cardio-ballistic artifact may be seen during central apnoea
	Oesophageal manometry	Intrathoracic pressure changes during breathing (Δp during in-/expiration)	Increases in respiratory effort (during obstruction) are seen as thoracic pressure becoming increasingly more negative during inspiration

Oxygen saturation	Pulse oximetry	Capillary blood oxygen saturation: desaturation due to respiratory events	Sometimes difficult interpretation of signal in relation to breathing; movements and arousals can be associated with hyperpnoea and subsequent saturation rises Photoplethysmogram signals may reflect autonomic arousals (with or without cortical arousal)
Body position	One sensor (different technologies)	Body position (left side, right side, upright, prone, supine)	Identification of positional-related changes in physiology or pathophysiology like position-related apnoeas, snoring, desaturations Note: verify the accuracy of the signal with video, as the sensor may shift position
ECG	Two ECG electrodes; Einthoven's lead II derivation	Cardiac rhythm changes; e.g. indicating autonomic arousals or rhythm disorders	Only cardiac frequency and rhythm can be commented on (due to the limited montage)

Different other sensors and electrodes can be applied, according to the clinical question, as modern PSG recorders offers various 'redundant' amplifier and recording channels.

Scoring Sleep Stages

Sleep scoring is based on splitting the recording into 30-second epochs. Each epoch is scored as a particular sleep stage, taking into account additional rules for sleep stage transitions, as well as age-specific characteristics. In healthy adults, non-REM sleep stages N1, N2 and N3 are recognised, in addition to stage R (rapid eye movement (REM) sleep) and W (wake). Up until 2012 slow wave sleep was divided into non-REM stages 3 and 4 based on the amount of delta activity in the EEG, but this distinction is now considered obsolete and these stages have been combined.

General Scoring Rules

Table 2.2 summarises the overall characteristics of each sleep stage.

With regard to sleep stage transitions, a general AASM-defined principle is that a switch between non-REM sleep stages occurs when specific EEG activity of this new sleep stage occurs in the first half of the new epoch. In the case of suspected REM sleep, one should 'look ahead' to scan for following epochs with rapid eye movements, and return, epoch by epoch, scoring R as long as EEG activity and chin EMG correspond to the R definition.

Arousals are scored alongside sleep stages. AASM defines arousals as sudden changes in EEG frequency with a duration of at least 3 seconds, with at least 10 seconds of prior stable sleep. In REM, an increase in chin EMG tone accompanying the EEG change is required to score an arousal. Note that this approach of scoring does not take into consideration so-called 'subcortical' or autonomic arousals which may be of clinical relevance. Arousals can then be further specified to the presumed causative factors, for example respiratory-related arousals (RERAs).

Table 2.2 Summary of characteristics used to identify sleep stages.

Stage	Dominant EEG activity	Sleep-specific grapho-elements	Eye movements	Chin-EMG tone
N1	Low amplitude, mixed-frequency; mostly theta	Vertex waves	Slow	Normal (i.e. as in rest during wake)
N2	Low amplitude theta, some delta possible	K-complex (not part of arousal) Sleep spindles	None (sometimes slow)	Normal
N3	High voltage delta	None	None	Normal (or low)
R	Low voltage, mixed-frequency; no delta	Sawtooth waves	Rapid	Atonia; some EMG bursts/twitches
Wake	Low amplitude, mixed-frequency; alpha (posterior dominant rhythm) with eyes closed	—	Slow and rapid eye movements; eye blinking	Normal (high during activity)

Cyclic Alternating Pattern

Visual analysis of the non-REM EEG over a longer time frame of several minutes may reveal a pattern of short frequency changes (K-complexes, delta-theta or alpha activity) without obvious sleep disruption. These patterns have been termed a cyclic alternating pattern (CAP) and may represent a form of sleep instability, which may 'open a window' for pathology to occur, such as epileptic events [6]. The scoring of CAP patterns is labour intensive, and the clinical value has still not been confidently determined. It does, however, underscore the dynamics of sleep regulation.

Sleep Related Movement Patterns

The assessment of movements during sleep is of prime importance, especially in the setting of neurological sleep medicine. A great number of sleep disorders are accompanied by specific patterns of movements and/or behaviours during sleep. However, these must be distinguished from physiological phenomena such as so-called 'sleep starts' or infrequent myoclonic twitches. Video recordings are of prime importance in confirming the body part involved and the precise nature of any movement, helped in certain situations by EMG recording. Movements are also frequently seen in other channels as prominent signal artifacts. While tibialis anterior EMG is part of the standard PSG montage, for specific indications additional muscle groups should be recorded.

In the AASM manual, several different PSG-based movement patterns are described, either as isolated phenomena, a specific syndrome or a combination of both. These are Periodic Limb Movements in Sleep (PLMs), Alternating Leg Muscle Activation (ALMA), Hypnagogic Foot Tremor (HFT), Excessive Fragmentary Myoclonus (EFM), Sleep Bruxism, REM Sleep Behaviour Disorder (RBD) and Rhythmic Movement Disorder. ALMA, HFT and EFM most likely do not have significant clinical consequences and a specific relationship with other disorders is not established. Criteria for these phenomena can be found in the manual though although their scoring is considered optional.

Periodic Limb Movements in Sleep

The scoring of periodic limb movements depends on recording individual EMG bursts in the limbs and evaluating if they occur in a consecutive regular sequence or series. The recommended PSG montage considers only the tibialis anterior site to define PLMs. A significant leg movement is defined as an EMG burst with a duration of 0.5–10 seconds with at least an 8-microvolt increase in amplitude above the resting EMG tone. Leg movements appearing between 0.5 seconds before and after a sleep-disordered breathing event should not be scored.

It is important to note that leg 'movements' may be recorded in the absence of clinical or visible movement of the body part and that isometric contractions may generate EMG activity fulfilling the scoring criteria.

The leg movements are considered as being part of a PLM series when there are at least four leg movements with a regular gap between the consecutive movements of 5–90 seconds. Both body sides are considered together. When bilateral bursts are separated by less than 5 seconds, they are counted as a single leg movement in the definition of a PLM series. When a leg movement is part of a PLM series, it is called periodic leg movement. Over the night, the PLM index (also generally known as PLM-i) can be calculated as the total number of PLMs dived by the total sleep time. Although PLM index above 15 is generally considered abnormal in the literature, any associated disturbance of sleep continuity is clinically much more important. Therefore, it may be useful to score whether PLMs are associated with arousals which, by definition, occur when there is less than 0.5 seconds between the end of either event and the start of the other. This may yield an overnight PLM arousal index with more clinical relevance although a threshold value above which there are clinically effects remains undetermined.

REM Sleep Behaviour Disorder

The polysomnographic hallmark of RBD is the presence of REM sleep without its normal physiological muscle atonia and is defined as sustained tonic chin EMG activity and/or excessive phasic muscle activity in chin or limb EMG. In addition, the video recording of specific dream enacting behaviour allows more confident diagnosis. The precise definition of 'REM sleep without atonia' in the absence of overt motor behaviours remains a little controversial. Without being validated for clinical use, AASM adopted the scoring of phasic activity during 3-second mini-epochs as 'recommended'. The manual also mentions the option to add additional EMG recording of other muscles such as flexor digitorum superficialis of the arm in order to increase sensitivity [7] (Figure 2.1).

Bruxism

Bruxism can be seen as phasic and/or tonic elevations of EMG activity of the chin EMG channel or from the masseter. Because the EEG electrodes are referenced towards the mastoid, characteristic bruxism-related artifacts are often prominent in the EEG channels.

The AASM manual states that bruxism can be reliably scored by audio analysis in combination with the EMG activity. As sound is often recorded using an ambient microphone, bruxism sounds are not always picked up. As the EMG-pattern is so characteristic, it is recommended to mention them in the report even when sounds themselves are not recorded.

Rhythmic Movement Disorder

The various expressions of Rhythmic Movement Disorder (RMD) such as body rolling and head banging are typically picked up as large rhythmic movement artifacts in the various PSG channels. Head rolling in the absence of body movements generates typical rhythmic high-voltage EEG artifacts. In the AASM manual, the defined EMG criteria are unfortunately very general and not accompanied by clarification of the specific muscles to be examined in the different RMD variants. Analysis of the video recording is therefore necessary to clarify the final diagnosis. Many RMD patients also vocalise and a typical 'humming' sound may accompany the rhythmic movements.

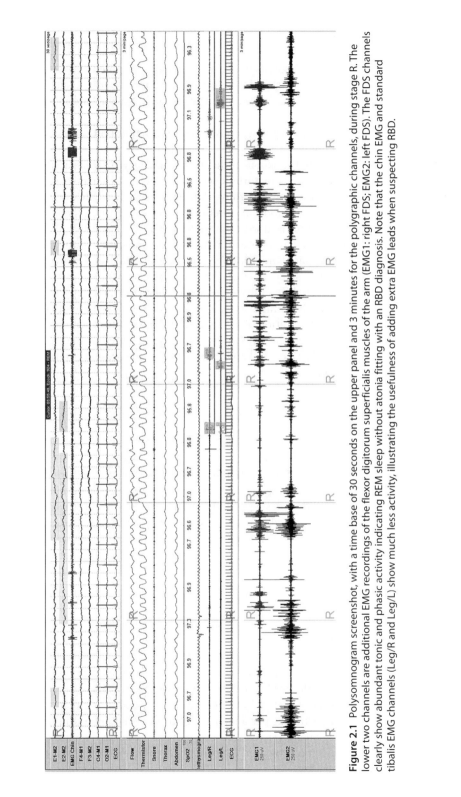

Figure 2.1 Polysomnogram screenshot, with a time base of 30 seconds on the upper panel and 3 minutes for the polygraphic channels, during stage R. The lower two channels are additional EMG recordings of the flexor digitorum superficialis muscles of the arm (EMG1: right FDS; EMG2: left FDS). The FDS channels clearly show abundant tonic and phasic activity indicating REM sleep without atonia fitting with an RBD diagnosis. Note that the chin EMG and standard tibialis EMG channels (Leg/R and Leg/L) show much less activity, illustrating the usefulness of adding extra EMG leads when suspecting RBD.

Sound Registration

The recording of sounds during PSG is a very important tool potentially serving multiple purposes. It detects snoring patterns, other breathing disorders such as stridor, vocal parasomnias such as catathrenia and vocalisations during motor parasomnias such as RBD.

Sounds can be recorded in several ways. A visual representation of sounds (the 'snore signal') on the polysomnogram is typically generated by a microphone or vibration detector attached directly to the skin near the trachea and larynx. A visual 'sound signal' may be generated indirectly from turbulence in the oronasal airflow which can be detected as an 'artifact' in the flow recording. Although not achievable during an ambulatory recording, more information and better quality can be obtained by using an ambient microphone synchronised with the video signal.

A contact sensor gives only an impression of loudness indicated by the amplitude of the signal whereas an ambient microphone can be calibrated and provide accurate measures of loudness expressed in decibels. With a contact sensor it is generally impossible to distinguish between different types of sounds and their aetiology. Indeed, snoring, stridor, groaning and humming will all look visually the same. When analysing sleep-related sounds, the respiration phase from which the sound is generated is important. For example, changes in the amplitude of the sound signal during an event that otherwise could be scored as a central apnoea may actually represent expiratory groaning, so-called 'catathrenia'.

Cardiac Function

Electrocardiographic recording is included in the AASM recommended parameters of PSG but only a limited (lead II) derivation is required as standard, in order to exclude certain arrhythmias. The following parameters are suggested worthy of reporting: average and highest heart rate during sleep; bradycardia, asystole, sinus tachycardia during sleep, narrow complex tachycardia, wide complex tachycardia, atrial fibrillation, and other arrhythmias. As always in the assessment of sleep recordings, it is of paramount importance to link any cardiac events to other observations from the sleep recordings, such as the occurrence in specific sleep stages or a relation with events like arousals or apnoeas.

Respiratory Scoring

Given the scope of this book, only a simplified overview of respiratory scoring is provided. Table 2.3 outlines the AASM criteria to score the various respiratory events. When two sets of criteria are listed, both definitions may count as equal. A non-filled box indicates that that particular parameter is not used in the definition of the event. Percent changes in a signal are related to the 'pre-event' baseline. The indication of an alternative sensor means it can be used to score the event even though this may lead to some under- or over-scoring.

Table 2.3 AASM criteria for scoring of respiratory events.

Event	Airflow pressure sensor	Airflow thermal Sensor	Respiratory inductance plethysmography	Oxygen saturation	EEG
Obstructive apnoea	(*Alternative sensor*) ≥90% drop peak signal during ≥10 seconds	≥90% drop peak signal during ≥10 seconds	Continued or increased inspiratory effort (entire period of absent airflow)		
Central apnoea	*Alternative sensor* ≥90% drop peak signal during ≥10 seconds	≥90% drop peak signal during ≥10 seconds	Absent inspiratory effort (entire period of absent airflow)		
Mixed apnoea	*Alternative sensor* ≥90% drop peak signal during ≥10 seconds	≥90% drop peak signal during ≥10 seconds	Initial part: (duration is not important) absent inspiratory effort / Second part: resumption of inspiratory effort		
Hypopnoea	≥30% drop peak signal during ≥10 seconds	*Cannot be used to score hypopnoeas*		≥3% desaturation	
	≥30% drop peak signal during ≥10 seconds	*Cannot be used to score hypopnoeas*			Arousal
Respiratory-related arousal	Flattening of the signal ≥10 seconds (not reaching criteria of hypopnoea or apnoea)		Increasing respiratory effort		Arousal
	No change or change but not reaching criteria of hypopnoea or apnoea				Arousal

While the determination of a full-blown apnoea to be either obstructive or central in nature is usually straightforward, it may not be as easy with regards to hypopnoeas. The presence of snoring, a flattening of the airflow pressure signal, out-of-phase thoracic and abdominal effort (paradoxical breathing) all point to an obstructive origin. Scoring respiratory related arousals (RERAs) is optional and labour-intensive, so is usually done specifically at the request of the physician ordering the sleep study. A cardio-ballistic 'artifact' can sometimes be seen in the flow or effort signals during a central apnoea, confirmed by the time-overlap with the ECG.

Important parameters to document in a report include the AHI, apnoea index, and the oxygen desaturation index (ODI, typically reported as desaturation events with a drop of either 3 or 4% from baseline). When RERAs are scored, the total event index is designated the respiratory disturbance index (RDI). Overall indications of oxygen saturation are also useful, such as average oxygen saturation (SaO_2) during wake and sleep, and the time spent at levels below 90 and 80%. It is usual to report values according to sleep stage and, importantly, body position (supine versus non-supine).

A General Approach to Analysis and Interpretation

Before reaching a final conclusion from PSG, an overall or holistic analysis of the data is necessary to interpret the study appropriately. Often, this is an intuitive process but a systematic approach is recommended. Parameters can be seen from a 'static' perspective, down to the event level, or viewed as 'dynamic' in relation to timing through the study. Information from as many sources or sensors needs to be considered. Ideally, scoring itself or review of a technologist's scoring, analysis and signal interpretation should all be undertaken by a single somnologist.

Analysis

Data from a polysomnogram can be analysed in at least two ways. Typically, changes in biological signals such as electrical activity, sound, movement, or pressure are represented graphically with continuous variability between certain upper and lower limits. *Signal analysis* refers to the act of putting a meaning to the signal, understanding the underlying processes that generate it. The physical process that a sensor or electrode is intended to record has to separated from unwanted or unintended signals (artifacts). The signal can also be changed or distorted downstream from the sensor by digital sampling and filtering. Visualisation of the signal will also depend on limitations in display resolution.

Trend analysis refers to the analysis of the recorded data and the associated scored events when the time scale is compressed across several minutes or ultimately the whole night. The x-axis always represents time, whilst the y-axis obviously depends on the particular signal displayed. Sometimes, calculations are performed to show changes across time by plotting, for example, the beat-to-beat variation of heart rate. Plotting the various signals together in one overview will often reveal clinically relevant clustering or evolution of events. Common examples include apnoeas solely occurring in supine position or during REM sleep (Figure 2.2), increases in heart rate in response to PLMs, or steady low oxygen saturation caused by hypoventilation. Some of the associations can also be expressed numerically such as the AHI in supine position.

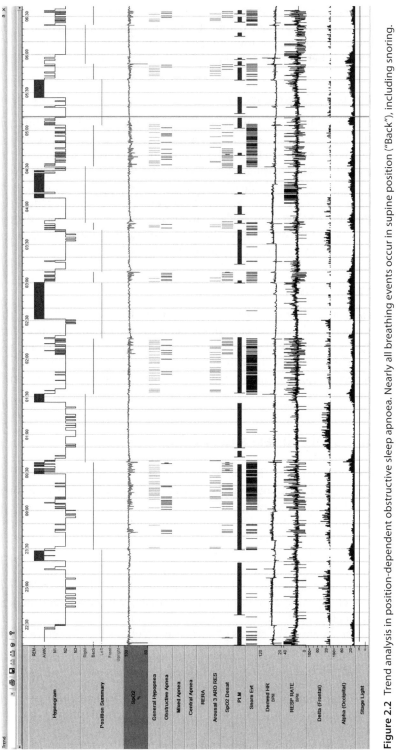

Figure 2.2 Trend analysis in position-dependent obstructive sleep apnoea. Nearly all breathing events occur in supine position ("Back"), including snoring.

Signal and trend analysis may provide considerable insights into the physiology and pathophysiology of sleep, usually demonstrating the superiority of digital to analogue PSG. Changing filter settings, reframing the time window, zooming in or out of details in relation to the other findings are all possible and often reveal useful information.

Interpretation of the Polysomnogram

All the information obtained from the sleep recording then needs to be interpreted in light of both physiology and pathophysiology, incorporating clinical information provided by the physician ordering the polysomnogram. However, caution is necessary to prevent clinical suspicion biasing interpretation and leading to false positive results. Some may prefer simply to provide factual data from the polysomnogram, leaving it for the clinician to interpret the data as more background is available. A report should at least provide the AASM recommended parameters whenever possible, together with graphical depiction of the data. The overnight trend graph is very useful in this respect with screenshots of key events as an important addition.

Conclusion of the Polysomnogram

The conclusion of the polysomnogram can be short and limited to addressing the question of the clinician although other findings should be mentioned if clinically relevant. However, PSG is never fully diagnostic in isolation. It is important to refrain from general statements on sleep quality without a clear underlying pathological substrate, as low levels of deep sleep, for example, may simply reflect an unfamiliar or uncomfortable recording environment.

Some Additional Pointers and Pitfalls

Issues around sensitivity and specificity of PSG mean that care is needed not to exaggerate the importance of findings such as periodic limb movements that may not always be clinically relevant. Interpreting data in the context of the presenting complaint is crucial, especially when fatigue, for example, rather than sleepiness is a main concern. An overall analysis of the polysomnogram is often useful, particularly when PLMs or other phenomena consistently lead to arousals and/or an overall fragmentation of the sleep structure, indicating they may be more likely to be clinically relevant and warranting treatment (Figure 2.3). In general, care is needed with conclusions on 'sleep quality' in the absence of a specific sleep disorder. For example, reduced amounts of deep sleep due to a fragmented night in a noisy hospital environment may often lead to unnecessary further assessments. The effects of normal aging on sleep architecture also need to be taken into consideration.

After sleep staging, the interpretation is usually taken further and parameters recorded such as arousal index, total sleep time, wake after sleep onset (WASO), sleep latency, REM-sleep latency, and sleep efficiency. The hypnogram also gives a further clear indication of overall sleep structure. The accepted normal pattern is based on four or five 90-minute sleep cycles each night, consisting of consecutive periods of N1, N2, N3 and R sleep with a small number of awakenings. The N3 sleep is expected to

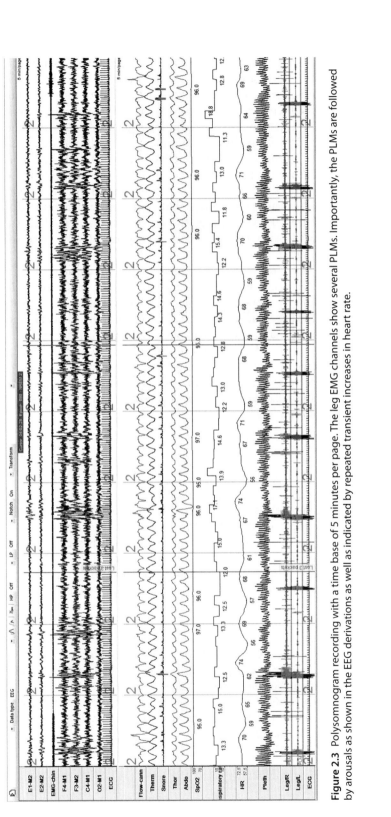

Figure 2.3 Polysomnogram recording with a time base of 5 minutes per page. The leg EMG channels show several PLMs. Importantly, the PLMs are followed by arousals as shown in the EEG derivations as well as indicated by repeated transient increases in heart rate.

dissipate over consecutive cycles whereas REM sleep increases through the night. Importantly, however, there are no strict, validated criteria to define sleep quality from this perspective and changes in sleep stage are not considered as pathognomonic findings. Analysis should therefore take into account other findings such as apnoeas. Ideally a patient's subjective experience of the recording night should also be recorded.

Some typical findings in the hypnogram may provide diagnostic clues or relate to medication effects. Examples include a reduction in N3 with benzodiazepine use, absence of REM sleep in the first part of the night due to antidepressants, direct awakenings from N3 in non-REM parasomnias. A sleep-onset REM period within 15 minutes is a finding that may suggest narcolepsy but can also occur as a rebound phenomenon after sleep deprivation. Highly fragmented sleep with frequent sleep stage changes is also seen in narcolepsy but is a relatively non-specific finding, also seen in sleep-disordered breathing

There is a wide range of activities during sleep that are considered normal variants and some EEG patterns may mistakenly be misinterpreted as a sleep disorder. Although there is also considerable potential for inter-observer variation in the analysis of polysomnographic recordings, 'manually' scored recordings are generally more accurate and preferred to purely automated or computerised reporting systems.

Simply inadequate sleep during the recording night may hamper a clear diagnosis, especially if the stage of sleep from which events of interest are most likely to occur is absent or curtailed. Nocturnal epilepsy, for example, arises most frequently from stage 2 NREM sleep and any epileptic features may be absent if this is shortened or fragmented by obstructive sleep apnoeas.

Key Points

- Polysomnography enables information to be acquired simultaneously about the precise sleep stage together with many other physiological parameters.
- Interpretation requires an understanding of technical issues, prior sleep history and assessment of other medical disorders and medication.
- While ambulatory recording in the home environment may result in more 'natural' sleep, PSG in the clinical setting has important advantages, such as the possibility for time-synchronised audiovisual recordings and close observation by clinical staff.
- PSG can be used to show the presence of a suspected disorder or additional 'co-morbid' sleep disorders as well as indicate the clinical severity or relevance of sleep-related events. Therapeutic responses can also be assessed if resources allow.
- The American Academy of Sleep Medicine has provided detailed standards on the technical aspects of the sleep recording, analysis and reporting.
- Information obtained from any sleep recording needs to be interpreted in light of both physiological and pathophysiological factors, and, most importantly, the specific clinical question that is being addressed.

References

1 Rechtschaffen A, Kales A, et al. (eds) A Manual of Standardized Terminology, Techniques and Scoring System for Sleep stages of Human Subjects. Public Health Service, U.S. Government Printing Office, 1968.
2 Berry R, Brooks R, Gamaldo C, et al. The AASM Manual for the Scoring of Sleep and Associated Events. American Academy of Sleep Medicine, vol. 2.3, 2016.
3 Aurora RN, Lamm CI, Zak RS, et al. Practice parameters for the non-respiratory indications for polysomnography and multiple sleep latency testing for children. *Sleep* 2012;35(11):1467–73.
4 Aurora RN, Zak RS, Karippot A, et al. Practice parameters for the respiratory indications for polysomnography in children. *Sleep* 2011;34(3):379–88.
5 Kushida CA, Littner MR, Morgenthaler T, et al. Practice parameters for the indications for polysomnography and related procedures: an update for 2005. *Sleep* 2005;28(4):499–521.
6 Parrino L, Ferri R, Bruni O, Terzano MG. Cyclic alternating pattern (CAP): The marker of sleep instability. *Sleep Med Rev* 2012;16(1):27–45. doi:10.1016/j.smrv.2011.02.003.
7 Frauscher B, Högl B. REM Sleep Behavior Disorder. In: Sleep and Movement Disorders (Chokroverty S, Allen RP, Walters AS, Montagna P, eds). Oxford University Press, 2013, pp. 406–22.

Further Reading

Basner RC. (ed.) Case Studies in Polysomnography Interpretation. Cambridge University Press, 2012.
Geyer JD, Carney PR. Atlas of Polysomnography. Wolters-Kluwer, Lippincott Williams & Wilkins, 3rd edn, 2017.
Scholle S, Feldmann-Ulrich E. Polysomnographic Atlas of Sleep-Wake States During Development from Infancy to Adolescence. Ecomed, 2012.

3

Daytime Tests for Sleepiness and Vigilance

Indications, Interpretation and Pitfalls

Gert Jan Lammers[1,2], Mojca van Schie[1] and J. Gert van Dijk[1]

[1] *Department of Neurology and Clinical Neurophysiology, Leiden University Medical Centre, Leiden, The Netherlands*
[2] *Sleep Wake Centre SEIN Heemstede, Heemstede, The Netherlands*

Introduction

This chapter focuses on the two most widely used polysomnography-based objective tests for the measurement of sleepiness, the Multiple Sleep Latency Test (MSLT) and Maintenance of Wakefulness Test (MWT). It will also discuss a test of vigilance that has been reasonably well validated in primary or central hypersomnias, the Sustained Attention to Response Task (SART). The MSLT is currently mainly used for diagnostic purposes whilst the MWT and SART for the quantification of sleepiness and vigilance, potentially after treatments.

What is Sleepiness?

During normal daytime hours healthy adults are generally expected to stay awake, even in monotonous situations. In this idealised view, sleepiness should only occur before habitual nocturnal sleep. Excessive sleepiness can accordingly be defined as sleepiness and/or sleep occurring during the daytime in a situation when an individual desires and would be expected to stay awake. Excessive daytime sleepiness (EDS) affects approximately 5–15% of the general population in Western countries [1,2] although it is important to realise that it is a symptom and not a diagnosis. It is not even necessarily a symptom of a sleep disorder, as external factors leading to sleep deprivation and/or disruption may, for example, induce sleepiness that is perceived as 'excessive'.

EDS can present in two qualitatively different ways. The first is an increased duration of sleep over a 24-hour day–night cycle, for which the word 'hypersomnia' was originally coined. It is characterised by an extended nocturnal sleep period and also a complaint of daytime sleepiness. The second pattern concerns the inability to stay awake during daytime, usually without an increased amount of sleep over the 24-hour period, for which the term 'EDS' was originally used. Unfortunately, there is a tendency to use hypersomnia and EDS interchangeably, obscuring a possibly essential difference in pathophysiology.

More correct use may provide important diagnostic clues and may, to a certain extent, predict the result of tests such as the MSLT or MWT.

Testing Sleepiness

An ideal objective test for daytime sleepiness should not only have diagnostic value but should also quantify the severity of sleepiness and be easy both to apply and replicate. Furthermore, there should be reliable normative data. Not surprisingly, there is no such ideal test. The currently available tests (MSLT and MWT) are troublesome: they may leave considerable diagnostic uncertainty, do not reliably predict complaints that patients experience in daily life, and do not reliably predict the risk for accidents [3]. The most plausible explanation for these limitations is that 'sleepiness' is essentially subjective in nature and too complex to be represented by the prime parameter the MSLT and MWT rely on, namely, the time taken to fall sleep. Nevertheless, both tests have some value in the evaluation of sleepiness.

What is Vigilance?

In contrast to sleepy people, fully awake and attentive people are expected to be aware of potential changes in their environment. This capability is called vigilance [4]. Theoretically, tests assessing vigilance should reflect complaints associated with sleepiness more accurately than the previously discussed tests focusing on sleep latency, although this has yet to be fully proven. Vigilance comprises two dimensions: a quantitative dimension, describing the level of vigilance, from low to high; and a temporal dimension which describes changes over time. A high level of vigilance is a prerequisite for a high level of attention. The difference between both concepts is that vigilance, in contrast to attention, lacks a direction. Therefore, vigilance is not a synonym for sustained attention, although many authors use the terms interchangeably. Instead, sustained attention represents an executive function that can be regarded as an operationalised aspect of vigilance.

Testing Vigilance

Several methods are available for the measurement of vigilance, such as subjective visual-analogue scales, pupillography [5], quantified electroencephalography (EEG) [6] and a variety of response tasks assessing sustained attention, such as the psychomotor vigilance test (PVT) and the sustained attention to response task (SART), described in detail later.

The MSLT

The MSLT was introduced in 1977 with standardisation and general acceptance in 1986 [7–9]. Originally, the clinical protocol differed from the research one. In a nap opportunity, the clinical variant allowed subjects a period of sleep after sleep onset, to permit rapid eye movement (REM) sleep to emerge, whereas the research protocol was designed to limit the occurrence of sleep by waking up the subject immediately after sleep onset to prevent any recovery of sleepiness.

Clinical Protocol

The clinical version is performed as follows: after having electrodes attached for standard sleep recording, subjects are requested to try to fall asleep in a quiet and dimmed room. Four or five sessions (sleep latency tests or nap opportunities) are performed throughout the day, starting typically at 9 a.m., with 2-hour intervals. The subject is asked to stay in bed for 20 minutes when no sleep occurs. When the subject falls asleep the duration is altered to allow recording for 15 minutes after the onset of sleep. Sleep onset is defined as the first epoch of any sleep stage, including stage I. The sleep onset latency is the time from 'lights-out' until the criterion of sleep onset is met, or is noted as 20 minutes when sleep did not occur. The final score is the average of values of the separate sleep latency tests over the day. The MSLT should ideally be performed the day after nocturnal polysomnography. For a detailed description see Table 3.1.

Validation

The capability of the MSLT to measure sleepiness was established by applying the test to a group of healthy young volunteers who were sleep-deprived [10]. Significant correlations between the severity of deprivation and sleep latency the next day were found. Moreover, there was a significant correlation between subjective sleepiness scales such as the Stanford Sleepiness Scale and sleep latency (SL) [11,12]. Test–retest reliability, inter- and intra-rater reliability were all high [13–15]. Hypnotic drugs also produced the expected changes [16]. These findings led to the conclusion that SL as assessed with a MSLT represented an objective quantitative measure of sleepiness although studies to obtain normative data in large population based cohorts were not undertaken initially. Another consequence was that the MSLT was accepted as the main diagnostic test for sleep disorders characterised by EDS and to quantify the severity of sleepiness. Because of the pronounced influence of sleep deprivation, it became customary to precede the MSLT by a night in which the subject slept at least 6 hours, as recorded with a polysomnogram.

Initially, validation studies were largely limited to narcolepsy. It was found that the vast majority of narcoleptic patients was characterised not only by short SL but also by the occurrence of multiple sleep onset REM periods (SOREMs), that is, REM occurring within 15 minutes of sleep onset. However, multiple SOREMs were not exclusively found in narcolepsy but also occasionally in other disorders, particularly OSAS [17–19]. Test–retest reliability of SOREMs in patients with narcolepsy was found to be high [20]. Only very recently has it been shown that test–retest reliability is low in other disorders of central hypersomnia [21].

The MWT

The usefulness of the MSLT as an objective test to quantify improvement in sleepiness after therapeutic interventions turned out to be disappointing, particularly in narcolepsy [22]. Typically, MSLT results did not correlate well with reported dramatic subjective improvements in sleepiness and a 'floor effect' was hypothesised. Put simply, in very sleepy patients objective improvements were not detected because the test lacked sensitivity to tell severe and moderate sleepiness apart. It was also argued that the test

Table 3.1 Guideline from the American Academy of Sleep Medicine for the performance of the MSLT.

1) The MSLT consists of five nap opportunities performed at 2-hour intervals. The initial nap opportunity begins 1.5 to 3 hours after termination of the nocturnal recording. A shorter four-nap test may be performed but this test is not reliable for the diagnosis of narcolepsy unless at least two sleep onset REM periods have occurred.

2) The MSLT must be performed immediately following polysomnography recorded during the individual's major sleep period. The use of MSLT to support a diagnosis of narcolepsy is suspect if TST on the prior night sleep is less than 6 hours. The test should not be performed after a split-night sleep study (combination of diagnostic and therapeutic studies in a single night).

3) Sleep logs may be obtained for 1 week prior to the MSLT to assess sleep–wake schedules.

4) Standardisation of test conditions is critical for obtaining valid results. Sleep rooms should be dark and quiet during testing. Room temperature should be set based on the patient's comfort level.

5) Stimulants, stimulant-like medications, and REM suppressing medications should ideally be stopped 2 weeks before MSLT. Use of the patient's other usual medications (e.g. antihypertensives, insulin, etc.) should be thoughtfully planned by the sleep clinician before MSLT testing so that undesired influences by the stimulating or sedating properties of the medications are minimised. Drug screening may be indicated to ensure that sleepiness on the MSLT is not pharmacologically induced. Drug screening is usually performed on the morning of the MSLT but its timing and the circumstances of the testing may be modified by the clinician. Smoking should be stopped at least 30 minutes prior to each nap opportunity. Vigorous physical activity should be avoided during the day and any stimulating activities by the patient should end at least 15 minutes prior to each nap opportunity. The patient must abstain from any caffeinated beverages and avoid unusual exposures to bright sunlight. A light breakfast is recommended at least 1 hour prior to the first trial, and a light lunch is recommended immediately after the termination of the second noon trial.

6) Sleep technologists who perform MSLTs should be experienced in conducting the test.

7) The conventional recording montage for the MSLT includes central EEG (C3-A2, C4-A1) and occipital (O1-A2, O2-A1) derivations, left and right eye electro-oculograms (EOGs), mental/submental electromyogram (EMG), and electrocardiogram (EKG).

8) Prior to each nap opportunity, the patient should be asked if they need to go to the bathroom or need other adjustments for comfort. Standard instructions for bio-calibrations (i.e. patient calibrations) prior to each nap include: (1) lie quietly with your eyes open for 30 seconds, (2) close both eyes for 30 seconds, (3) without moving your head, look to the right, then left, then right, then left, right and then left, (4) blink eyes slowly 5 times, and (5) clench or grit your teeth tightly together.

9) With each nap opportunity the subject should be instructed as follows: 'Please lie quietly, assume a comfortable position, keep your eyes closed and try to fall asleep.' The same instructions should be given prior to every test. Immediately after these instructions are given, bedroom lights are turned off, signalling the start of the test. Between naps, the patient should be out of bed and prevented from sleeping. This generally requires continuous observation by a laboratory staff member.

10) Sleep onset for the clinical MSLT is determined by the time from lights out to the first epoch of any stage of sleep, including stage 1 sleep. Sleep onset is defined as the first epoch of greater than 15 seconds of cumulative sleep in a 30-second epoch. The absence of sleep on a nap opportunity is recorded as a sleep latency of 20 minutes. The latency is included in the calculation of mean sleep latency (MSL). In order to assess for the occurrence of REM sleep, in the clinical MSLT the test continues for 15 minutes from after the first epoch of sleep. The duration of 15 minutes is determined by 'clock time', and is not determined by a sleep time of 15 minutes. EM latency is taken as the time of the first epoch of sleep to the beginning of the first epoch of REM sleep regardless of the intervening stages of sleep or wakefulness.

11) A nap session is terminated after 20 minutes if sleep does not occur.

12) The MSLT report should include the start and end times of each nap or nap opportunity, latency from lights out to the first epoch of sleep, mean sleep latency (arithmetic mean of all naps or nap opportunities), and number of sleep-onset REM periods (defined as greater than 15 seconds of REM sleep in a 30-second epoch).

13) Events that represent deviation from standard protocol or conditions should be documented by the sleep technologist for review by the interpreting sleep clinician.

Source: Ref. [3]. Reproduced with permission of Oxford University Press.

simply measured 'sleepability' and did not reflect normal daily life: patients with EDS try to stay awake instead of trying to fall asleep, and they also do not spend their time in darkness without alerting factors. A new test dealing with these shortcomings was developed in 1982: the MWT [23].

Clinical Protocol

During the MWT, the subject has to sit up in a chair in a quiet and dimly lit room with the instruction to stay awake, a situation which better reflects normal daily life. Speaking and moving are not allowed. The rest of the procedure is comparable with the MSLT: usually comprising four sessions in a day with the occurrence of sleep recorded in all. To increase the sensitivity the recommended duration of each session is generally increased from 20 to 40 minutes in accordance with the most recent guideline in 2005. For a detailed description see Table 3.2.

Validation

The MWT indeed detected treatment effects more clearly than the MSLT but the measured correlation with subjective experienced improvements and performance was still only moderate. An exception may be driving performance in untreated obstructive sleep apnoea syndrome (OSAS) patients [24]. Another problem is the large variation in methodology between various studies. Test periods are either 20 or 40 minutes, and there are different definitions of sleep onset. These differences may profoundly affect the outcome and normative values (see the section on 'Normative data'). The MWT is not used for the diagnosis of a specific sleep disorder but is used to quantify sleepiness. In narcolepsy there are only data from pharmacological trials, which usually recruit selected patient groups. Baseline values in narcolepsy in these trials show mean SL values below 11 minutes, independent of the 20- or 40-minute protocol and the definition of sleep onset.

Sustained Attention to Response Task

Although the MWT appeared useful in detecting and quantifying treatment effects in central hypersomnias, it also turned out to have serious limitations. Complexity, costs, and motivational influences are particular drawbacks. Researchers were therefore prompted to search for more practical vigilance tests which, in addition, might be more accurate in predicting actual real-life performance. The SART has been studied most extensively although more validation studies have to be performed to determine its exact role and value in clinical sleep medicine.

The SART is a go/no-go task in which the no-go target appears unpredictably and rarely, and in which both accuracy, assessed through commission and omission errors, and response speed, quantified as reaction time (RT), are important. The SART was developed to investigate lapses of sustained attention in individuals with neurological impairment but proved to be a useful tool to investigate sustained attention in a number of other clinical conditions, including sleep disorders.

Table 3.2 Guideline from the American Academy of Sleep Medicine for the performance of the MWT.

1) The four-trial MWT 40-minute protocol is recommended. The MWT consists of four trials performed at 2-hour intervals, with the first trial beginning about 1.5–3 hours after the patient's usual wake-up time. This usually equates to a first trial starting at 09:00 or 10:00 hours.

2) Performance of a PSG prior to MWT should be decided by the clinician based on clinical circumstances.

3) Based on the Rand/UCLA Appropriation Method, no consensus was reached regarding the use of sleep logs prior to the MWT; there are instances, based on clinical judgement, when they may be indicated.

4) The room should be maximally insulated from external light. The light source should be positioned slightly behind the subject's head such that it is just out of his/her field of vision, and should deliver an illuminance of 0.10–0.13 lux at the corneal level (a 7.5 W night light can be used, placed 1 foot off the floor and 3 feet laterally removed from the subject's head). Room temperature should be set based on the patient's comfort level. The subject should be seated in bed, with the back and head supported by a bedrest (bolster pillow) such that the neck is not uncomfortably flexed or extended.

5) The use of tobacco, caffeine and other medications by the patient before and during MWT should be addressed and decided upon by the sleep clinician before MWT. Drug screening may be indicated to ensure that sleepiness/wakefulness on the MWT is not influenced by substances other than medically prescribed drugs. Drug screening is usually performed on the morning of the MWT but its timing and the circumstances of the testing may be modified by the clinician. A light breakfast is recommended at least 1 hour prior to the first trial, and a light lunch is recommended immediately after the termination of the second noon trial.

6) Sleep technologists who perform the MWT should be experienced in conducting the test.

7) The conventional recording montage for the MWT includes central EEG (C3-A2, C4-A1) and occipital (O1-A2, O2-A1) derivations, left and right eye electro-oculograms (EOGs), mental/submental electromyogram (EMG), and electrocardiogram (ECG).

8) Prior to each trial, the patient should be asked if they need to go to the bathroom or need other adjustments for comfort. Standard instructions for bio-calibrations (i.e. patient calibrations) prior to each trial include: (1) sit quietly with your eyes open for 30 seconds, (2) close both eyes for 30 seconds, (3) without moving your head, look to the right, then left, then right, then left, right and then left, (4) blink eyes slowly five times, and (5) clench or grit your teeth tightly together.

9) Instructions to the patient consist of the following: 'Please sit still and remain awake for as long as possible. Look directly ahead of you, and do not look directly at the light.' Patients are not allowed to use extraordinary measures to stay awake such as slapping the face or singing.

10) Sleep onset is defined as the first epoch of greater than 15 seconds of cumulative sleep in a 30-second epoch.

11) Trials are ended after 40 minutes if no sleep occurs, or after unequivocal sleep, defined as three consecutive epochs of stage 1 sleep, or one epoch of any other stage of sleep.

12) The following data should be recorded: start and stop times for each trial, sleep latency, total sleep time, stages of sleep achieved for each trial, and the mean sleep latency (the arithmetic mean of the four trials).

13) Events that represent deviation from standard protocol or conditions should be documented by the sleep technologist for review by the sleep specialist.

Source: Ref. [3]. Reproduced with permission of Oxford University Press.

Clinical Protocol

This test, lasting 4 minutes and 19 seconds, displays the numbers 1–9 a total of 25 times (225 numbers in all) in random order on a black computer screen. Subjects have to respond to the appearance of each number by pressing a button, except when the number is a 3, which occurs 25 times in all. The button has to be pressed before the next number appears. Protocols differ in the instruction provided to subjects: some instruct to give equal importance to accuracy and speed in performing the task, others prioritise accuracy over speed. At least two SART sessions with a 1-hour break in between are required for a reliable measurement, preceded by a full training session. The primary outcome measure is the error count, consisting of key presses when no key should be pressed (i.e. commission errors), and absent presses when a key should have been pressed (i.e. omission errors). For a detailed description see Table 3.3.

Validation

To date, the validation of the SART as a tool to measure sustained attention in sleep-disordered patients is based on a comparison of SART results between patients with narcolepsy and healthy controls. The SART discriminated well between these groups, indicating good construct validity. Between-subjects variability in SART performance was higher in the narcolepsy group than in the control group. No correlations were found between SART performance and subjective sleepiness (ESS) or between SART performance and the average sleep onset latency during the MSLT. In other words, the SART showed discriminant validity with these measures of sleepiness [25].

Table 3.3 Recommendations for the SART protocol.

1) The five-trial protocol prior to each of five MSLT sessions is recommended to quantify the level of vigilance in the diagnostic phase.

2) In any other phase, it is recommended to administer at least two SART sessions with 1.0–1.5 hour in between, preceded by a full training session.

3) The use of tobacco, caffeine and other medications by the patient before and during the SART should be addressed and decided upon by the sleep clinician before SART.

4) Subjects are seated on a chair in front of a computer screen in a dimly lit room.

5) The font size is chosen at random from 26, 28, 36, or 72 points. The numbers are presented in a predetermined and quasirandom way so that identical numbers are not clustered. Each number is presented for 250 milliseconds, followed by a blank screen for 900 milliseconds.

6) Instructions to the patient consist of the following: 'A number from 1 to 9 will be shown 225 times in random order. You have to respond to the appearance of each number by pressing a button, except when the number is a 3. You have to press the button before the next number appears, but note that accuracy is more important than speed.'

7) The following data should be recorded: the number of times a key was pressed when a 3 was presented (commission errors), the times when no key was pressed when it should have been (omission errors), and the reaction time of every correct press.

8) The SART error score consists of the total number of errors, expressed as the sum of the commission and omission errors.

Previous sleep studies administered the SART four to five times per day prior to each session of an MSLT or MWT. This design showed a higher error score on the first session compared with subsequent sessions in healthy controls [25] and in patients with excessive daytime sleepiness [26] which was caused by a repetition effect. This beneficial effect of repetition is more pronounced when instructing subjects to prefer accuracy to speed, but is neutralised by a full training session [27]. A study in healthy controls indicated that time of day (morning versus afternoon) did not influence SART performance, nor did napping between sessions when the SART is administered 1 hour after the nap (as in an MSLT design). However, these findings have not yet been replicated in patients with sleep disorders.

Normative Data

MSLT

Normative values for the MSLT depend on a variety of small studies often with unclear selection criteria and protocol details. Moreover, many factors influence the results of the MSLT: age (perhaps counterintuitively, in adults latency reliably increases with age), sex, number of naps (five SLTs versus four), use of psychotropic medication, anxiety, depression, and HLA DQB1*0602 positivity [27–29]. Inadvertent naps in-between the scheduled SLTs of the MSLT do not seem to influence the sleep latency of the scheduled naps significantly [30]. Healthy subjects may increase their SL by trying to stay awake during the test [31]. The degree of physical activity between the tests may substantially influence SL, at least in healthy subjects before and after sleep deprivation [32]. The occurrence of SOREMs is influenced by age, circadian rhythm and use of certain psychotropic drugs such as tricyclic antidepressants and the majority of SSRIs [27–29].

The pooled data of all these studies resulted in the following 'normal values': a mean SL of 10.4 ± 4.3 minutes for the 4 SLT protocol and 11.6 ± 5.2 minutes for the 5 SLT variant [3]. Note that the above-mentioned influences were not taken into account, except for one: subjects were free of psychotropic medication. Due to a large variability the distributions of patient and control values overlap substantially. Furthermore, a recent community-based study in over 500 subjects found that a mean $SL \leq 8$ minutes and ≥ 2 SOREMPs (i.e. the diagnostic criteria for narcolepsy) were observed in 5.9% of males and 1.1% of females, confirming findings in some earlier, largely neglected, small studies [28]. None of the subjects had cataplexy and the majority had an Epworth Sleepiness score ≤ 10. SOREMPs were not related to age, body mass index, depression and apnoeic events during sleep, but were associated with shift work, short sleep and decreased mean lowest oxygen saturation in males. Assuming that these subjects did not suffer from narcolepsy, which is probable in view of low Epworth Sleepiness Scale scores and the absence of cataplexy, this finding has consequences for the interpretation of MSLT results. Although 6% of all men may not seem much for a false positive result, this should be compared with common standards for many laboratory tests, in which a 2 or 3 standard deviation (SD) threshold is used to delineate abnormality. For a 2 SD threshold, a false positive rate of 2.5% may be expected. Compared with this a value of 6% is appreciably higher. It may well be wondered if such a rate is not too high for a test considered to be the 'gold' standard for a particular diagnosis. Moreover, taking into account that the estimated prevalence of narcolepsy is less than 0.05%, a group of people with a SL < 8 minutes and ≥2 SOREMPs, will contain only a very small proportion of people with narcolepsy.

Even more worrying were the results of a follow up study in this cohort, published in 2014, studying the stability over time of a positive MSLT including SOREMPs [33]. The prevalence of multiple SOREMPs was 7%, MSL < 8 minutes 22%, and a combination of both 3.4%, again the percentages were higher in males when compared with females. Shift work had a major impact on the results. Sleep deprivation only influenced sleep latencies and not SOREMPs. However, the stability over time of these abnormal results, which was the reason to perform this study, was very low: kappa <2 and not significant. Only 10–20% of subjects with abnormal MSLT findings in the first study showed them again during follow up after several years. The main conclusion to be drawn seems that before performing an MSLT, sleep deprivation and shift work in the week(s) prior to the test should be ruled out. Actigraphy is probably the most reliable tool to exclude significant sleep deprivation and shift work.

MWT

As with the MSLT, there is no large multicentre systematically collected set of normative data nor a large population based study. An additional complicating factor is that different protocols have been used. Normative data has been calculated from the available literature for the various protocols [27]:

- 20 minutes protocol; four nap opportunities; sleep onset defined by three epochs of stage 1 sleep or one epoch of any other sleep stage: 18.8 ± 3.3 minutes sleep latency.
- 40 minutes protocol; four nap opportunities; sleep onset defined by three epochs of stage 1 sleep or one epoch of any other sleep stage: 35.2 ± 7.8 minutes sleep latency.
- 40 minutes protocol; four nap opportunities; sleep onset defined by first epoch of sleep including stage 1: 30.4 ± 11.20 minutes sleep latency.

The MWT is significantly influenced by psychotropic medications, the prior amount of sleep, physical activity, motivational factors and age. As with the MSLT, sleep latency increases with age [3,30,31,34]. There is limited impact of inadvertent sleep between the sessions or the duration of previous nocturnal sleep. Similar to the MSLT there is a large overlap between findings in patients and the normal population. It has been suggested that 8 minutes should be considered as the lower limit of normal (for the 40 minutes; four nap first epoch variant) [3,27]. This would correspond to a false positive rate of 2.5% in the normal population.

Sustained Attention to Response Task

As with the MSLT and MWT, there is no large systematically collected set of normative data for the SART. A complicating factor is that different instructions have been used. An example of the latter factor is that the instruction to give equal importance to accuracy and speed results in higher error rates and a larger between-subjects variability in healthy subjects, due to the so-called 'speed–accuracy trade-off'. Normative data based on a small study are only available for the instruction to prefer accuracy over speed in a five-session protocol [25]: the median SART error score was 10.6 (6.1–18.7) errors for narcolepsy patients and 2.0 (1.3–4.0) errors for controls. Based on the 95th percentile in controls (5.4 errors), a five-error cut-off point was proposed. There is no direct comparison between patients and controls for the instruction to pay equal importance to accuracy and speed: the median SART error score was 11.1 (6.0–17.4) for narcolepsy patients in a five-session protocol compared with 9.3 (6.1–14.8) for healthy subjects in a two-session protocol. Data from the SART measuring treatment effects in narcolepsy are available for the instruction to pay equal importance to accuracy and speed: an average improvement from 11.6 to 10.4 errors was detected after treatment with modafinil, from 12.5 to 10.0 errors after treatment with the novel wake-promoting drug pitolisant, and no improvement was observed in the placebo group (from 11.5 to 11.4 errors) [35].

Diagnostic Criteria

There have been some changes in diagnostic criteria in consecutive versions of the International Classification of Sleep Disorders, ICSD (1990, 2005, 2014) [36,37]. For example, a pathological level of sleepiness was first assigned to a mean SL of less than 5 minutes, and later changed to less than 8 minutes in the second edition of ICSD. In the third edition (ICSD-3) the names for 'narcolepsy with cataplexy' and 'narcolepsy without cataplexy' have been changed to 'Narcolepsy type 1' and 'Narcolepsy type 2', accompanied by a minor change in the MSLT criteria: a sleep onset REM period during the night before the MSLT counts as a SOREM during the MSLT. In Idiopathic Hypersomnia the distinction between a subgroup characterised by long sleep versus one characterised by EDS has been removed, and a MSLT is no longer mandatory for the diagnosis. Below, we list the current criteria for the most important sleep disorders characterised by daytime sleepiness.

Narcolepsy with Cataplexy (Narcolepsy Type 1) and Narcolepsy Without Cataplexy (Narcolepsy Type 2)

According to the ICSD-3, apart from meeting clinical criteria, a MSLT is mandatory to diagnose narcolepsy without cataplexy. In narcolepsy with (typical) cataplexy, the MSLT is potentially optional if hypocretin levels are shown to be extremely low. Criteria for the diagnosis of narcolepsy with and without cataplexy are a mean SL ≤8 minutes *and* ≥2 SOREMs (a SOREM during polysomnography the night before the MSLT may count as a SOREM during the MSLT). It is important to realise that up to 10% of patients suffering from narcolepsy with cataplexy and who are likely to be hypocretin deficient, do not fulfil these criteria [38].

Idiopathic Hypersomnia

Besides the required clinical criteria, a SL during MSLT testing of ≤8 min and <2 SOREMs is required. As an alternative, the registration of >11 hours of sleep during a 24-hour polysomnogram, or a week of actigraphy are considered to be diagnostic as well. Sleep deprivation before these procedures should be ruled out. Note that these criteria are not evidence based but are deemed more realistic than the criteria listed in the second edition.

Hypersomnia Due to Medical Conditions

An MSLT is not required for the diagnosis. However, when a MSLT is performed, the mean SL should be ≤8 minutes. In neurodegenerative disorders, the EEG may occasionally be difficult to interpret. Comparing signals obtained during nocturnal sleep with those found during MSLT testing may sometimes facilitate the interpretation.

Parkinson's Disease
The MSLT frequently shows a short SL, and less frequently SOREMs. Correlations with subjective complaints are not consistent however, and dopaminergic medication may contribute to EDS [39–42]. Data on the use of the MWT in Parkinson's disease are scarce. One small study (20 patients in a tertiary-care centre) showing a high percentage of patients fulfilling criteria for EDS on the MSLT, but with relatively long latencies during MWT testing. The mean SL of the MSLT was 3.1 minutes, for the MWT it was 20.9 minutes (40-minute variant) in patients with a complaint of EDS. Respective values were 10.9 and 33.3 minutes in patients without a complaint of EDS [42]. Another study showed broadly similar results but patients were allowed to stay asleep during the MWT [43].

Myotonic Dystrophy
The MSLT is frequently abnormal showing a short SL. SOREM occurs relatively frequently, usually in association with complaints of subjective sleepiness [44].

Traumatic Brain Injury
In a cohort study, 28% of traumatic brain injury patients had complaints of EDS besides complaints of fatigue, and 25% showed a mean SL < 5 min on MSLT testing, 6 months after the trauma [45].

Insufficient Sleep Syndrome/Behaviourally Induced Insufficient Sleep Syndrome

A MSLT is not mandatory for the diagnosis. There are few studies; a SL ≤ 8 min and SOREM was reported to occur without estimates of its frequency. The recent findings that shift work and sleep deprivation may induce the MSLT findings characteristic for narcolepsy underline that MSLT abnormalities are often found in this situation. There are indications that in contrast to the findings in narcolepsy, where SOREMs are usually preceded by N1 sleep, in insufficient sleep syndrome they are more often preceded by stage N2 [46].

Sleep-related Breathing Disorders

Neither the MSLT nor the MWT or SART are required for the diagnosis of any sleep-related breathing disorders [1].

Recommendations for Use and Interpretation

Clinical Shortcomings

A diagnostic test should ideally be directly related to the pathophysiological process under study. This is not the case with the MSLT, the MWT, or the SART. Both sleep tests use SL as a surrogate marker for sleepiness but in different predefined circumstances. This use of SL as a surrogate marker is based on several assumptions, including the one that subjectively experienced sleep and sleep as measured by polysomnography correlate well, or are even identical. Another assumption is that the SL is only influenced by the degree of sleepiness. However, these assumptions need to be critically assessed. The use of stage I as 'sleep' is also controversial, and it has been shown that individuals who are 'polysomnographically asleep' are not necessarily fully asleep by their own subjective experience [47]. Importantly, sleep onset is not only influenced by sleepiness, but also by motivational and environmental factors. Likewise, the use of sleep latency as a diagnostic measure prevents a distinction between sleep deprivation and a (primary) sleep disorder. Importantly, sleep deprivation is not always easy to identify because of the large inter-individual variation in sleep need.

Finally, there may be a difference between sleepiness and the ability to make the transition from wake into sleep. Sleepiness may cause people to fall asleep quickly but some subjects may make the transition quickly without suffering from EDS. This point is largely neglected in the literature. Narcolepsy is often considered primarily as a 'transition disorder', characterised by an inability to sustain either the waking or the sleeping state for any length of time [48].

Sustained attention tasks also have limitations. A poor performance on the SART does not necessarily correspond to a vigilance problem, but may also be attributed to the inability to focus attention or to respond in a timely manner. Accordingly, the importance of the SART does not lie in the diagnostic aspect of performance impairment but in the quantification of such impairment and its comparison between different situations, such as before and on treatment. As with SL, performance on the SART is presumably influenced by motivational and environmental factors.

The SART is susceptible to voluntary efforts to perform poorly, but there is not much gain to be obtained from falsifying the test in that direction. For matters such as driving, performing better than usual is wanted. The SART is quite robust against attempts in that direction though, in contrast to the MWT, in which patients can use strategies to stay awake. Hence, the SART is suitable in situations where patients have a vested interest in performing well.

The MSLT in Practice

The MSLT is, despite its shortcomings, a valuable test in the diagnosis of hypersomnia and disorders characterised by EDS. Apart from CSF hypocretin levels, it is in fact the only objective test used for the diagnosis of narcolepsy without cataplexy. The test does not stand on its own: it is of major importance to interpret the results in any patient in the context of the patient's symptoms and of other tests. Recent studies show that it is mandatory to rule out sleep deprivation and particularly shift work as explanation for sleep complaints and/or abnormal MSLT findings [33]. One should also keep in mind that a negative test result may be found in disorders characterised by a need for increased sleep duration, the classical hypersomnias. Even in typical cases of narcolepsy with cataplexy with proven hypocretin deficiency it may occasionally be negative. The MSLT also has a very limited role as tool to detect improvement of sleepiness in therapeutic trials, particularly in narcolepsy.

The MWT in Practice

The MWT has no diagnostic value for a specific sleep disorder. Its main application is the quantification of sleepiness. Compared with the MSLT, the MWT is more sensitive to detect improvement in pharmacological trials for EDS, for example. The MWT may also be indicated in assessment of individuals in whom the inability to remain awake constitutes a safety issue. There is little hard evidence however, that links mean SL on the MWT with risk of accidents in real world circumstances. For this reason, the sleep clinician should not rely solely on mean sleep latency as a single indicator of impairment or risk for accidents, but should also rely on clinical judgement [3].

The SART in Practice

Similar to the MWT, the SART has no diagnostic value for a specific sleep disorder, but it is sensitive to detect improvement in pharmacological studies. In contrast to the MWT, it is not applied to quantify sleepiness, but to quantify vigilance. As such, it seems to be a better predictor of performance and has been proposed a more reliable estimator of the risk of accident in the real-world situation than the MWT. To date, however, scientific data to support this hypothesis have not yet been published.

Key Points

- The MSLT is the most widely used objective test for the assessment of daytime sleepiness. It is mainly used for diagnostic purposes.
- The MWT is used for the quantification of daytime sleepiness and the assessment of treatment effects.
- Although the MSLT is recognised as the best available test for the assessment of pathological sleepiness, its sensitivity and specificity are too low to use it as the sole diagnostic test. Results should always be interpreted in the clinical context.
- The SART may be used for the quantification of daytime vigilance and is sensitive to treatment effects.

References

1 Bixler, E.O., Kales, A., Soldatos, C.R., et al. (1979). Prevalence of sleep disorders in the Los Angeles metropolitan area. *Am. J. Psychiatry* 136: 1257–1262.
2 Joo, S., Baik, I., Yi, H., et al. (2008). Prevalence of excessive daytime sleepiness and associated factors in the adult population of Korea. *Sleep Med.* 10: 182–188.
3 Littner, M.R., Kushida, C., Wise, M., et al. (2005). Practice parameters for clinical use of the multiple sleep latency test and the maintenance of wakefulness test. *Sleep* 28: 113–121.

4 Lim, J., Dinges, D.F. (2008). Sleep deprivation and vigilant attention. *Ann. NY Acad. Sci.* 1129: 305–322.

5 Morad, Y., Lemberg, H., Yofe, N., et al. (2000). Pupillography as an objective indicator of fatigue. *Curr. Eye Res.* 21: 535–542.

6 Coenen, A M. (1995). Neuronal activities underlying the electroencephalogram and evoked potentials of sleeping and waking: implications for information processing. *Neurosci. Biobehav. Rev.* 19: 447–463.

7 Carskadon, M.A., Dement, W. (1977). Sleep tendency: an objective measure of sleep loss. *Sleep Res.* 6: 200.

8 Carskadon, M.A., Dement, W.C., Mitler, M.M.. et al. (1986). Guidelines for the multiple sleep latency test (MSLT): a standard measure of sleepiness. *Sleep* 9: 519–524.

9 Thorpy, M.J. (1992). The clinical use of the Multiple Sleep Latency Test. *The Standards of Practice Committee of the American Sleep Disorders Association. Sleep* 15: 268–276.

10 Carskadon, M.A., Dement, W.C. (1979). Effects of total sleep loss on sleep tendency. *Percept. Mot. Skills* 48: 495–506.

11 Carskadon,M.A., Dement, W.C. (1977). Sleepiness and sleep state on a 90-min schedule. *Psychophysiology* 14: 127–133.

12 Carskadon, M.A., Dement, W.C. (1982). The multiple sleep latency test: what does it measure? *Sleep* 5(Suppl. 2): S67–S72.

13 Zwyghuizen-Doorenbos, A., Roehrs, T., Schaefer, M., et al. (1988). Test-retest reliability of the MSLT. *Sleep* 11: 562–565.

14 Drake, C.L., Rice, M.F., Roehrs, T.A., et al. (2000). Scoring reliability of the multiple sleep latency test in a clinical population. *Sleep* 23: 911–913.

15 Benbadis, S.R., Qu, Y., Perry, M.C., et al. (1995). Interrater reliability of the multiple sleep latency test. *Electroencephalogr. Clin. Neurophysiol.* 95: 302–304.

16 Bliwise, D., Seidel, W., Karacan, I., et al. (1983). Daytime sleepiness as a criterion in hypnotic medication trials: comparison of triazolam and flurazepam. *Sleep* 6: 156–163.

17 Reynolds, C.F., III, Coble, P.A., Spiker, D.G., et al. (1982). Prevalence of sleep apnea and nocturnal myoclonus in major affective disorders: clinical and polysomnographic findings. *J. Nerv. Ment. Dis.* 170: 565–567.

18 Zorick, F., Roehrs, T., Koshorek, G., et al. (1982). Patterns of sleepiness in various disorders of excessive daytime somnolence. *Sleep* 5(Suppl. 2): S165–S174.

19 Walsh, J.K., Smitson, S.A., Kramer, M. (1982). Sleep-onset REM sleep: comparison of narcoleptic and obstructive sleep apnea patients. *Clin. Electroencephalogr.* 13: 57–60.

20 Folkerts, M., Rosenthal, L., Roehrs, T., et al. (1996). The reliability of the diagnostic features in patients with narcolepsy. *Biol. Psychiatry* 40: 208–214.

21 Trotti, L.M., Staab, B.A., Rye, D.B. (2013). Test-retest reliability of the multiple sleep latency test in narcolepsy without cataplexy and idiopathic hypersomnia. *J. Clin. Sleep Med.* 9(8):789–795.

22 Lammers,G.J., van Dijk, J.G. (1992). The Multiple Sleep Latency Test: a paradoxical test? Clin. Neurol. *Neurosurg.* 94(Suppl.): S108–S110.

23 Mitler, M.M.,Gujavarty, K.S., Browman, C.P. (1982). Maintenance of wakefulness test: a polysomnographic technique for evaluation treatment efficacy in patients with excessive somnolence. *Electroencephalogr. Clin. Neurophysiol.* 53: 658–661.

24 Philip, P., Sagaspe, P., Taillard, J., et al. (2008). Maintenance of Wakefulness test, obstructive sleep apnea syndrome, and driving risk. *Ann. Neurol.* 64(4): 410–416.

25 Fronczek, R., Middelkoop, H.A., van Dijk, J.G., et al. (2006). Focusing on vigilance instead of sleepiness in the assessment of narcolepsy: high sensitivity of the Sustained Attention to Response Task (SART). *Sleep* 29: 187–191.

26 van Schie, M.K.M., Thijs, R.D., Fronczek, R., et al. (2012). Sustained attention to response task (SART) shows impaired vigilance in a spectrum of disorders of excessive daytime sleepiness. *J. Sleep Res.* 21: 390–395.

27 Arand, D., Bonnet, M., Hurwitz, T., et al. (2005). The clinical use of the MSLT and MWT. *Sleep* 28: 123–144.

28 Mignot, E., Lin, L., Finn, L., et al. (2006). Correlates of sleep-onset REM periods during the Multiple Sleep Latency Test in community adults. *Brain* 129: 1609–1623.

29 Dauvilliers, Y., Gosselin, A., Paquet, J., et al. (2004). Effect of age on MSLT results in patients with narcolepsy-cataplexy. *Neurology* 62: 46–50.

30 Kasravi, N., Legault, G., Jewell, D., et al. (2007). Minimal impact of inadvertent sleep between naps on the MSLT and MWT. *J. Clin. Neurophysiol.* 24: 363–365.

31 Bonnet, M.H., Arand, D.L. (2005). Impact of motivation on Multiple Sleep Latency Test and Maintenance of Wakefulness Test measurements. *J. Clin. Sleep Med.* 1: 386–390.

32 Bonnet, M.H., Arand, D.L. (1998). Sleepiness as measured by modified multiple sleep latency testing varies as a function of preceding activity. *Sleep* 21: 477–483.

33 Goldbart, A., Peppard, P., Finn, L., et al. (2014). Narcolepsy and predictors of positive MSLTs in the Wisconsin Sleep Cohort. *Sleep* 37(6): 1043–1051.

34 Shreter, R., Peled, R., Pillar, G. (2006). The 20-min trial of the maintenance of wakefulness test is profoundly affected by motivation. *Sleep Breath.* 10: 173–179.

35 Dauvilliers, Y., Bassetti, C., Lammers, G.J., et al. (2013). Pitolisant versus placebo or modafinil in patients with narcolepsy: a double-blind, randomised trial. *Lancet Neurol.* 12: 1068–1075.

36 American Academy of Sleep Medicine (2005). International Classification of Sleep Disorders, 2nd edn. Westchester, IL.

37 American Academy of Sleep Medicine (2014). International Classification of Sleep Disorders, 3rd edn. Darien, IL.

38 Aldrich, M.S., Chervin, R.D., Malow, B.A. (1997). Value of the multiple sleep latency test (MSLT) for the diagnosis of narcolepsy. *Sleep* 20: 620–629.

39 Arnulf, I. (2005). Excessive daytime sleepiness in parkinsonism. *Sleep Med. Rev.* 9: 185–200.

40 Baumann, C., Ferini-Strambi, L., Waldvogel, D., et al. (2005). Parkinsonism with excessive daytime sleepiness – a narcolepsy-like disorder? *J. Neurol.* 252: 139–145.

41 Shpirer, I., Miniovitz, A., Klein, C., et al. (2006). Excessive daytime sleepiness in patients with Parkinson's disease: a polysomnography study. *Mov. Disord.* 21: 1432–1438.

42 Stevens, S., Cormella, C.L., Stepanski, E.J. (2004). Daytime sleepiness and alertness in patients with Parkinson disease. *Sleep* 27: 967–972.

43 Bliwise, D.L., Trotti, L.M., Juncos, J.J., et al. (2013). Daytime REM sleep in Parkinson's disease. *Parkinsonism Relat Disord.* 19(1): 101–103.

44 Gibbs, J.W., III, Ciafaloni,E., Radtke, R.A. (2002). Excessive daytime somnolence and increased rapid eye movement pressure in myotonic dystrophy. *Sleep* 25: 662–665.

45 Baumann, C.R., Werth, E., Stocker, R., et al. (2007). Sleep-wake disturbances 6 months after traumatic brain injury: a prospective study. *Brain* 130: 1873–1883.

46 Marti, I., Valko, P.O., Khatami, R., et al. (2009). Multiple sleep latency measures in narcolepsy and behaviourally induced insufficient sleep syndrome. *Sleep Med.* 10: 1146–1150.

47 Weigand, D., Michael, L., Schulz, H. (2007). When sleep is perceived as wakefulness: an experimental study on state perception during physiological sleep. *J. Sleep Res.* 16: 346–353.

48 Overeem, S., Mignot, E., van Dijk, J.G., et al. (2001). Narcolepsy: clinical features, new pathophysiologic insights, and future perspectives. *J. Clin. Neurophysiol.* 18: 78–105.

4

Diagnostic Strategies and Classification

Geert Mayer[1] and Dirk Pevernagie[2]

[1] *Sleep Disorders Unit, Hephata Klinik, Schwalmstadt-Treysa, Germany*
[2] *Centre for Sleep Medicine 'Kempenhaeghe', Heeze, The Netherlands*

Introduction

In the previous three chapters, the basic elements have been described to achieve a diagnosis for specific sleep disorders. However, it is often not straightforward to put together all the information provided by a detailed history, nocturnal sleep studies as well as daytime tests. In particular, sleep disorders are not always seen in a 'pure' state. Given the high prevalence of sleep-disordered breathing for example, it is not uncommon to encounter a patient with psychophysiological insomnia who also suffers from sleep apnoea. Complex symptomatology and pathophysiology are even more common in sleep disorders associated with neurological diseases. Moreover, people exposed to substantial socio-professional stress may suffer from sleep disturbances and may have daytime symptoms that are similar to those reported in primary sleep disorders, e.g. daytime fatigue and excessive sleepiness. These functional complaints may persist even if an associated sleep disorder is adequately treated.

This chapter introduces the current classification of sleep disorders: the third edition of the International Classification of Sleep Disorders (ICSD-3) [1]. Published in 2014, this publication constitutes a useful and comprehensive framework to direct diagnostic efforts.

An increasing number of sleep questionnaires are becoming available. These can sometimes be of help at the start of the diagnostic process and some of the more widely used questionnaires are discussed. However, questionnaires primarily aim to measure markers of certain conditions in target groups. Most questionnaires have therefore limited validity to accurately assess symptoms or other disease characteristics in individual patients. As such they may be used for screening of populations at-risk, but they are certainly not a proxy for appropriate history taking, on which the eventual diagnosis is based.

A final diagnosis and management plan will often depend on clinical data together with information provided by sleep studies. The importance of a systematic approach will be illustrated by case examples.

Sleep Disorders in Neurology: A Practical Approach, Second Edition.
Edited by Sebastiaan Overeem and Paul Reading.
© 2018 John Wiley & Sons Ltd. Published 2018 by John Wiley & Sons Ltd.

Classifications

The International Classification of Sleep Disorders is a concise reference book with information on the presently known disorders of sleep. The diagnostic framework of the previous (2nd) and highly influential edition resulted from consensus meetings of a large group of professionals selected by the American Academy of Sleep Medicine [2]. The ICSD-2 classified the various sleep disorders based on the following categories: insomnias, sleep-related breathing disorders, central hypersomnias, circadian rhythm disorders, parasomnias, and sleep-related movement disorders. In 2011, a detailed revision of the ICSD was undertaken, resulting in ICSD-3 [1]. The general categories were retained, but in several areas the complexity of the nosological classification of sleep disorders was reduced (Table 4.1). Symptoms that were separately classified as 'isolated symptoms' in ICSD-2 (e.g. primary snoring, sleep talking) have in the third edition been added to the chapters to which they are most applicable. Neurological disorders that are specifically sleep-related are listed in Appendix A of the ICSD-3 (i.e. fatal familial insomnia, fibromyalgia and sleep-related epilepsy).

The coding framework of the ICSD-3 is essentially different from more widely used general medical classification systems, such as the International Classification of Diseases (currently in its 10th edition – ICD-10). In ICD-10, the neurological disease should be coded as the primary diagnosis. Furthermore, not all sleep disorders are represented in ICD-10. Although by nature, important discrepancies will persist between these classification systems, the ICSD-3 manual provides corresponding or appropriate ICD codes (both ICD-9 and -10) for every diagnosis. At present, many neurological disorders with prominent sleep–wake symptoms are not specifically mentioned in ICSD-3. Table 4.2 lists most of these disorders, the majority of which are discussed in detail in other chapters of this book.

Sleep Questionnaires

A detailed sleep history is clearly crucial in achieving an accurate diagnosis, but time constraints and inexperience with managing sleep-disordered patients may pose problems for general neurologists. In selected patients, therefore, standard questionnaires may be usefully applied to estimate whether certain sleep disorders could be present. When the results are confirmative, the diagnosis should be established by formal history taking, and, if appropriate, by additional diagnostic tests. Many such questionnaires are available (Table 4.3). Some of these focus on a single symptom such as daytime sleepiness, whilst others attempt to aid diagnosis of specific disorders such as obstructive sleep apnoea. However, as stated previously, many questionnaires are not developed and/or validated for diagnostic use in individual patients, and the limitations of such an approach are illustrated in Case 1.

Some of the questionnaires used both in clinical practice and in scientific studies are discussed below.

The *Epworth Sleepiness Scale* (ESS) is by far the most frequently used self-administered questionnaire to evaluate daytime sleepiness [3]. Patients are asked to rate the

Table 4.1 Main diagnostic entities in the ICSD-3.

Insomnia
  Short term insomnia disorder
  Other insomnia disorder
  Isolated symptoms and normal variants
      Excessive time in bed
      Short sleeper

Sleep-related breathing disorders
  Obstructive sleep apnoea disorders
      Obstructive sleep apnoea, adult (OSA)
      Obstructive sleep apnoea, pediatric
  Central sleep apnoea syndromes
      Central sleep apnoea (CSA) with Cheyne–Stokes breathing
      Central sleep apnoea due to a medical disorder, without Cheyne–Stokes breathing
      Central sleep apnoea due to high altitude periodic breathing
      Central sleep apnoea due to a medication or substance
      Primary central sleep apnoea
      Primary central sleep apnoea of infancy
      Primary central sleep apnoea of prematurity
      Treatment-emergent central sleep apnoea
  Sleep-related hypoventilation disorders
      Obesity hypoventilation syndrome
      Congenital central alveolar hypoventilation syndrome
      Late-onset central hypoventilation with hypothalamic dysfunction
      Idiopathic central alveolar hypoventilation
      Sleep related hypoventilation due to a medication or substance
      Sleep related hypoventilation due to a medical disorder
  Sleep-related hypoxaemia disorder
      Sleep related hypoxaemia
  Isolated symptoms and normal variants
      Snoring
      Catathrenia

Central disorders of hypersomnolence
  Narcolepsy type 2
  Idiopathic hypersomnia
  Kleine–Levin syndrome (KLS)
  Hypersomnia due to a medical disorder
  Hypersomnia due to a medication or substance
  Hypersomnia associated with a psychiatric disorder
  Insufficient sleep syndrome
  Isolated symptoms and normal variants
      Long sleeper

Circadian rhythm sleep–wake disorders
  Advanced sleep–wake phase disorder (ASPS)
  Irregular sleep–wake rhythm disorder
  Non-24-hour sleep–wake rhythm disorder
  Shift work disorder
  Jet lag disorder
  Circadian sleep–wake disorder not otherwise specified

(Continued)

Table 4.1 (Continued)

Parasomnias

NREM-related parasomnias
   Disorders of arousal (from NREM sleep)
   Confusional arousals
   Sleepwalking
   Sleep terrors
   Sleep related eating disorder

REM-related parasomnias
   REM Sleep Behaviour Disorder (RBD)
   Recurrent isolated sleep paralysis
   Nightmare disorder

Other parasomnias
   Exploding head syndrome
   Sleep related hallucinations
   Sleep enuresis
   Parasomnias due to a medical disorder
   Parasomnias due to a medication or substance
   Parasomnia, unspecified
Isolated symptoms and normal variants
   Sleep talking

Sleep-related movement disorders
   Periodic Limb Movement Disorder (PLMD)
   Sleep related leg cramps
   Sleep related bruxism
   Sleep related rhythmic movement disorder
   Benign sleep myoclonus of infancy
   Propriospinal myoclonus at sleep onset
   Sleep related movement disorder due to a medical disorder
   Sleep related movement disorder due to a medication or substance
   Sleep related movement disorder, unspecified
Isolated symptoms and normal variants
   Excessive Fragmentary Myoclonus (EFM)
   Hypnagogic Foot Tremor (HFT) and Alternating Leg Muscle Activation (ALMA)
   Sleep starts (hypnic jerks)

Other sleep disorders

Appendix: Sleep-related medical and neurological disorders
   Sleep-related epilepsy
   Sleep-related headaches
   Sleep-related laryngospasm
   Sleep-related gastroesophageal reflux
   Sleep-related myocardial ischaemia

---

likelihood of dozing off in eight different situations on a four-point scale. The total score, therefore, potentially ranges from 0 to 24. Generally, a score above 10 is regarded to indicate significant and excessive daytime sleepiness, although several authors feel that a cut-off of 12 provides a better trade-off between sensitivity and specificity. Scores of 0 or 24 should generally arouse suspicion about the reliability.

The ESS measures daytime sleepiness over the past month. In contrast, another commonly used scale, the *Stanford Sleepiness Scale* (SSS), is designed to probe the contemporaneous feeling of sleepiness [4].

Table 4.2 Sleep disorders classified in the ICD-10 as 'neurological', together with neurological diseases that are very often accompanied by sleep disturbances; not all of which are mentioned in ICSD-3.

Neurological disease	ICD-10 code
Narcolepsy	G47.4
Idiopathic hypersomnia	G47.1
Kleine Levin syndrome	G47.8
Fatal familial insomnia	A81.8
RLS	G25.8
PLMD	G25.8
RBD	G47.8
Fibromyalgia	M79.6-/70
Sleep-related epilepsies	G40.2 - 40.8 + G47.0/1
Status epilepticus in sleep (CSWS)	G41.8
Sleep-related headaches:	
Migraine	G43.x
Cluster headache	G44.0
Chronic paroxysmal hemicrania	G44.0
Hypnic headache	G44.81
Neuromuscular diseases:	
Dystrophia myotonica Curschmann–Steinert	G71.1
Myopathies	G71.2-73.7
Myasthenia gravis	G70.x
Amyotrophic lateral sclerosis	G12.2
Guillain–Barré syndrome	G61.0
Polyneuropathies	G60-63
Multiple sclerosis	G35.x
Cerebellar ataxias:	
Spinocerebellar ataxia, SCA 1-6	G11.x
Hereditary ataxia	G11.x
Extrapyramidal diseases:	
Parkinson´s disease	G20
Chorea Huntington	G10
Dystonias	G24.x
Multi system atrophy (MSA)	G23.2/8, G90.3
Corticobasal degeneration (CBD)	G23.8
Progressive supranuclear palsy (PSP)	G23.1
Dementia of Lewy-body type (DLB)	G31.88
Alzheimer dementia (AD)	G30.x
Cerebrovascular diseases	I60-68
Head trauma	S06.x
CNS tumours	C70-72, D32-33D42-43

Table 4.3 Questionnaires often used in sleep medicine.

Name	Abbreviation	Diagnostic targets	Reference
Epworth Sleepiness Scale	ESS	Evaluation of daytime sleepiness	[3]
Stanford Sleepiness Scale	SSS	Evaluation of daytime sleepiness on a continuous, hourly scale	[4]
Pittsburg Sleep Quality Index	PSQI	Severity of sleep disorders	[5]
Berlin Questionnaire		Prediction of sleep apnoea	[6]
Ulanlinna Narcolepsy Scale	UNS	Distinguishes narcolepsy from sleep apnoea, multiple sclerosis and epilepsy	[7]
REM sleep behaviour disorder screening questionnaire	RBDSQ	REM Sleep Behaviour Disorder	[8]
Munich Parasomnia Screening	MUPS	Parasomnias	[9]
Sleep EVAL		Assessment of sleep disorders according to ICSD and DSM-IV	[10]
Structured interview for sleep disorders according to DSM-III-R	SKID	Provides interview techniques to obtain correct diagnosis according to DSM-III-R	[11]
SF-36	SF-36	Health-related quality of life	[12]

Case 1 Be careful with questionnaires

A 56-year-old man with Parkinson's disease was referred for problems with sleep mainte-nance. He did not indicate specific nocturnal events on a general sleep questionnaire but scored very high on the REM Sleep Behaviour Disorder (RBD) Screening Questionnaire. A detailed history, however, revealed that he was most likely suffering from sleep walking. The information in the questionnaire turned out to reflect 'second hand details' from his wife because he, himself, was totally amnesic for his nocturnal disturbances. The wife's report on his nocturnal actions had been very dramatic with descriptions of aggressive behaviours. The patient himself had no recall of his recent nocturnal actions but recalled that he fre-quently wandered around at night as a child. In particular, his mother had told him that his eyes were always open and he looked very 'blunt', typical of sleepwalking. This case shows that questionnaires can give wrong directions, especially in cases where a specific diagnosis such as RBD is quite likely a priori. Historical details that are the clue to the right diagnosis are usually only picked up in a clinical interview by an experienced physician. In this case, the lack of dream recall on apparent arousal, the detailed nature of the motor disturbance, the fact that he frequently left the bed together with a prior history of likely sleep walking all made RBD less likely than a non-REM parasomnia as a working diagnosis.

The *Pittsburg Sleep Quality Index* (PSQI) is a detailed questionnaire evaluating nocturnal sleep quality over the past month [5]. It comprises 18 self-rating questions and 5 questions to be filled in by the partner, if present. The 18 questions are divided into seven compo-nents which each yield a component-score between 0 and 3, which are then added for a global score. The components probe subjective sleep quality, sleep latency, sleep duration, sleep efficiency, several symptoms of specific sleep disorders such as sleep apnoea, consumption of hypnotics and daytime sleepiness. An empirical cut-off score of 5 allows discrimination of 'bad' from 'good' sleepers. However, note that the PSQI is not suited for differential diagnosis in clinical practice. Evaluation at a group level however, allows the component scores to have value assessing different aspects of nocturnal sleep quality.

The *Berlin Questionnaire* is a validated explorative tool of 13 questions designed to identify patients with obstructive sleep apnoea. The questions are targeted toward key symptoms such as snoring, witnessed apnoeas, daytime sleepiness and obesity [6]. The questionnaire has been shown to identify patients with a respiratory disturbance index of >5/hour with good reliability.

The *Ulanlinna Narcolepsy Scale* was designed to probe the two core symptoms of narcolepsy, excessive daytime sleepiness and cataplexy [7]. It has good discriminative properties, at least in a validation study against patients with sleep apnoea, multiple sclerosis and epilepsy.

The Munich Chronotype Questionnaire (MCTQ) focuses on the personal preferences of the sleep phase and the impact of week and weekend days on sleep and daytime functioning [13]. It provides new information about the influences of external factors and allows an insight into the function of biological clocks in social life. The results of the MCTQ allow each participant to be assigned into one of seven chronotype groups.

Other questionnaires directed towards specific sleep disorders are: the *International Restless Legs Severity Scale* [14]; the *Munich parasomnia screening* [9]; and the *REM Sleep Behaviour Disorder Screening Questionnaire* [8].

A different approach is taken by the *Sleep EVAL* system, a knowledge-based computerised expert system that allows the diagnosis of the main sleep disorders from the ICSD [10]. The system uses the interviewees' response as direct input, rather than the interviewer's judgement. Depending on the answers given, a decision-tree is systematically followed. The time needed to complete a Sleep EVAL interview therefore varies widely with a range from 10 minutes to more than an hour.

Sleep disorders often co-occur with psychiatric disease. The *SKID* is a validated diagnostic based on the DSM-III-R psychiatric classification system [11]. Finally, health-related quality of life can be assessed by specific questionnaires such as the *EQ-5D* or *SF-36* [12].

Reaching a Diagnosis

Perhaps more than most medical specialties, reaching a reliable diagnosis in sleep medicine can be less straightforward than anticipated. Symptoms are often more complex than at first appears and uncertainties frequently lead to 'probable' diagnoses.

A common first hurdle is for the patient actually to *acknowledge* there is a sleep problem, as symptoms are frequently misinterpreted. For example, excessive daytime sleepiness is regularly dismissed as tiredness which could, in theory, be solved by going to bed a little earlier.

On the other hand, patients may significantly *overestimate* problems with sleep. Paradoxical insomnia, for instance, is a condition in which a complaint of severe insomnia cannot be corroborated by objective sleep testing. Polysomnography in these patients often shows a normal sleep architecture.

Not infrequently, patients seek a medical explanation or diagnosis for functional complaints that are difficult to explain from a medical point of view. Comprehensive laboratory testing often fails to demonstrate a plausible cause for syndromes characterised by unrelenting fatigue and diffuse bodily pain. Moreover, the association between functional complaints and an established sleep disorder may still be coincidental. In such a case, treatment of the primary sleep disorder will not (or only temporarily) result in symptomatic relief.

Agreement between the patient and the physician that there is some form of sleep–wake pathologic process is key to the successful management of the sleep disorder. In many cases, the medical history with or without the addition of questionnaires, is sufficient to establish an initial working hypothesis along with a differential diagnosis. Diagnostic doubt in more difficult cases usually requires one or more objective sleep tests such as polysomnography. The diagnosis of certain sleep disorders, especially if there is combined or complex pathology, often requires specific attention and investigation in a specialised sleep centre.

The data gathered by questionnaires, the clinical interview and additional technical procedures should be integrated into a logical framework that provides a working hypothesis, differential diagnosis, and eventually a final, confirmed diagnosis. In this process, medical co-morbidity should always be taken into account. This holds not only true for a primary neurological disorder, but also for many other diseases such as psychiatric, endocrine or pulmonary disturbances.

Translating the Complaints

From the medical history (detailed in Chapter 1), a list of reported complaints is compiled, such as 'falling asleep during activity', 'inability to concentrate upon awakening', or 'itching of the legs'. These complaints should then be translated into formal symptoms: 'excessive daytime sleepiness', 'sleep inertia or drunkenness', 'restless legs'. The next step is to formulate a working hypothesis that points to a disease according to the ICSD-3 criteria: possible obstructive sleep apnoea syndrome, restless legs syndrome.

Sometimes the array of symptoms seems so classical that a specific diagnosis jumps out very early in the interview. However, it is generally recommended to follow a structured examination of all general aspects of sleep and address symptoms that could indicate other sleep disorders. For example, information on normal bed times and sleep hygiene should always be sought. Routine screening for restless legs, nocturnal movements and sleep apnoea symptoms are also mandatory. Finally, a drug history may reveal agents potentially disturbing sleep or masking certain complaints. If the diagnostic trajectory is focused towards one specific disorder too soon, one may easily miss the correct diagnosis (see Case 2). In addition, the information from the general sleep interview may be of help with treatment. For example, even though narcolepsy patients usually merit drug treatment, improving ingrained bad sleep habits such as an irregular sleep–wake schedule may be very beneficial to individual subjects.

The Need for Additional Tests

Sleep tests are not only potentially useful when a clinical diagnosis is uncertain. Besides clarifying a differential diagnosis, sleep-related investigations may be required to assess the presence and degree of co-morbid sleep disorders. At the very least, tests usually

---

Case 2 A sleep disorder may not come alone

A 40-year-old male presented in the sleep clinic because of persisting severe daytime sleepiness despite continuous positive airway pressure (CPAP) therapy for earlier diagnosed obstructive sleep apnoea. For the first time, at the age of 36, the patient had consulted a physician in a pulmonary sleep laboratory to assess his longstanding sleepiness. The referral had been prompted by a number of failed exams after a management course at work. In a state of severe drowsiness, he had written nonsense prose in a presumed state of automatism and, as a consequence, had failed.

A polygraphic study revealed severe obstructive sleep apnoea (apnoea–hypopnoea index, AHI = 56/hour). Nasal CPAP treatment at a pressure of 11 cm H_2O was initiated and the patient showed good compliance. He felt that his sleepiness had improved during the initial 4 months after the start of the treatment. He had another polygraphic study at the age of 38, which did not show any apnoeas under CPAP treatment. However, he still complained about severe excessive daytime sleepiness at that time. Furthermore, he reported 'breaking away of legs', when scolding his children or telling jokes. He was then referred to a general sleep clinic.

A thorough medical history revealed that, even at the age of 19, when joking around with friends, he would buckle at the knees. In addition, he often felt asleep at school and classmates regularly had to waken him during lessons. In the clinic, several other complaints were picked up:

- suddenly falling asleep during the daytime;
- recognising his sleepiness only by looking at mistakes made whilst writing, often illegibly;
- buckling of the legs one or two times a day, sometimes with falls;
- frequent short nocturnal awakenings, even with CPAP treatment;
- nocturnal talking, sometimes accompanied by aggressive movements of the arms and legs, disturbing the sleep of his wife.

A Multiple Sleep Latency Test was performed, showing a mean sleep latency of 4.4 minutes and three sleep onset REM periods. This confirmed a diagnosis of narcolepsy/cataplexy, and treatment with stimulants and antidepressants for cataplexy was initiated.

This patient shows that complaints not recognised as part of a sleep disorder may be present for many years before a sleep doctor is consulted. Even then, only the most prominent complaints are spontaneously reported. To establish a final diagnosis, the whole array of symptoms of a suspected sleep disorder has to be scrutinised. Furthermore, in every patient a general sleep history has to be taken. Given the high prevalence of certain sleep disorders such as sleep apnoea, it is not uncommon to encounter patients with more than just one disease. In this case, the recognition of cataplexy would have prevented the considerable delay of over 4 years before appropriate treatment was started.

---

provide insight into the severity of the disorder in a relatively objective way. Furthermore, the diagnosis of certain primary sleep disorders such as narcolepsy may have important psychosocial, legal and treatment consequences. This stresses the importance of making every effort to reach a certain and objective diagnosis.

The performance and interpretation of sleep investigations are covered in Chapters 2 and 3. It should again be emphasised, however, that the interpretation of polysomnographic recording never stands alone. Failing to include relevant information from the medical history is almost guaranteed to produce erroneous conclusions (Case 3).

Case 3 History, history, history

A 42-year-old man was referred from a peripheral hospital to the sleep clinic. He had been a normal sleeper until 10 months previously. At that time, he experienced a traffic accident whilst biking. He was hit by a car and was flung onto the hood of the car, receiving a blow to the back of the head. He was rendered unconscious for several minutes. He was examined during a short hospital admission for a mild traumatic brain injury, requiring only relative rest. After a few weeks, he began to suffer from insomnia with initially problems of sleep maintenance. Later, the initiation of sleep became a major issue as well. This condition progressively worsened to the extent that he was unable to go to work. Whilst his sleep was reportedly very bad, he was not particularly sleepy during the daytime. A polysomnogram scheduled in the general hospital showed a long sleep latency but a relatively normal sleep architecture thereafter. There were no frank apnoeas but frequent hypopnoeas with an index of 17.8/hour (Figure 4.1).

The polysomnogram was separately reviewed by a neurologist and a pulmonologist. The former established a diagnosis of delayed sleep phase syndrome based on the long sleep latency and the subsequent stretch of relatively stable sleep. The neurologist prescribed melatonin 3 mg before bedtime. The pulmonologist diagnosed obstructive sleep apnoea syndrome and recommended treatment with nasal CPAP.

Melatonin resulted in better sleep initiation although this effect was lost after 2 weeks. The patient could not tolerate nasal CPAP as it worsened his insomnia. He was then referred to the sleep clinic because of treatment failure. All necessary diagnostic steps for diagnosis were repeated, starting with a thorough history of the actual symptoms.

The history revealed an acute-onset insomnia evolving into a progressive chronic course. The accident served as the primary triggering event. The delay of several weeks between the event and the onset of sleep symptoms also suggested a psychological

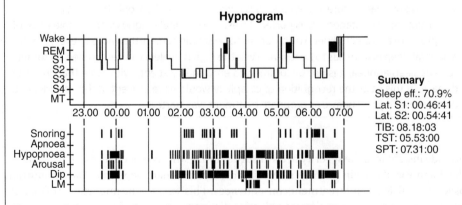

Figure 4.1 Polysomnography results of the patient described in Case 3.

rather than a physical ('organic') consequence of the accident. When the patient could not fall asleep, or woke up after sleep onset he would start to worry. Ruminations about his health and fitness to continue his job were the main recurrent themes. When unable to sleep, he became very tense and restless with a tendency to turn to his alarm clock. Overall, the history was consistent with psychophysiological insomnia.

The insomnia culminated in absence from work for 3 months. A course of zoplicone 7.5 mg at bedtime gave temporary relief. It was not until he received cognitive behavioural therapy that his condition improved substantially. He gradually slept better and was able to fall asleep faster after nocturnal awakenings. He had learned not to watch the clock and had reduced sleeping pills to one or two times a week, taking them when he had a bad night before. He had resumed his work on a part-time basis.

It appeared that the history was not taken well into consideration in the initial assessment at the peripheral hospital. The delay in sleep onset on the polysomnographic recording actually reflected sleep-onset insomnia, rather than being a sign of a circadian rhythm disorder. The elevated number of hypopnoeas was obtained from automated scoring by which the hypopnoea index was probably overestimated. Most importantly, the patient's actual history was not suggestive for sleep-related breathing problems.

This case illustrates that all pieces of diagnostic information must be taken into account. A detailed history is clearly the starting point. In this case, the working hypothesis should have been 'psychophysiological insomnia' right from the beginning. This would have changed the conclusions inferred from the polysomnographic recording and may have obviated the need for doing this test in the first place.

'Diagnostic Treatment'

Sometimes it can be helpful to start a treatment in the context of a working diagnosis, not only for the benefit of the patient but also as a diagnostic aid.

For example, if bad sleep hygiene is picked up in a patient with excessive somnolence, this should be initially addressed and appropriate advice given. The same holds true when withdrawing or changing medications or substances that are likely to disturb sleep. When these measures do not lead to resolution of daytime somnolence, further testing can then be considered.

Another situation is the sleepy patient with reported snoring but a low apnoea index recorded on nocturnal polysomnography. If a trial of CPAP treatment is undertaken for a few weeks and leads to clear improvement of nocturnal sleep with disappearance of daytime sleepiness, significant sleep-related breathing disorder can be assumed. In contrast, when patients with suspected sleep-disordered breathing and a high apnoea index do not report subjective improvement following adequate CPAP therapy, other causes for their complaints must be sought.

Although this empirical approach can be helpful, it is essential to discuss and decide beforehand how long a treatment trial will be attempted and what parameters for treatment success or failure will be used. This helps to avoid unnecessary continued treatments in patients when beneficial effects are – at best – doubtful.

The Sleep Specialist

It should be within the scope of most general neurologists to diagnose many sleep disorders with confidence. However, when diagnostic doubt remains, it is advisable to consult a sleep specialist at an early stage so that specific sleep tests can be considered. A sleep physician may also be required when the presence of another medical disorder interferes with the diagnostic process. This also holds true for – often rare – primary sleep disorders in which a definite diagnosis has severe consequences for daily activities such as narcolepsy, or if potentially complex treatments need consideration. Following diagnosis, a sleep specialist is best placed to decide on the most appropriate therapeutic strategy whether this is positive-airway pressure therapy for sleep-disordered breathing, multidrug regiments for narcolepsy, cognitive behavioural therapy for insomnia, or even a combination of all three.

It is increasingly common for a sleep specialist to uncover a previously unrecognised neurological or other medical disorder. For example, RBD is now considered to be a reliable pre-motor manifestation of a parkinsonian syndrome. Therefore, the sleep specialist should consider the potential presence of a neurodegenerative disorder, in a patient with RBD, and refer appropriately. Another example is excessive daytime sleepiness as a sign of nocturnal hypercapnia in patients with undiagnosed neuromuscular disease. Close collaboration between the sleep specialist and the neurologist may not only yield a complete and proper diagnosis but also enhances the quality of management. Treating the symptoms of sleep-disordered patients not only improves quality of life but may also help to circumvent significant medical consequences. For example, it is likely that in the case of sleep-related breathing disorders, morbidity and mortality due to potential cardiovascular sequelae such as stroke and ischaemic heart disease can be positively influenced by the use of nasal ventilation therapy [15,16].

Key Points

- The International Classification of Sleep Disorders provides a comprehensive framework for the diagnosis of sleep disorders, although it does not always highlight a sleep disorder when embedded in a neurological syndrome.
- Sleep questionnaires are never a substitute for a detailed history but may provide a useful and efficient screening tool to pick up sleep-related symptoms in a variety of populations.
- Sleep investigations may provide additional information to improve diagnostic confidence and reveal unsuspected or co-morbid sleep pathologies.
- It is sometimes appropriate to consider a treatment trial as part of the diagnostic process, provided clear guidelines for gauging effects are in place.
- Many patients benefit from the involvement of both a sleep physician and a neurologist in the management of sleep-related symptoms within neurological disease.

References

1 American Academy of Sleep Medicine. The International Classification of Sleep Disorders, 3rd edn. Darien, IL: American Academy of Sleep Medicine, 2014.
2 American Academy of Sleep Medicine. ICSD-2 – International Classification of Sleep Disorders, 2nd edn: Diagnostic and Coding Manual. Westchester, IL: American Academy of Sleep Medicine, 2005.

3 Johns MW. Reliability and factor analysis of the Epworth Sleepiness Scale. *Sleep* 1992;15:376–381.

4 Hoddes E, Zarcone V, Smythe H, et al. Quantification of sleepiness: a new approach. *Psychophysiology* 1973;10:431–436.

5 Buysse DJ, Reynolds CF, Monk TH, et al. The Pittsburgh Sleep Quality Index: a new instrument for psychiatric practice and research. *Psychiatry Res* 1989;28:193–213.

6 Netzer NC, Stoohs RA, Netzer CM, et al. Using the Berlin Questionnaire to identify patients at risk for the Sleep Apnea Syndrome. *Ann Intern Med* 1999;131:485–491.

7 Hublin C, Kaprio J, Partinen M, et al. The Ullanlinna Narcolepsy Scale: validation of a measure of symptoms in the narcoleptic syndrome. *J Sleep Res* 1994;3:52–59.

8 Stiasny-Kolster K, Mayer G, Schäfer S, et al. The REM Sleep Behavior Disorder Screening Questionnaire (RBDSQ) – a new diagnostic instrument. *Mov Disord* 2007;22(16):2386–2393.

9 Fulda S, Hornyak M, Müller K, et al. Development and validation of the Munich Parasomnia Screening (MUPS). A questionnaire for parasomnias and nocturnal behaviour. *Somnologie* 2008;12(1):56–65.

10 Ohayon MM. Sleep-EVAL, Knowledge Based System for the Diagnosis of Sleep and Mental Disorders, Copyright Office, Canadian Intellectual Property Office [English Finnish, French, German, Italian, Portuguese, and Spanish versions]. Ottawa, ON: Industry Canada, 1994.

11 Schramm E, Hohagen F, Grasshoff U, et al. Test-retest reliability and validity of the structured interview for sleep disorders according to DSM-III-R. *Am J Psychiatry* 1993;150:867–872.

12 Ware Jr JE, Gandek B. Overview of the SF-36 health survey and the international quality of life assessment (IQOLA) project. *J Clin Epidemiol* 1998;51(11):903–912.

13 Zavada A, Gordijn MC, Beersma DG, et al. Comparison of the Munich Chronotype Questionnaire with the Horne-Ostberg's Morningness-Eveningness Score. *Chronobiol Int* 2005;22:267–278.

14 Walters AS, LeBrocq C, Dhar A, et al. Validation of the International Restless Legs Syndrome Study Group rating scale for restless legs syndrome. *Sleep Med* 2003;4(2):121–132.

15 Marin JM, Carrizo SJ, Vicente E, Agusti AG. Long-term cardiovascular outcomes in men with obstructive sleep apnoea-hypopnoea with or without treatment with continuous positive airway pressure: an observational study. *Lancet* 2005;365:1046–1053.

16 Yaggi HK, Concato J, Kernan WN, et al. Obstructive sleep apnea as a risk factor for stroke and death. *N Engl J Med* 2005;353:2034–2041.

5

Pharmacological Treatment of Insomnia and Parasomnias

Paul Reading[1] and Sue J. Wilson[2]

[1] Department of Neurology, James Cook University Hospital, Middlesbrough, UK
[2] Psychopharmacology Unit, Dorothy Hodgkin Building, University of Bristol, Bristol, UK

Introduction

In neurological clinical practice the full range of sleep disorders are commonly encountered either in combination with a neurological disorder or as a consequence of it. This chapter will focus on the pharmacological treatment of nocturnal sleep problems of which chronic insomnia, as defined by impaired sleep onset and/or maintenance, is by far the commonest. Despite the lack of a credible evidence base, drug treatment, if required, of parasomnias will also be covered. Although parasomnias are generally divided into those arising from either non-rapid eye movement (non-REM) or REM sleep, treatment options in practice do not differ greatly.

Sleep-onset and Sleep-maintenance Insomnia

Overall, insomnia is the most common sleep disorder in the general population with approximately 10–15% of the adult population reporting chronic symptoms [1,2]. The latest formal symptom-based definition of chronic insomnia in the International Classification of Sleep Disorders (3rd edition) remains somewhat arbitrary and refers to 'chronic insomnia disorder' [3]. In brief, to fulfil the criteria, sleep initiation, consolidation, duration, or quality needs to be disrupted at least three nights a week and be present for over 3 months, despite the opportunity to sleep adequately in an appropriate environment [3]. The inadequate night-time sleep quality must adversely impact on daytime performance with fatigue, poor attention, mood disturbance, increased errors and reduced motivation as common associations.

Traditionally, insomnia has been considered as being 'primary' or 'secondary' to identifiable external or internal factors that fuel or even cause the sleep disturbance. Most authorities now tend to avoid this distinction although it is accepted that around 85% of insomniacs may have potentially reversible factors contributing to their sleep

Sleep Disorders in Neurology: A Practical Approach, Second Edition.
Edited by Sebastiaan Overeem and Paul Reading.
© 2018 John Wiley & Sons Ltd. Published 2018 by John Wiley & Sons Ltd.

disturbance. These include neurological, psychiatric and other medical conditions, substance abuse, as well as lifestyle factors. Normal age-related deterioration in sleep quality also contributes to the increasing prevalence of chronic insomnia in the elderly, particularly if there is the additional component of a neurodegenerative condition. Indeed, all neurodegenerative diseases have been reported to include significant sleep disturbance as an early or even prodromal feature (see Chapters 14 and 15).

Increasingly, assuming provoking factors have been adequately addressed, treatment approaches to all forms of chronic insomnia are broadly similar. It is generally accepted that the most effective treatment for the commonest forms of chronic insomnia are behavioural or non-pharmacological (see Chapter 9). In particular, so-called 'psychophysiological insomnia', characterised by heightened arousal and learned sleep-preventing associations, responds best to cognitive behaviour therapy, specifically tailored for insomnia (CBT-I) [4]. This can be delivered by a variety of methods but availability in the majority of health services is generally very poor. The alternative option of using hypnotic medication remains the most practical option to the vast majority of patients despite considerable controversies and concerns, particularly over long-term adverse consequences [5]. If a drug treatment is considered appropriate, however, it is important to recognise the precise nature of a patient's insomnia with respect to sleep onset or sleep maintenance as this will influence the choice of drug.

Increasingly it is recognised that insomnia is a major and often neglected issue not only because of the huge negative impact it can have on quality of life but also because of its implications for public health. For instance, subjects with insomnia have up to a fourfold risk of subsequently developing depression [6]. Unfortunately, there are often numerous problems faced by doctors attempting to treating insomnia. First, drug treatments are often subject to guidelines or protocols recommending strict restrictions on the length of prescribing, conflicting with the long-term and persistent nature of most patients' symptoms. Secondly, the treatment pathways for non-pharmacological therapies such as CBT-I are generally poorly developed or not recognised by health commissioning bodies, partly due to inadequate data on the cost effectiveness of such therapies.

Choice of Hypnotic Medication

Many patients will have tried over the counter (OTC) sleep remedies before consulting the medical profession. These usually contain antihistamines with a relatively long duration of action and the subsequent potential for daytime sedation. Regarding herbal sleep aids, such as lavender, there are very few randomised clinical trials [7] and, so far, convincing evidence for efficacy is inconsistent.

In the clinical setting, an appropriate choice of hypnotic would be a drug whose absorption and elimination characteristics suit or match the patient's problem: that is, a fast-acting and short-lasting drug for someone whose only problem is falling asleep, or a slower-acting and longer-lasting agent for someone who has problems with sleep interruptions later in the night (Figure 5.1 and Table 5.1).

Specifically, in a neurological setting, where the sleep symptoms may be more complex, an empirical approach is often required. Furthermore, if an extended duration of treatment is anticipated, it is often more acceptable to recommend drugs not considered typical 'hypnotics'. For example, if sleep maintenance is a major symptom and

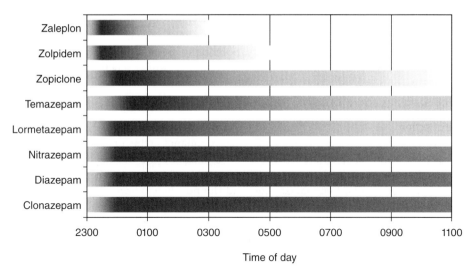

Figure 5.1 Graphic depiction of plasma levels of some typical hypnotic drugs, taken at 23:00 hours. The depth of shading corresponds to plasma levels.

Table 5.1 Benzodiazepines and benzodiazepine receptor-agonist ('z') hypnotic drugs.

	Usual dose (mg)	Rapid onset	Elimination half-life (h)	Daytime (hangover) effects	Safety
Zopiclone	7.5	+	3.5–6	?Yes	✓
Zolpidem	10	++	1.5–3	No	✓
Zaleplon	10	++	1–2	No	✓
Temazepam	20		5–12	?Yes	✓
Loprazolam	1		5–13	?Yes	✓
Lormetazepam	1	+	8–10	?Yes	✓
Nitrazepam	5–10	+	20–48	Yes	✓
Lorazepam	0.5–1	+	10–20	Yes	✓
Diazepam	5–10	+	20–60	Yes	✓
Oxazepam	15–30		5–20	Yes	✓
Alprazolam	0.5	+	9–20	Yes	✓
Clonazepam	0.5–1	+	18–50	Yes	✓
Chloral hydrate/ betaine	700–1000	+	8–12	?Yes	X
Chlormethiazole	192	+	4–8	?Yes	X
Barbiturates	Varies	+	Varies	Yes	X

reduced levels of presumably restorative deep slow wave sleep are thought likely, then an agent that increases the relative amount of deep slow wave sleep would be a logical suggestion. The concept that sleep quality, potentially defined by the total amount of slow wave sleep, is as important as simple sleep quantity is relatively new.

Benzodiazepines and 'z' Drugs

Mode of Action

Most hypnotic drugs used to aid sleep onset act by enhancing the function of the inhibitory neurotransmitter γ-aminobutyric acid (GABA) in the brain. The associated increased inhibitory transmission can lead to a combination of sedative, anticonvulsant and anti-anxiety effects. Benzodiazepines and the non-benzodiazepine 'z' drugs (primarily zopiclone and zolpidem) are generally effective hypnotics [8] that have an agonist effect at a modulatory site on the GABA-A receptor, effectively enhancing the inhibitory effects of GABA. Taken in overdose they have favourable safety characteristics since they enhance the effect of an endogenous transmitter. As a result, their sedative and respiratory depressant effects are limited by the availability of this transmitter such that they are not lethal when taken alone. However, with the addition of alcohol or other drugs which have the ability to directly affect the GABA-A receptor, this relative safety in overdose is compromised.

The shortest-acting benzodiazepines are temazepam, loprazolam and lormetazepam with half-lives of up to 12 hours. Zopiclone has a half-life of 6–8 hours, and is usually an effective drug both for initiating and maintaining sleep. Zolpidem has a fast onset (30–60 minutes) and short duration of action, with a half-life of 3 hours. A longer acting extended release formulation of zolpidem is available in some countries. Studies in volunteers have shown that zolpidem has no effect on psychomotor performance including driving skills when taken at least 5 hours before testing. This means that it can be taken during the night, either when patients have tried getting off to sleep for a long time, or if they wake during the night and cannot return to sleep, without hangover effect. It is the only prescribable hypnotic that can be used in this way. Patients find it reassuring because it means that they do not have to take a drug every night but feel they have medication potentially available, increasing confidence about sleeping and reducing associated worry.

Objective measures of sleep show that these hypnotics decrease the time to sleep onset and reduce waking during the night. The subjective effects of improved sleep are usually greater than the objective changes, probably because of the anti-anxiety properties of these drugs. Other changes in sleep architecture are dependent on duration of action, with the very short-acting compounds having the least effect. Usually very light (stage 1) sleep is decreased and stage 2 sleep is increased. Higher doses of longer acting drugs partially suppress slow wave sleep.

Other drugs that act on the GABA-A benzodiazepine receptor and enhance GABA function are chloral hydrate, chlormethiazole and barbiturates. However, at high doses they have the additional capacity directly to open the membrane chloride channel. This may lead to potentially lethal respiratory depression and explains their low therapeutic ratio. These drugs also have a propensity for misuse and are therefore considered very much as second-line treatments.

Side Effects and Other Issues

GABA-ergic drugs have side effects which include muscle relaxation, memory impairment, and ataxia. These may not be a problem when the patient is asleep but if it is necessary to get up during the night, especially if elderly or physically disabled, or if the action of the drug is prolonged past the time of arousal, then these effects can become very important. Any adverse effects are likely to be magnified in those with cognitive impairment. Those drugs with longer duration of action are likely to affect memory, concentration and performance in skills such as driving the next day. However, the daytime anxiolytic and muscle-relaxing effects which also persist can be helpful in some people.

Care should be taken in prescribing GABA-ergic drugs to patients with co-morbid sleep-related breathing disorders, such as obstructive sleep apnoea syndrome, which may be exacerbated by benzodiazepines in particular. Another very important point is that alcohol potentiates the effects of these drugs, and patients should be made aware that if they have had a drink in the evening, their sleeping pill will have greater and longer-lasting effects, possibly impacting on driving or work performance the next day.

Topics which worry patients and particularly their doctors when considering the use of hypnotics are those of tolerance, dependence, and withdrawal. Hypnotic drugs are licensed for short-term use and we have found that many insomnia patients can be frightened by their experience of stopping sleeping pills. There is almost always a short-term rebound of poor sleep, interpreted as a pressing need to start taking them again. When it is explained that this rebound is likely even in good sleepers in research studies, they often respond positively.

For patients who wish to stop their hypnotics there are various strategies. One is to encourage intermittent use of short-acting hypnotics, so that the patient knows they will get a good night's sleep two or three times a week with medication, helping them to cope with the bad nights. Another is to encourage dose tapering over a short period with education of the patient about rebound insomnia. Psychological interventions such as those involving cognitive behaviour therapy (CBT-I) may also provide the patient with strategies which will make stopping their tablets easier.

There will be some patients in whom it is difficult to ameliorate the sleep-disruptive factors which perpetuate their insomnia, or who continue to complain that their insomnia responds only to drugs. In such cases, the patient and clinician together need to weigh up the risks and benefits of remaining on medication, bearing in mind the possible risk of the patient using alcohol or unprescribed drugs as an alternative. There is emerging data on continuing long-term efficacy of the active (S) enantiomer of zopiclone (eszopiclone) for 6 months [9] and 12 months [10] and also for extended-release zolpidem for 6 months [11].

Antidepressants

Particularly in primary care, antidepressant classes of drug are commonly used as surrogate hypnotic agents, often in patients without significant mental health problems and usually at doses lower than those recommended for mood control. Antidepressants such as the selective serotonin reuptake inhibitors (SSRIs) which have good efficacy in anxiety disorders are often helpful in reducing anxious ruminations about poor quality sleep. If a typical hypnotic drug is used in combination and is to be withdrawn, the patient should be stabilised on a standard antidepressant dose before withdrawal of the hypnotic is started.

In depression, mirtazapine is useful in patients with marked insomnia as a major symptom because of its sleep-promoting properties. It has a receptor antagonist profile which includes blocking histamine H1 and serotonin 5HT2 receptors [12].

Trazodone also blocks 5HT2 receptors and is also often used in depressed patients with prominent insomnia. There has not been a controlled study of its use in insomniac patients who are not clinically depressed although it is widely used for this purpose in the USA. It may also increase slow wave sleep in both healthy volunteers and depressed patients (for review see Ref. [13]). When formally assessed, trazadone increases total sleep time and efficiency, reduces awakenings, increases slow wave activity and decreases sleep spindles [14]. Furthermore, it appears to improve sleep in a model of insomnia in healthy volunteers [15].

There is a small amount of data on the use of low doses of the antipsychotic quetiapine to improve sleep. It is primarily an atypical neuroleptic but also acts as a H1/5HT2 blocker with α1-adrenoceptor antagonism. However, drugs of this class may have long-lasting actions on sedation and have effects beyond the sleep-inducing brain systems producing potential unfavourable side effect profiles.

An alternative but non-recommended strategy used by many general practitioners, at least in the UK, is to prescribe low doses of sedating tricyclic antidepressants (TCAs), usually amitriptyline, for improving sleep. However, there is no objective evidence that very low doses of tricyclic antidepressants improve sleep long-term in primary insomnia. Doxepin 25 mg was shown to have a modest efficacy in a 4-week study [16], attributed to its anti-histamine effects. One reason for not using tricyclics is that these drugs are the commonest cause of suicide by self-poisoning with drug [17]. The side effect profile of weight gain and dry mouth is often also prohibitive. Furthermore, if restless legs or periodic leg movements are partly fuelling insomnia, these drugs are likely to worsen the situation.

Melatonin

Melatonin is the natural hormone produced by the pineal gland during darkness. Administration of exogenous melatonin has been investigated for insomnia because it assists sleep in circadian rhythm disorders when phase is altered such as during jet lag. However, its efficacy in primary insomnia is questionable [18], perhaps because it is very quickly metabolised. A modified release formulation of synthetic melatonin that prolongs the effective half-life has shown significant effects to improve subjective quality of sleep and daytime function in insomniacs over 55 years old [19]. In this age group there is some evidence of reduced endogenous melatonin rhythm. There were no significant daytime sedation or withdrawal effects. This new synthetic melatonin agonist, ramelteon [20], produces shortening of sleep latency in sleep onset insomnia, and shows no cognitive, motor or respiratory-related side-effects.

Another melatonin compound, Circadin, has been approved in several countries as a licensed agent for insomnia in the elderly and is now widely used. It is a slow-release preparation containing synthetically produced melatonin and is available in a 2 mg dose.

Melatonin is well tolerated although some patients report significant body cooling, perceived an hour or two after ingestion. This presumably reflects a physiological action of the drug on circadian temperature control.

Other Drugs to Improve Sleep Maintenance

Sodium Oxybate

Sodium oxybate is generally regarded as the most effective treatment for cataplexy and the other core symptoms of narcolepsy. Given before bed, it has marked and interesting effects on sleep quality, subjectively and objectively. It is the sodium salt of gamma-hydroxybutyric acid (GHB) which probably acts mainly through GABA-B receptors in the brain. However, a neurotransmitter system with specific GHB receptors has also been described [21]. The drug may also be metabolised to GABA thereby affecting GABA-A receptors too. Outside medical practice, it is a drug that is abused for its euphoric, intoxicating and growth-hormone promoting effects. Its half-life in plasma is very short but its central effects are somewhat longer lasting.

Its effects on sleep are to shorten sleep latency, reduce waking and markedly increase slow wave sleep. In narcolepsy, it appears to reduce the characteristically fragmented nocturnal sleep pattern and may 'normalise' sleep architecture, consolidating both non-REM and REM sleep elements [22]. Certainly, in healthy volunteers it has the effect of decreasing stage shifts, particularly from REM sleep [23].

In narcolepsy it is given in doses of up to 9 g per day in two doses, one at bedtime and one around 2–4 hours later. It is a controlled drug in most countries and dispensing is regulated largely due to its perceived abuse liability, particularly as a 'date rape' drug.

Because of its properties, sodium oxybate is also under investigation for a variety of sleep-related conditions, including fibromyalgia, Parkinson's disease [24] and REM sleep behaviour disorder (RBD). In a small series of patients with RBD and narcolepsy, the RBD episodes disappeared during routine treatment with sodium oxybate [25]. Despite its potency and likely effectiveness, it is unlikely that sodium oxybate will be used for uncomplicated chronic insomnia for the foreseeable future.

Gabapentin and Pregabalin

Although not licensed primarily for sleep-related problems, gabapentin and, in particular, pregabalin, are increasingly used by sleep physicians to treat sleep maintenance insomnia, especially if anxiety or pain symptoms predominate. These drugs are more commonly used as neuropathic pain agents but have the relatively rare pharmacological property of enhancing slow wave non-REM sleep [26]. This may improve subjective feelings of morning refreshment for patients in whom sleep is generally fragmented and/or dominated by light stage 2 non-REM sleep.

Parasomnias

Recognition and diagnosis of these nocturnal disturbances are described fully in Chapter 12. Simply having a formal diagnosis of parasomnia is often reassuring to patients, as they often fear epilepsy or that their nocturnal disturbances somehow reflect insufficient self-control. They also report both guilt about the effect the night-time disturbance has on family or housemates and fear regarding the potential harm they may inflict on themselves or others. Indeed, there is an increasing medico-legal literature as testament to this rare but distinct latter possibility.

Many subjects report increasing parasomnia activity in times of stress and it is likely that reducing anxiety levels may be particularly helpful for night terrors and other agitated parasomnias. However, the evidence base for behavioural therapies such as CBT, mindfulness or hypnosis remains rudimentary.

With regards to drug therapy, the majority of parasomnias do not justify treatment, especially if the patient is young and the disturbances are either mild or infrequent. However, particularly if violence and injury are feared or have occurred, pharmacological treatment should be discussed and potentially offered, if only on an intermittent basis. Unfortunately, there is an extremely small evidence base to guide choice as severe examples are relatively rare or, at least, unpredictable, making controlled studies very difficult. However, there are enough case series and small studies to provide a basis for empirical therapeutic trials.

Non-REM Parasomnias – Night Terrors and Sleepwalking

A first step should assess and treat potential trigger factors for any parasomnia. Most non-REM parasomnias are considered as 'disorders of arousal' in which a behavioural event occurs when a subject arouses abnormally and partially from the first cycle of deep slow wave sleep. Episodes therefore tend to arise either if sleep is abnormally deep, especially following sleep deprivation, or if there are particular arousing factors such as an uncomfortable sleeping environment, severe snoring or restless legs. Attention to issues of sleep hygiene may prove very helpful, especially in young adult populations. Unfortunately, sleep deprivation may be difficult to address if it is secondary to an arduous (night) shift work pattern.

Although a very controversial area, alcohol may increase the risk of an episode of night terror or sleep walking, probably because it deepens slow wave sleep, especially at the beginning of the night. However, it is equally likely that the secondary effects of high alcohol intake such as a full bladder or increased snoring may also act as an arousing stimulus to trigger events.

Anecdotally, episodes are more common and potentially more dangerous when sleeping in a strange or uncomfortable environment. For instance, escape behaviour is a common manifestation of non-REM parasomnias and is dependent on the door being in its familiar place in the bedroom. In this situation, an attempted escape via stairs or a window may cause injury. Many people prepare for this possibility by taking locks with them to secure doors and windows when sleeping away from home. Similarly, patients not keen on regular medication to treat their parasomnia often prefer to take it intermittently, at times of perceived higher risk.

Our precise knowledge of the underlying neurobiological mechanisms behind non-REM parasomnias remains limited such that it is difficult to provide a scientific rationale for a specific drug treatment. In general terms, it is accepted that agents which increase the depth of slow wave sleep, including alcohol, have the potential for triggering events and should be avoided if possible. Anecdotally, sodium oxybate used in narcolepsy may precipitate parasomnia activity and agents such as zolpidem or atypical neuroleptics are sometimes culpable. Given that natural ageing is usually the most effective 'cure' for non-REM sleep parasomnias, it might be surmised that an agent which moderately suppresses slow wave sleep activity without major adverse effects on overall sleep quality would be a suitable candidate. This is perhaps why the available evidence suggests benzodiazepines as first-line therapy, particularly nightly clonazepam [27], a drug with a long duration of action which decreases arousals from sleep and probably decreases slow wave sleep intensity. A dose of 0.5 mg is typically used with the aim of halving or doubling according to effectiveness and tolerability. Smaller studies have confirmed the efficacy of other benzodiazepines such as diazepam [28], alprazolam [29] and the very short-acting midazolam in children [30]. However, none of the patients in the clonazepam studies managed to reduce their dose of benzodiazepines without reappearance of the episodes, and withdrawal from clonazepam can cause a rebound worsening of night terrors.

Paroxetine, an SSRI antidepressant which increases serotonin function through blocking the reuptake site is also reportedly effective [31]. It can work even after the first dose implying that the mechanism cannot be the same as that for lifting mood, which usually takes 3–4 weeks. The most likely explanation is a direct pharmacological action to increase serotonin in brainstem regions suppressing ascending arousal pathways. In support of this theory is a controlled study reporting successful suppression of night terrors after daily use of 5-hydroxytryptophan, the serotonin precursor, in children with night terrors [32]. It remains speculative but likely that other SSRIs would also work in night terrors.

Some patients with severe or nightly terrors will be happy to take drugs such as paroxetine on a long-term basis. Some wish to try for a few months, and see if the terror 'habit' can be broken, which in some of our patients does seem to happen. Medication should be tailed off gradually because there is a risk of rebound after long-term dosing.

Anecdotal evidence suggests that other drugs that manipulate sleep architecture or potentially reduce anxiety may be effective in individual patients. Commonly used agents are clomipramine (25–75 mg) or melatonin (2–4 mg). If night eating as a manifestation of non-REM sleep parasomnia is the main concern, a number of case reports suggest topiramate (25–50 mg) may suppress events, potentially by its apparent effects on appetite suppression [33].

REM Sleep Behaviour Disorder

RBD, either in the context of a parkinsonian syndrome or as the idiopathic form, is worthy of treatment as it often poses a significant risk of injury to subjects and bed partners alike, particularly in the elderly with co-morbidities. Antidepressants, particularly SSRIs, TCAs, mirtazapine and mixed reuptake inhibitors such as venlafaxine are generally observed to make RBD worse or even cause it and should be discontinued if possible. Bupropion may not have this effect but evidence is anecdotal so far.

If RBD is non-violent or predominantly vocal, active treatment is usually not appropriate, especially if there is no bed partner. Similarly, some prefer simply to adjust the sleeping environment, potentially sleeping on a low bed away from furniture or using a sleeping bag. However, if there is risk of injury or significant sleep disruption in the subject or partner, nightly clonazepam is effective in the majority of cases in doses of 0.5–2.0 mg [34]. Unfortunately, adverse effects are not rare with daytime sedation or even confusion in elderly subjects, particularly if there is associated advanced Parkinson's disease. There is also a risk that underlying sleep-disordered breathing will be exacerbated or unmasked. To limit the risk of tolerance, some practitioners advocate drug-free days each week.

Increasingly, case reports and small series have shown some benefit from melatonin 5–10 mg [35], and some will use this as a first-line agent. More limited evidence exists for the dopamine agonist pramipexole [36] and the alpha-2 adrenoceptor agonist clonidine [37] which probably acts pre-synaptically to switch off noradrenaline activity. For symptom control, patients will usually have to take their medication for the foreseeable future and this should be emphasised to the patient and their treating physician.

Key Points
• Chronic insomnia is disabling to many patients and confers a risk of depression.
• If clear secondary causes have been addressed and drug treatment is considered, it should be tailored to the type of insomnia experienced by the subject.
• Zolpidem is the shortest acting generally available agent and can probably be used effectively in the middle of the night to improve sleep maintenance.
• Drugs increasing the slow wave elements of non-REM sleep such as pregabalin may have a useful role in some insomniacs.
• Tricyclic antidepressants are widely used as surrogate hypnotic agents but may worsen overall sleep quality and be dangerous in overdose.
• Most of the common parasomnias do not merit regular drug treatment.
• Clonazepam can be used intermittently for non-REM parasomnias and more persistently for REM sleep behaviour disorder.
• Paroxetine may help non-REM parasomnias by a mechanism separate to its antidepressant effects.

References

1 Ohayon MM, Caulet M, Priest RG, Guilleminault C. DSM-IV and ICSD-90 insomnia symptoms and sleep dissatisfaction. *Br. J. Psychiatry* 1997;171:382–388.

2 Roth T. Prevalence, associated risks, and treatment patterns of insomnia. *J. Clin. Psychiatry* 2005;66(Suppl. 9):10–13.

3 American Academy of Sleep Medicine. The International Classification of Sleep Disorders, 3rd edn. Darien, IL: American Academy of Sleep Medicine, 2014.

4 Morgenthaler T, Kramer M, Alessi C, et al. Practice parameters for the psychological and behavioural treatment of insomnia: an update. An American Academy of Sleep Medicine report. *Sleep* 2006;29:1415–1419.

5 Wilson SJ, Nutt DJ, Alford C, et al. British Association for Psychopharmacology consensus statement on evidence-based treatment of insomnia, parasomnias and circadian rhythm disorders. *J. Psychopharmacology* 2010;23:1577–1601.

6 Nutt DJ, Wilson SJ, Paterson LM. Sleep disorders as core symptoms of depression. *Dialogues Clin. Neurosci.* 2008;10(3):329–336.

7 Gyllenhaal C, Merritt SL, Peterson SD, et al. Efficacy and safety of herbal stimulants and sedatives in sleep disorders. *Sleep Med. Rev.* 2000;4:229–251.

8 Buscemi N, Vandermeer B, Friesen C, et al. The efficacy and safety of drug treatments for chronic insomnia in adults: a meta-analysis of RCTs. *J. Gen. Intern. Med.* 2007;22:1335–1350.

9 Krystal AD, Walsh JK, Laska E, et al. Sustained efficacy of eszopiclone over 6 months of nightly treatment: results of a randomized, double-blind, placebo-controlled study in adults with chronic insomnia. *Sleep* 2003;26:793–799.

10 Roth T, Walsh JK, Krystal A, et al. An evaluation of the efficacy and safety of eszopiclone over 12 months in patients with chronic primary insomnia. *Sleep Med.* 2005;6:487–495.

11 Krystal AD, Erman M, Zammit GK, et al. Long-term efficacy and safety of zolpidem extended-release 12.5 mg, administered 3 to 7 nights per week for 24 weeks, in patients

with chronic primary insomnia: a 6-month, randomized, double-blind, placebo-controlled, parallel-group, multicenter study. *Sleep* 2008;31:79–90.

12 Winokur A, DeMartinis NA, III, McNally DP, et al. Comparative effects of mirtazapine and fluoxetine on sleep physiology measures in patients with major depression and insomnia. *J. Clin. Psychiatry* 2003;64:1224–1229.

13 Wilson S, Argyropoulos S. Antidepressants and sleep: a qualitative review of the literature. *Drugs* 2005;65:927–947.

14 Kaynak H, Kaynak D, Gozukirmizi E, Guilleminault C. The effects of trazodone on sleep in patients treated with stimulant antidepressants. *Sleep Med.* 2004;5:15–20.

15 Paterson LM, Wilson SJ, Nutt DJ, et al. A translational, caffeine-induced model of onset insomnia in rats and healthy volunteers. *Psychopharmacology (Berl.)* 2007;191:943–950.

16 Hajak G, Rodenbeck A, Voderholzer U, et al. Doxepin in the treatment of primary insomnia: a placebo-controlled, double-blind, polysomnographic study. *J. Clin. Psychiatry* 2001;62:453–463.

17 Nutt DJ. Death by tricyclic: the real antidepressant scandal? *J. Psychopharmacol.* 2005;19:123–124.

18 Buscemi N, Vandermeer B, Hooton N, et al. The efficacy and safety of exogenous melatonin for primary sleep disorders. *A meta-analysis. J. Gen. Intern. Med.* 2005;20:1151–1158.

19 Wade AG, Ford I, Crawford G, et al. Efficacy of prolonged release melatonin in insomnia patients aged 55-80 years: quality of sleep and next-day alertness outcomes. *Curr. Med. Res. Opin.* 2007;23:2597–2605.

20 Erman M, Seiden D, Zammit G, et al. An efficacy, safety, and dose-response study of Ramelteon in patients with chronic primary insomnia. *Sleep Med.* 2006;7:17–24.

21 Crunelli V, Emri Z, Leresche N. Unravelling the brain targets of gamma-hydroxybutyric acid. *Curr. Opin. Pharmacol.* 2006;6:44–52.

22 Robinson DM, Keating GM. Sodium oxybate: a review of its use in the management of narcolepsy. *CNS Drugs* 2007;21:337–354.

23 Lapierre O, Montplaisir J, Lamarre M, Bedard MA. The effect of gamma-hydroxybutyrate on nocturnal and diurnal sleep of normal subjects: further considerations on REM sleep-triggering mechanisms. *Sleep* 1990;13:24–30.

24 Ondo WG, Perkins T, Swick T, et al. Sodium oxybate for excessive daytime sleepiness in Parkinson's disease: an open-label polysomnographic study. *Arch. Neurol.* 2008;65:1337–1340.

25 Kosky C, Bonakis A, Merritt S, et al. Sodium oxybate improves coexisting REM behavior disorder in narcolepsy with cataplexy. *J. Sleep Res.* 2008;17:97.

26 Hindmarsh I, Dawson J, Stanley N. A double-blind study in healthy volunteers to assess the effects on sleep of pregabalin compared with alprazolam and placebo. *Sleep* 2005;28:187–193.

27 Schenck C, Mahowald M. Long-term,nightly benzodiazepine treatment of injurious parasomnias and other disorders of disrupted nocturnal sleep in 170 adults. *Am. J. Med.* 1996;100:333–337.

28 Allen RM. Attenuation of drug-induced anxiety dreams and pavor nocturnus by benzodiazepines. *J. Clin Psychiatry* 1983;44:106–108.

29 Cameron OG, Thyer BA. Treatment of pavor nocturnus with alprazolam. *J. Clin. Psychiatry* 1994;46:504.

30 Popoviciou L, Corfariou O. Efficacy and safety of midazolam in the treatment of night terrors in children. *Br. J. Clin. Pharmacol.* 1983;16(Suppl. 1):97S–102S.

31 Wilson SJ, Lillywhite AR, Potokar JP, et al. Adult night terrors and paroxetine. *The Lancet* 1997;350:185.

32 Bruni O, Ferri R, Miano S, Verrillo E. L-5-Hydroxytryptophan treatment of sleep terrors in children. *Eur. J. Pediatr.* 2004;163:402–407.

33 Milano W, de Rosa M, Milano L, Capasso A. Night eating syndrome: an overview. *J. Pharm. Pharmacol.* 2012;64:2–10.

34 Gagnon JF, Postuma RB, Montplaisir J. Update on the pharmacology of REM sleep behavior disorder. *Neurology* 2006;67:742–747.

35 Boeve BF, Silber MH, Saper CB, et al. Pathophysiology of REM sleep behaviour disorder and relevance to neurodegenerative disease. *Brain* 2007;130:2770–2788.

36 Fantini ML, Gagnon JF, Filipini D, Montplaisir J. The effects of pramipexole in REM sleep behaviour disorder. *Neurology* 2003;61:1418–1420.

37 Nash JR, Wilson SJ, Potokar JP, Nutt DJ. Mirtazapine induces REM sleep behavior disorder (RBD) in parkinsonism. *Neurology* 2003;61:1161.

6

Pharmacological Treatment of Excessive Daytime Sleepiness

Karel Šonka

Department of Neurology, 1st Medical Faculty, Charles University and General Teaching Hospital, Prague, Czech Republic

Introduction

An ability to maintain adequate alertness for sufficient periods of time is, in every respect, essential for good quality of life. When alertness is insufficient, there are major potential effects on learning, general performance, efficiency, and safety. Excessive daytime sleepiness (EDS) is simply defined as a reduced ability to maintain continuous wakefulness during the day. EDS may present as brief lapses into sleep, imperative in some cases. However, it may also manifest as longer periods of somnolence leading to frank naps in favourable circumstances. The presence of unplanned naps whilst performing activities or otherwise occupied usually indicates severe symptoms. It is important to distinguish EDS from fatigue although this can clinically be difficult at times. The most defining question is simply to ask: 'do you fall asleep unintentionally during the day?', as a hallmark characteristic of EDS (see Chapters 1 and 8).

Several questionnaires have been developed to assess the presence of EDS, and its severity. The most well-known is the Epworth Sleepiness Scale (ESS), which rates the chance of falling asleep in eight everyday situations. ESS scores higher than 10 are generally considered to indicate significant subjective EDS. The ESS can also be used to evaluate treatment effects. Objective techniques for the diagnosis of EDS include the Multiple Sleep Latency Test and the Maintenance of Wakefulness Test (see Chapter 3), both of which have their advantages and disadvantages. Importantly, there often is only a limited correlation between the subjective beneficial effects that certain drugs provide and changes observed in quantitative objective tests.

Underlying causes of EDS are numerous. Most common, especially in the young, is self-imposed sleep deprivation. It can also be a side effect of many widely used classes of drugs, notably anxiolytics. Clearly, nocturnal sleep disturbances can ultimately lead to daytime sleepiness, and should always be assessed and actively treated if possible. However, in several conditions, EDS is not a consequence of night-time sleep loss, and should be considered a primary symptom. These disorders include narcolepsy type 1 and 2 (i.e. narcolepsy with and without cataplexy), idiopathic hypersomnia, Kleine–Levin

Sleep Disorders in Neurology: A Practical Approach, Second Edition.
Edited by Sebastiaan Overeem and Paul Reading.

syndrome (recurrent hypersomnia) and a variety of medical and neurological conditions including Parkinson's disease and other neurodegenerative conditions.

General Aspects of Treatment

Any treatment of EDS should always be preceded by concerted attempts to identify the underlying cause (Figure 6.1). Sleep deprivation, in particular, should be addressed and corrected. If there is a suspicion that EDS is secondary to sedative medication, it is often necessary to re-evaluate the patient once the drug in question has been discontinued, if possible. If night-time sleep disturbances are present, these should be treated accordingly (see Chapter 5). However, in many conditions such as Parkinson's disease, there may be an underlying primary form of EDS accentuated by nocturnal sleep disorders and/or medication. Therefore, when improvement of night-time sleep does not lead to resolution of daytime sleepiness, further symptomatic treatment should be considered.

In many conditions, EDS may respond adequately to planned daytime naps. In narcolepsy, the beneficial effects of multiple short naps are established [1,2]. In many other conditions, if practically possible, it is often worthwhile assessing the effects of a planned daytime nap. When limited to around 30 minutes, there often is no major detrimental effect on night-time sleep quality.

If reversible causes have been addressed and planned naps, if appropriate or possible, have failed to help and EDS still poses important limitations, symptomatic drug treatment should be considered. Although the available drugs have important drawbacks,

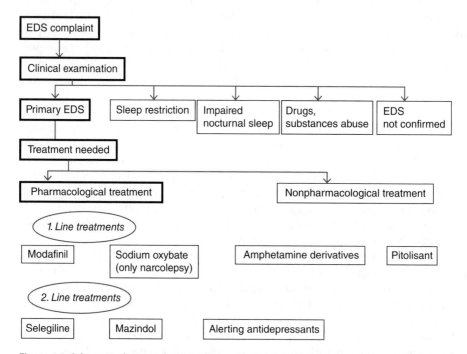

Figure 6.1 Schematic diagram showing diagnostic and therapeutic steps and considerations when dealing with excessive daytime sleepiness.

the influence of EDS on daytime functioning can be disabling and it is likely that under-treatment is more of an issue for public health than over-treatment.

The objective of any drug treatment is to eliminate EDS and to produce the fullest possible normal function for patients whether at work, school or home, and allow normal social interactions. Before starting treatment with stimulants, the patient should be informed of the likely time course of treatment effects and that sleepiness will most likely return once the therapeutic levels of any drug drop below a threshold. Patients stabilised on therapy should ideally be monitored at least once a year by a specialist for treatment efficacy, side effects, including night sleep disturbances, mood changes, and cardiovascular or metabolic abnormalities, and also for the development of tolerance. Tolerance can sometimes be avoided by taking 'drug holidays' in periods when absolute wakefulness is not required or, in the case of less severely affected patients, on days having a more relaxed regime, potentially weekends. Patients who fail to respond to adequate doses of stimulant medication should be carefully reassessed for other co-morbid sleep disorders that may contribute to EDS. The possibility of stimulant abuse or misuse may also need to be addressed in occasional seemingly resistant cases.

Effectiveness, side effects, and tolerability of stimulant medication can be difficult to predict in individuals. Therefore, knowledge of effectiveness of a certain stimulant as assessed in groups is of relative importance when making a choice for an individual. The delayed or immediate action of a drug and its duration of action may be of more importance than its expected overall effectiveness.

Despite a lack of controlled evidence from trials, traditionally, the most established and effective compounds to treat EDS remain the amphetamine-like central nervous system (CNS) stimulants. However, in the last two decades, use of the non-amphetamine stimulant modafinil has considerably increased, based on the more favourable side-effect profile and several large controlled trials. Alternative treatment options remain limited but include sodium oxybate and pitolisant (both for narcolepsy only), the MAO-B inhibitor selegiline, antidepressants with stimulating properties, or caffeine. Note that no stimulant drug is considered entirely safe in pregnancy or during breast-feeding. Furthermore, neither modafinil nor sodium oxybate are currently indicated for children, despite promising clinical experience.

Abrupt changes of differing types of stimulant medication should present few problems. However, for patients taking high doses of sympathomimetic medications, a gradual weaning period may be prudent. Furthermore, if the patient is switching from amphetamine to modafinil, then the qualitative difference in their alerting effects and the difference in peripheral side effects usually necessitates a 3- to 4-week adjustment period. The long-term parallel treatment by two stimulants has not been tested formally except for the combination of sodium oxybate and modafinil [3,4].

Indications

Narcolepsy is the 'prototype' sleep disorder for which treatment with stimulants is considered most appropriate and has provided most of the clinical experience and evidence from (limited) randomised controlled trials. The management of narcolepsy , idiopathic hypersomnia [5] and other central hypersomnias is discussed in Chapter 8. Although formal data are limited, EDS is also often treated when present in other neurological disorders. Beneficial effects of modafinil have been reported in myotonic dystrophy (see Chapter 16), extrapyramidal disorders [6,7] (see Chapter 14), multiple sclerosis [8] (see Chapter 22), and traumatic brain injury [9] (see Chapter 20). In these forms of 'secondary' EDS, the distinction from fatigue is very important, as this symptom is generally much less responsive to pharmacological treatment. Trials to date of modafinil for fatigue and EDS associated with Parkinson´s disease, multiple sclerosis, traumatic brain injury and post-polio syndrome have provided inconsistent results [10] and the clinician must take this into consideration. One must also take into consideration that central stimulants are in many countries indicated for the treatment of EDS in narcolepsy only and that other indications are off-label.

Amphetamine Derivatives

Amphetamines

Amphetamines have been used as a stimulant from the early twentieth century [1–4,11]. There are several compounds in this class that differ in potency, duration of action, and side-effect profile. The mode of action of these drugs is complex, but the central mechanism depends on catecholamine reuptake and transport inhibition (mainly dopamine and, to a lesser degree, noradrenaline) as well as the indirect enhancement of dopamine release. In higher doses, other mechanisms start to play a role, including interaction with monoamine transporters. Because of the side effects and the potential for widespread abuse, amphetamines such as methamphetamine are less often used nowadays and are even unavailable in some countries. Dextroamphetamine is still in relatively common use, however. Duration of its action is relatively long, in the range of 6–10 hours. The typical dosing schedule for dextroamphetamine is between 1 and 12 of the 5 mg tablets spread through the day with many patients responding well to the lower end of the dose range. Increases in dose should always be slowly titrated. Side effects are typically related to alpha-adrenergic stimulation, and include tachycardia and increased blood pressure, restlessness, irritability and agitation. Appetite suppression may cause unacceptable weight loss in some. Psychotic symptoms may also appear, albeit rarely. Dextroamphetamine is contraindicated in advanced arteriosclerosis, symptomatic cardiovascular disease, moderate to severe hypertension, hyperthyroidism, known hypersensitivity to the sympathomimetic amines, thyrotoxicosis, psychosis, glaucoma, in patients with a history of drug and alcohol abuse and during or within 14 days following the administration of monoamine oxidase inhibitors because of the risk of hypertensive crises. Dextroamphetamine is also not recommended in patients younger than 6 years old. One potential undesirable effect of amphetamines in childhood, known from the treatment of attention deficit and hyperactivity disorder, is growth retardation.

Pemoline, a drug used in the past, has been withdrawn due to cases of lethal hepatotoxicity.

Methylphenidate

Methylphenidate is a piperazine derivative of amphetamine, with a comparable mode of action [1–3,12,13]. The stimulant efficacy approximates to amphetamine but may be slightly less. The most important difference is the duration of action, which is considerably shorter, in the order of 3–4 hours. Together with the rapid onset of effect, it makes methylphenidate suitable not only for regular treatment but also for use 'on demand', in acute situations where sleepiness is likely to cause a problem. Typical total daily doses are in the range 10–60 mg with 10–20 mg taken three times daily. Long-acting methylphenidate is available in some countries. Clinical impression suggests that the side-effect profile is comparable with the amphetamines and the safety profile slightly better although proper safety studies are lacking. The contraindications are similar to those of amphetamines and the drug is not recommended in children under 6 years old.

Modafinil

Modafinil was developed in France in the 1980s as a stimulant not chemically related to the amphetamines [1,2,4]. Initially, an alpha-1 agonist action was presumed, but this was subsequently questioned. Recent studies point to an increasing effect on dopamine and noradrenaline signalling, although the exact mechanism of action remains unknown. The starting dose is usually 100 mg per day, either once in the morning, or divided in two doses. If not efficacious, one should titrate up to 400 mg per day, although higher doses have been reported to have good effects and are generally well tolerated. The duration of action is relatively long (elimination half-life is 10–15 hours), so one or two doses (in the morning and at noon) typically cover the whole day. Generally speaking, the overall stimulant effect of modafinil is somewhat less than the amphetamines. On the other hand, side effects are usually mild. The most important undesirable effects include headache, nausea, loss of appetite, and nervousness, depression and psychotic episodes but they are infrequent and seldom lead to therapy withdrawal. Tolerance is not common, although some reports do require increases in doses over time. Modafinil induces P450 activity to some extent and for this reason women of childbearing age who continue taking low-dose oestrogen contraception should be informed of the small possibility of an unwanted pregnancy. It is recommended to reduce the dosage in elderly patients and in hepatic insufficiency. In the European Union the use of modafinil has been recently restricted only to adult patients suffering from narcolepsy only largely because of reports of serious skin and allergic reactions. The age limitation has been criticised by expert group based on their own experience [14]. In opposition to the European Union warning, modafinil was found to be as efficient and safe as a treatment option in idiopathic hypersomnia as compared with narcolepsy [15]. In the United States, modafinil is indicated to improve wakefulness in adult patients with EDS associated with narcolepsy, obstructive sleep apnoea/hypopnoea syndrome (as an adjunct to standard treatment for the underlying obstruction), and shift work sleep disorder. Modafinil is contraindicated in patients with known hypersensitivity to the drug which usually manifests as a rash, occurring mostly in children under 17 years old. There are no known risk factors that might predict the occurrence or severity of rash associated with modafinil. Nearly all cases of serious rash associated with modafinil occurred within 1–5 weeks after the treatment initiation.

Armodafinil [16] is the R-enantiomer of modafinil which has a longer action but similar efficacy and safety profile. Armodafinil is given in smaller dose than modafinil and only once a day in the morning. The indications and contraindications of armodafinil are identical to those of modafinil. No serious skin rashes have been reported in clinical trials of armodafinil. However, because armodafinil is the R-isomer of racemic modafinil, a similar risk of serious rash with armodafinil cannot be ruled out.

Caffeine

Caffeine acts as a (relatively mild) stimulant although its usefulness in this respect may be under-recognised in practice [4]. Caffeine is a xanthine derivative, and a nonspecific adenosine receptor antagonist. Adenosine is an interesting neurotransmitter or neuro-modulator, the levels of which increase with prolonged wakefulness, potentially acting as a homeostatically driven 'sleep signal'. Caffeine is typically obtained from various drinks, notably coffee and cold stimulant preparations, but is also sold over the counter in many countries as an oral preparation. Twice daily doses of 100 mg seem to have a rather favourable effect/side-effect ratio.

Sodium Oxybate

Sodium oxybate (sodium salt of gamma-hydroxybutyrate) given in a total dose of 4.5–9 g divided over two night-time doses improves all symptoms of narcolepsy type 1 [1–4]. Sodium oxybate may also reduce EDS in Parkinson's disease [17]. The positive effects of sodium oxybate on alertness are noticeable within weeks of use. Other than improving the depth of overnight sleep, the mechanism by which EDS improves is not completely known. It is suggested that the effect may be mediated partly through interaction with GABA-B and gamma-hydroxybutyrate receptors and through indirect modulation of dopaminergic neuronal activity.

Long-term treatment by sodium oxybate is associated with few side effects, but sleep-walking and nocturnal enuresis have been reported. Sodium oxybate should not be used with alcohol or other CNS depressants. Its abuse potential seems mild with appro-priate use in clinical populations. In patients with comorbid sleep-related breathing disorders, treatment must be closely monitored since sodium oxybate may potentially worsen obstructive sleep apnoea. Because of the risk of CNS depression and abuse/misuse, sodium oxybate is often available only through a restricted distribution pro-gramme. Its high cost is also a prohibitive factor in many countries.

Pitolisant

Pitolisant is the inverse agonist of the H3 receptor which appears to improve wakeful-ness by facilitating histamine release via its effects on the posterior hypothalamus. Its efficacy and safety in narcolepsy have been recently documented in a large European multicentre double-blind, randomised controlled trial in narcolepsy [18]. It has recently gained approval for use in Europe for narcolepsy and its novel mode of action is likely to make it a useful addition to treatment options.

Selegiline

Selegiline is a potent specific monoamine oxidase B (MAO-B) inhibitor, which is metabolised into various compounds, including amphetamine and methamphetamine. There have been a number of reports showing a beneficial effect of 10–40 mg of selegiline on EDS and cataplexy in narcolepsy [1,2,4]. It can be a useful drug for patients who demonstrate an insufficient response to modafinil and who do not tolerate amphetamines well. However, potential dietary restrictions and incompatibility with triptans and selective serotonin reuptake inhibitors limit its routine use.

Mazindol

Mazindol is an imidazolidine derivative that was developed as an appetite suppressant [19]. It has a pharmacological profile that is comparable with amphetamines, with prominent dopamine and norepinephrine reuptake blocking properties. Side effects can be considerable, including nervousness, tachycardia, and anorexia. Mazindol has been taken off the market in many countries because of potential severe side effects (pulmonary hypertension and cardiac valvular regurgitation). Closely monitored treatment with annual cardiac checks including ultrasound may still be useful in those patients with a clear beneficial response.

Alerting Antidepressants

These include the dopamine reuptake inhibitor, bupropion; the combined serotonin-norepinephrine reuptake inhibitor, venlafaxine; and atomoxetine, a specific adrenergic reuptake blocker normally indicated for attention deficit hyperactivity disorder. The drugs have limited stimulating effects which can still be useful in some cases. However, side effects such as nausea, dry mouth, and other anticholinergic symptoms may limit their use [20,21].

Acknowledgement

Karel Šonka is supported by Charles University grant PROGRES Q27/LF1.

Key Points
• EDS should be distinguished from fatigue. 'Do you fall asleep unintentionally during the day?' is the key question to ask.
• EDS can have severe consequences on daily functioning. Active treatment should therefore always be considered.
• Always consider sleep deprivation and/or nocturnal sleep disturbances as a potential cause of EDS, and treat accordingly.
• Modafinil and amphetamine or methylphenidate are first-line pharmacological treatment options.
• Modafinil has a favourable side-effect profile and a relatively long duration of action.
• Amphetamine and methylphenidate are considered more potent and are most commonly used flexibly as add-on agents.

References

1 Billiard M, Bassetti C, Dauvilliers Y, et al. EFNS guidelines on management of narcolepsy. *European Journal of Neurology* 2006;13(10):1035–48.

2 Morgenthaler TI, Kapur VK, Brown T, et al. Practice parameters for the treatment of narcolepsy and other hypersomnias of central origin. *Sleep* 2007;30(12):1705–11.

3 Wise MS, Arand DL, Auger RR, et al. Treatment of narcolepsy and other hypersomnias of central origin. *Sleep* 2007;30(12):1712–27.

4 O´Malley MB, Gleeson SK, Weir ID. Wake-promoting medications: efficacy and adverse effects. In: Kryger MH, Roth T, Dement WC, editors. Principles and Practice of Sleep Medicine, 5th edn. St Louis, MI: Elsevier Saunders, 2011, pp. 527–41.

5 Evangelista E, Lopez R, Dauvilliers Y. Update on treatment for idiopathic hypersomnia. *Expert Opin Investig Drugs* 2018;27(2):187–92.

6 Hogl B, Saletu M, Brandauer E, et al. Modafinil for the treatment of daytime sleepiness in Parkinson's disease: a double-blind, randomized, crossover, placebo-controlled polygraphic trial. *Sleep* 2002;25(8):905–9.

7 Hauser RA, Wahba MN, Zesiewicz TA, et al. Modafinil treatment of pramipexole-associated somnolence. *Movement Disorders* 2000;15(6):1269–71.

8 Zifko UA, Rupp M, Schwarz S, et al. Modafinil in treatment of fatigue in multiple sclerosis. Results of an open-label study. *Journal of Neurology* 2002;249(8):983–7.

9 Jha A, Weintraub A, Allshouse A, et al. A randomized trial of modafinil for the treatment of fatigue and excessive daytime sleepiness in individuals with chronic traumatic brain injury. *The Journal of Head Trauma Rehabilitation* 2008;23(1):52–63.

10 Sheng P, Hou L, Wang X, et al. Efficacy of modafinil on fatigue and excessive daytime sleepiness associated with neurological disorders: a systematic review and meta-analysis. *PloS ONE* 2013;8(12):e81802.

11 Heal DJ, Smith SL, Gosden J, Nutt DJ. Amphetamine, past and present – a pharmacological and clinical perspective. *Journal of Psychopharmacology* 2013;27(6):479–96.

12 Spencer T, Wilens T, Biederman, J et al. A double-blind, crossover comparison of methylphenidate and placebo in adults with childhood-onset attention-deficit hyperactivity disorder. *Archives of General Psychiatry* 1995;52(6):434–43.

13 Feldman HM, Reiff MI. Clinical practice. Attention deficit-hyperactivity disorder in children and adolescents. *The New England Journal of Medicine* 2014;370(9):838–46.

14 Lecendreux M, Bruni O, Franco P, et al. Clinical experience suggests that modafinil is an effective and safe treatment for paediatric narcolepsy. *Journal of Sleep Research* 2012; 21(4):481–3.

15 Lavault S, Dauvilliers Y, Drouot X, et al. Benefit and risk of modafinil in idiopathic hypersomnia vs. narcolepsy with cataplexy. *Sleep Medicine* 2011;12(6):550–6.

16 Black JE, Hull SG, Tiller J, et al. The long-term tolerability and efficacy of armodafinil in patients with excessive sleepiness associated with treated obstructive sleep apnea, shift work disorder, or narcolepsy: an open-label extension study. *Journal of Clinical Sleep Medicine* 2010;6(5):458–66.

17 Ondo WG, Perkins T, Swick T, et al. Sodium oxybate for excessive daytime sleepiness in Parkinson disease: an open-label polysomnographic study. *Archives of Neurology* 2008;65(10):1337–40.

18 Dauvilliers Y, Bassetti C, Lammers GJ, et al. Pitolisant versus placebo or modafinil in patients with narcolepsy: a double-blind, randomised trial. *Lancet Neurology* 2013;12(11):1068–75.

19 Nittur N, Konofal E, Dauvilliers Y, et al. Mazindol in narcolepsy and idiopathic and symptomatic hypersomnia refractory to stimulants: a long-term chart review. *Sleep Medicine* 2013;14(1):30–6.

20 Cooper JA, Tucker VL, Papakostas GI. Resolution of sleepiness and fatigue: a comparison of bupropion and selective serotonin reuptake inhibitors in subjects with major depressive disorder achieving remission at doses approved in the European Union. *Journal of Psychopharmacology* 2014;28(2):118–24.

21 Mignot EJ. A practical guide to the therapy of narcolepsy and hypersomnia syndromes. *Neurotherapeutics* 2012;9(4):739–52.

7

The Effects of Medication on Sleep and Wakefulness

Gé S.F. Ruigt[1] and Joop van Gerven[2]

[1] Clinical Consultancy for Neuroscience Drug Development, Oss, The Netherlands
[2] Centre for Human Drug Research, Leiden, The Netherlands

Introduction

Sleep and wakefulness are processes governed by several partly overlapping neuroana-tomical and neurochemical systems in the brain. This chapter summarises the most important principles of sleep physiology and pharmacology, which hopefully will help the clinician to understand how sleep and wakefulness are affected not only by neuro-logical disorders, but also by their medical treatment. The latter is highly relevant since impairments of sleep or wakefulness, namely insomnia or hypersomnolence, are among the most frequently reported adverse events across the neurological pharmacopoeia. Understanding the pharmacological basis of sleep and wakefulness can also aid both the clinical analysis of sleep disorders and guide choices for appropriate medication in neu-rological and psychiatric practice. Further, with the recent elimination of the formal distinction between 'primary' and 'secondary' insomnia in classifications of insomnia, more attention is being paid to the medical relief of comorbid insomnia which is respon-sible for the majority of sleep problems encountered in the clinic.

Sleep and Wake Systems in the Brain

Historically, based largely on the original and prescient clinic-pathological observations of von Economo, a clear neuroanatomical distinction has been made between sleep and wake promoting systems. In particular, von Economo found that patients with encepha-litic lesions of the anterior hypothalamus appeared to develop severe insomnia whereas, more commonly, patients with lesions in the posterior hypothalamus became exces-sively somnolent. This suggested that centres in the anterior hypothalamus were involved in the generation and maintenance of sleep, a notion corroborated by early animal data.

Another early approach centred on animal models. Thus, cats with mid-pontine lesions were found to be extremely hypersomnolent prompting Moruzzi and Magoun to subsequently propose the existence of an ascending reticular activating system involved in the maintenance of wakefulness. They demonstrated that stimulation of the brainstem reticular formation converted the high-voltage synchronised electroencephalographic (EEG) activity, characteristic of sleep and anesthesia, into the desynchronised low amplitude activity of waking.

Neurophysiologically, sleep has been associated with an increased inhibitory drive, especially through activation of GABA-ergic systems arising predominantly from the lateral preoptic area of the anterior hypothalamus. Indeed, the bulk of current hypnotic medication, including benzodiazepines, consists of compounds facilitating GABA-ergic transmission. By contrast, waking has been associated with an increased excitatory drive through a number of neurotransmitter systems, particularly stimulant biogenic amines (noradrenaline, dopamine, histamine, serotonin) and acetylcholine (Ach), each emanating from specific nuclei in the brainstem and posterior hypothalamus. Wake-promoting systems are clearly essential for wakefulness but this implies also that sleep may be prevented if they are too active. Consequently, agonists of these biogenic amines, used in a variety of situations, often cause insomnia, whereas antagonists are frequently associated with sedation. Insomnia must therefore be assessed as a possible disorder of hyper-arousal rather than as a specific impairment of sleep mechanisms. This has fuelled developments in hypnotic medication and prompted a shift in emphasis from activation of sleep-inducing networks to the inhibition of arousal systems. It has also become evident that it is necessary for drugs to enhance both the restorative value of sleep as well as the quality of daytime functioning and that these two aspects are intimately linked.

Sleep-related Drug Side Effects

In this chapter, the most relevant neuropharmacological systems are presented, together with the routinely used medications that can have an impact on the sleep–wake cycle. Appendix 7.A provides an overview of several drug classes with their most important pharmacological mechanisms of action and how they impact on sleep or wakefulness. The overview is derived not so much from published polysomnography (PSG) studies but more from descriptions rooted in clinical practice and experience. Appendix 7.A lists many different drugs currently in use, but excludes general anaesthetics, locally applied medications, supplements such as enzymes, minerals or vitamins, as well as recreational or illicit drugs. The list provides general information on the severity of sleep–wake effects in the clinical dose range as derived from the frequency of adverse events mentioned in the labelling information.

Several drug classes not generally used to treat diseases of the nervous system, may still cause prominent sedation or insomnia. This can be due either to secondary pharmacological effects impacting on sleep–wake regulation, or to indirect physiological effects that affect circadian regulatory processes. The precise therapeutic indication of a drug may also have an effect on the type of adverse event reported. Sildenafil, for instance, is used to treat both pulmonary hypertension and erectile dysfunction. Insomnia is quite frequently reported with the former indication but not with the second, related potentially not only to differences in dosing but also to the fundamental differences in the treatment conditions. It should also be noted that some drugs with a pharmacological mechanism of action which might be expected to have an effect on sleep-regulatory systems, are not listed as having such effects in Appendix 7.A. This may be due to the limited therapeutic dose range of the drug, to inadequate blood–brain barrier (BBB) penetration, or because the disease and its treatment have contrasting effects on sleep and wakefulness. It should also be stressed that insomnia or sedation secondary to treatment effects may be exaggerated in some subjects due a variety of factors. These include high plasma levels as a result of reduced clearance or high doses, increased BBB penetration in severe systemic or brain disease, or an increased sensitivity of the central nervous system (CNS) in the very young or elderly. These factors are often brought about by drug interactions. Under these aggravating conditions, the severity or frequency of side effects of drugs with well known effects on sleep or wakefulness may also increase, sometimes to levels of delirium, hallucinations, stupor and even coma. An understanding of the pharmacology of the systems involved in the sleep–wake cycle can therefore also contribute to understanding impairment of consciousness. The emphasis of this chapter, however, is on excessive sleepiness, significant insomnia and abnormal dream or nightmare activity at dose levels considered therapeutic.

Neuropharmacology of Waking and Rapid Eye Movement Sleep

No single neurotransmitter system is required absolutely to keep a subject awake and there is redundancy in the wake-promoting systems. Rather, wakefulness is maintained by multiple parallel arousal systems (Figure 7.1). However, the different neurotransmitter systems implicated in wakefulness, such as Ach, histamine, noradrenaline, serotonin, dopamine, glutamate and hypocretin (orexin) may mutually excite each other and, as such, act in concert, each system potentially subserving different aspects of the wakeful state. To a large extent, these interactions have not yet been fully elucidated nor are the underlying mechanisms completely understood. A number of regulatory peptides such as substance P, thyrotropin releasing hormone (TRH), corticotrophin releasing hormone (CRH), vasoactive intestinal polypeptide (VIP), vasopressin and neurotensin further serve to enhance and prolong excitatory activity as co-agonists in the excitatory neurotransmitter pathways. This widespread diversity of pharmacological systems involved in sleep–wake regulation helps to explain why so many different treatments affect sleep and/or wakefulness.

Acetylcholine

Wakefulness

Ach plays a unique role in the sleep–wake cycle, since this neurotransmitter not only promotes wakefulness but also facilitates rapid eye movement (REM) sleep (Figure 7.2). Cholinergic neurons in the pedunculopontine (PPT) and latero-dorsal tegmental (LDT) nuclei have a major rostral pathway that projects densely onto medial and intra-laminar thalamic nuclei which, in turn, facilitate cortical activation. In particular, Ach activates nicotinic and muscarinic M_1 receptors on glutamatergic thalamocortical relay neurons

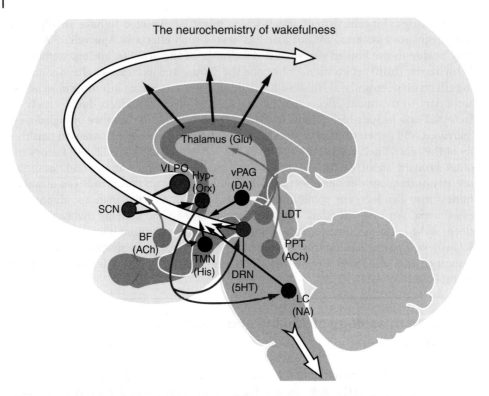

Figure 7.1 During wakefulness, brainstem ascending arousal systems activate the brain by stimulation of thalamocortical transmission and of attentional processes in frontal regions, which also leads to behavioural expressions (open white arrows). The activities of different stimulating neurotransmitter systems originating in specific brainstem nuclei (including noradrenergic, dopaminergic, histaminergic and cholinergic neurons) are modulated by peptidergic systems like orexin. In this way, wakefulness can be modified by physiological conditions and circadian rhythms. Brain regions: BF, basal forebrain; DRN, dorsal raphe nuclei; Hyp., hypothalamus; LC, locus coeruleus; LDT, laterodorsal tegmental nuclei; PPT, pedunculopontine tegmental nuclei; SCN, suprachiasmatic nucleus; TMN, tuberomammillary nucleus; VLPO, ventrolateral preoptic area; vPAG, ventral periaqueductal grey. Neurochemical: 5HT, serotonin; ACh, acetylcholine; DA, dopamine; Glu, glutamate; His, histamine; NA, noradrenaline; Orx, orexin. *Source:* Courtesy of Dr Kari L. Franson.

to facilitate cortical activation and fast cortical rhythms. This effect is further enhanced by M_2 receptor-mediated inhibition of gamma-aminobutyric acid (GABA)-containing thalamic reticularis neurons. A minor ventral projection pathway leads to the basal forebrain, posterior hypothalamus and brainstem reticular formation. From the basal forebrain there is also a dense cholinergic projection to the cortex, amygdala and hippocampus. The cholinergic tegmental and basal forebrain neurons are active during waking, while their firing is reduced with increasing depth of sleep. Ach or cholinergic agonists, both nicotinic and muscarinic, produce prolonged wakefulness when administered during the wake period, which is associated with cortical activation and desynchronised EEG activity. Muscarinic antagonists, however, enhance low frequency synchronised activity in the EEG. The cholinergic cell loss in the basal forebrain in Alzheimer's disease is also associated with EEG slowing.

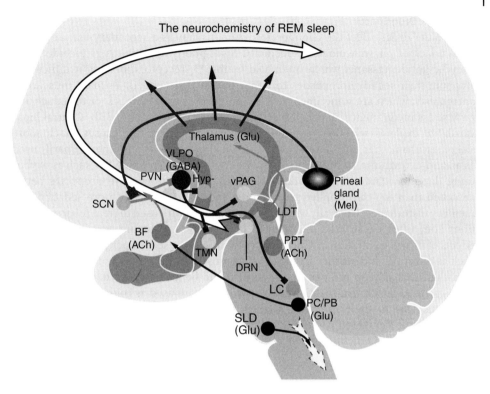

Figure 7.2 Acetylcholine is not only involved in waking, but is also important in REM sleep. Cholinergic neurons facilitate thalamocortical activation, which produces some of the characteristic cortical rhythms observed in the sleep EEG. This cortical stimulation does not lead to behavioural manifestations, because the brainstem systems that mediate motor activity are inhibited during physiological REM sleep (arrows to transparent nuclei). Muscle tone is further reduced by glutamatergic projections from the sublaterodorsal nucleus in the pons. Brain regions: BF, basal forebrain; DRN, dorsal raphe nuclei; Hyp., hypothalamus; LC, locus coeruleus; LDT, laterodorsal tegmental nuclei; PC/PB, pericoeruleus and parabranchial nuclei; PPT, pedunculopontine tegmental nuclei; PVN, paraventricular nucleus; SCN, suprachiasmatic nucleus; SLD, sublaterodorsal nucleus; TMN, tuberomammillary nucleus; VLPO, ventrolateral preoptic area; vPAG, ventral periaqueductal grey. Neurochemical: ACh, acetylcholine; GABA, gamma-aminobutyric acid; GLU, glutamate; Mel, melatonin. *Source:* Courtesy of Dr Kari L. Franson.

REM Sleep

The firing frequency of cholinergic LDT/PPT neurons is increased during REM sleep (Figure 7.2). In this state, there is striking cortical activation in the absence of behavioural arousal or consciousness. Cholinergic agonists such as carbachol injected into the ponto-mesencephalic tegmentum also produce cortical activation with muscle atonia, akin to a REM-like state. In the brainstem reticular formation, Ach excites glycinergic medullary neurons involved in motor inhibition, while inhibiting those reticulospinal neurons that excite motor neurons to produce the striking atonia of REM sleep. The REM-enabling cholinergic neurons are strongly inhibited by noradrenaline and to a lesser extent serotonin and histamine, explaining the REM-suppressant effects of noradrenergic and serotonergic antidepressants. During waking, there is a balance between ACh-mediated and noradrenaline-mediated neurotransmission, safeguarding a waking state with stimulation of both muscle tone and cortical activation.

Cholinergic Drug Effects

Many older drugs affect the cholinergic system, usually as a secondary feature arising from a lack of pharmacological specificity. Such poorly specific drugs include many tricyclic antidepressants which often also inhibit H_1-receptors, making it difficult to attribute their sedative properties to either one of these effects. Primary muscarinic antagonists, which are sometimes used as anti-emetics or mydriatics, or to reduce urinary stress incontinence, may cause sedation if they penetrate the BBB. Central bioavailability explains why scopolamine used for motion sickness causes much more sleepiness than other potent anti-muscarinergic drugs such as atropine, primarily used as an anti-arrhythmic, or most anti-muscarinergic bladder spasmolytics such as oxybutinin, dariphenacine and tolterodine. Similarly, cyclopentolate eye drops are better absorbed than topically applied tropicamide and therefore cause more sedation and memory disturbance. Centrally active nicotinic agonists are used to treat tobacco addiction. They often cause insomnia, related both to their stimulant activity and to the effects of nicotine withdrawal. Cholinesterase inhibitors used for peripheral indications such as intestinal and bladder atonia or neuromuscular transmission disorders such as myasthenia usually do not penetrate the BBB and hence generally do not impair the sleep–wake cycle. Centrally active cholinergic drugs are used as cognitive enhancers in dementia. Due to their stimulant actions, they might be expected to impair sleep although some demented patients, paradoxically, experience sedation and sleep more soundly, often with enhanced REM sleep.

Histamine

Histaminergic neurons in the mammillary bodies of the posterior hypothalamus stimulate cortical activation both through diffuse rostral projections and by depolarising or exciting multiple elements of the various arousal systems. They discharge during wakefulness, decrease firing during slow wave non-REM sleep (SWS) and cease firing altogether during REM sleep. A decrease in histaminergic brain activity appears to be linked to reduced consciousness and not to sleep-related loss of muscle tone. Evidence for the functional role of histamine in awakening as well as in the maintenance of waking also comes from histidine decarboxylase knockout mice, which are slower to wake than wild type mice and have more difficulty staying awake. Centrally acting H_1 antihistamines are universally known for their sedative and sleep-inducing properties. H_2 receptors do not appear to play a role in sleep and waking, whereas inhibition of H_3 receptors, located as autoreceptors on histaminergic terminals and as heteroreceptors on monoaminergic terminals, also reduce cortical activation and waking.

Histaminergic Drug Effects

H_1 antagonists are widely used to treat allergies. The older compounds in this class usually had such strong sedative properties that they were also widely used as surrogate hypnotics to treat insomnia. Although the use of sedating antihistamines to treat insomnia is no longer generally recommended, some older compounds such as diphenhydramine and doxylamine are still available as non-prescription sleeping pills. Newer so-called 'non-sedating' antihistaminergics do not penetrate the BBB as readily but are still often associated with sedation and sleepiness. In children, however, paradoxical insomnia can be observed. Many older and poorly selective CNS active drugs including some antipsychotics and anti-emetics have prominent secondary antihistaminergic properties that contribute to their sedative side effect profile. Particularly for some antidepressants, these sedative antihistaminergic effects override the stimulant pharmacological properties associated with other elements of their pharmacological profile (such as noradrenergic facilitation by noradrenaline α_2 blockade by mianserin, or noradrenalin reuptake inhibition by amitriptyline or clomipramine). Central H_2 receptors seem to be implicated in working memory (mediated by cholinergic activation), but their direct involvement in sleep is unclear. Still, a number of H_2 receptor blocking antacids such as famotidine cause mild insomnia in some patients. This may be related to a consequence of antacid activity itself, since most proton pump inhibitors can also cause mild sleep impairment through unclear (vagal?) mechanisms.

Noradrenaline

Noradrenergic cell bodies in the locus coeruleus (LC) stimulate cortical activation and behavioural arousal by diffuse projections through the cortex, hippocampus, thalamus, hypothalamus, brainstem and spinal cord, exciting wake-promoting target neurons through α_1 postsynaptic receptors. Inactivation of the noradrenergic LC leads to ipsilateral muscle atonia and to hippocampal theta activity, simplistically suggesting that noradrenaline may somehow play a role in connecting the brain to the body. This could be particularly relevant during REM sleep when brain activity is intense in the absence of conscious thought or movements. In keeping with this concept, LC neurons discharge during waking, particularly during high levels of activity, decrease firing during SWS and cease firing during REM sleep. Drugs that affect the noradrenergic system have contributed valuable information on the role of this system in the sleep–wake cycle. For example, noradrenergic α_1 antagonists facilitate sleep onset. Drugs with this mechanism of action such as doxazosin and prazosin are sometimes used clinically as vasodilating antihypertensives. Such agents not only cause sedation but may also be useful to treat insomnia and abnormal dreams in post traumatic stress syndrome. Peripheral α_1 antagonists such as alfuzosine and terazosine licensed to treat urinary retention may also cause sedation, probably because they penetrate the brain to some extent. Drugs blocking the presynaptic α_2 autoreceptor (yohimbine) delay sleep through noradrenergic disinhibition.

Adrenergic Drug Effects

Compounds such as clonidine that stimulate inhibitory α_2 autoreceptors on noradrenergic neurons reduce noradrenergic activity and are sometimes used for treatment-resistant hypertension or to prevent migraine attacks. Their use, however, is limited by their strong sedative effects. Presynaptic α_2 inhibition also reduces melatonin production which may explain why occasionally insomnia is paradoxically reported rather than sedation. Centrally acting antihypertensives such as rilmenidine and moclonidine that modulate the imidazoline receptor, related to the α_2 receptor, have similar effects. Drugs that either activate the release or block the reuptake of noradrenaline including amphetamines, viloxazine, reboxetine and modafinil, enhance or prolong wakefulness and can be used to treat hypersomnolence in primary sleep disorders such as narcolepsy. If used recreationally or for other indications such as depression or attention deficit disorder, these stimulant effects can lead to insomnia. This is also the case for methylphenidate, which is increasingly used for attention deficit and related disorders. Many older antidepressants also inhibit noradrenaline reuptake but often have other secondary more sedative, usually antihistaminergic, pharmacological properties that may either compensate for the activating effects of noradrenergic stimulation or cause mixed effects of sedation and insomnia in a clinical population or even in the same patient.

Beta adrenergic antagonists are widely used to treat hypertension, chronic heart failure, and certain types of cardiac arrhythmia. Beta-blockers are also prescribed for essential tremor and anxiety. These 'relaxing' effects are at least partly due to reduction of the peripheral associations of stress and anxiety, such as diminished tachycardia and palpitations. Many beta-blockers also penetrate the CNS where they may cause a reduction in the diurnal increase of melatonin in the afternoon and early evening, normally facilitating the sleep phase. Probably as a result, many beta-blockers cause sleep disturbances including abnormal and vivid dreams, particularly early during their treatment. These side effects are most frequent with lipophilic beta-blockers, although some typical hydrophilic drugs such as atenolol and celiprolol can also impair certain aspects of sleep.

Serotonin

In the 1960s, serotonin was postulated to be the most important neurotransmitter involved in sleep promotion, based largely on the observation that depletion of serotonin in cats resulted in sleep suppression. However, serotonergic neurons, concentrated in the brainstem dorsal raphe nuclei, discharge maximally during waking, decrease their discharge during SWS and virtually cease firing during REM sleep, suggesting that the highest extracellular 5-hydroxytryptamine (5-HT) levels should be found during waking. This neurophysiological finding has subsequently been corroborated by microdialysis studies. The notion that serotonin promotes wakefulness is also confirmed by drugs that enhance serotonergic transmission by inhibiting presynaptic serotonin reuptake. Sleep is generally promoted by inhibition of serotonergic activity by activating, for example, presynaptic inhibitory 5-HT_{1a} autoreceptors following direct injection of the 5-HT_{1a} agonist 8-OH-DPAT into the dorsal raphe nuclei. On the other hand, activation of postsynaptic 5-HT_{1a} by systemic exposure to 8-OH-DPAT enhances waking, while mixed antagonists of 5-HT_{2a} and 5-HT_{2c} receptors (ritanserin, ketanserin), selective 5-HT_{2a} antagonists and inverse 5-HT_{2a} agonists (primavanserin) increase SWS. Pharmacologically, (inhibitory) 5-HT_{1a} receptors have a higher affinity for serotonin than (stimulatory) 5-HT_{2a} receptors, which may underlie some of the biphasic or ambivalent dose-related effects of serotonergic drugs on sleep and waking.

Serotonergic Drug Effects

The important and complex role of serotonin in the regulation of the sleep–wake cycle is reflected by the fact that many serotonergic drugs have an unpredictable impact on sleep or wakefulness, frequently affecting both aspects. The serotonergic system is also involved in a wide range of other physiological functions and drugs that target this system are encountered in many different therapeutic areas. In addition, many of these drugs show only limited selectivity for the dozen or so different subtypes of serotonin receptors. Thus, triptans used for acute migraine are highly selective 5HT1b/d-receptor agonists but the fact that most of them can cause some sedation is probably mediated by other 5HT-receptor subtypes. Methysergide is an older ergotamine used for migraine and related headaches with inhibitory effects on $5HT_{2b}$ receptors that can lead to both insomnia and sedation. $5HT_2$ antagonists such as the vasodilator ketanserin promote sleep and cause sedation. Most atypical antipsychotic drugs are $5HT_2$ antagonists in addition to being dopamine antagonists. Although most of these drugs cause sleepiness, this property varies considerably, mainly depending on additional pharmacological characteristics such as antihistaminergic effects. Some $D_2/5HT_2$ inhibitors such as tiapride or the diphenylbutylpiperidenes (pimozide) do not cause significant sedation. Selective $5HT_3$ antagonists including ondansetron also do not affect sleep and waking, although less selective anti-emetics such as granisetron or metoclopramide, which also block D_2 receptors, can cause sedation.

After acute administration, almost all antidepressants cause a secondary or primary increase in synaptic serotonin levels, either by reducing degradation (MAO inhibitors), by inhibiting synaptic reuptake or by (indirectly) stimulating serotonin release. Antidepressants are well-known for their REM sleep reducing effects, a property that is sometimes used as a biomarker to predict the antidepressant properties of novel drugs in development, although it is still a subject of debate whether REM reduction per se contributes to the resolution of depression. The widespread and nonselective synaptic serotonin increase caused by most antidepressants can lead to a variety of sleep–wake abnormalities, including not only acute or withdrawal insomnia but also sedation and abnormal dreams, bruxism and yawning.

As a clinical guideline, serotonin activation will generally promote wakefulness while inhibition will cause sedation, particularly if $5HT_2$ receptors or higher activity levels are involved. Since many of the diseases themselves that are treated with serotonergic medications can also affect sleep or alertness, pragmatic dose reductions or switching to nonserotonergic alternative treatments can provide support for the involvement of a serotonergic drug if a patient complains of excessive sedation or insomnia.

Dopamine

Mesencephalic dopaminergic neurons in the ventral tegmental area and substantia nigra project to the striatum, basal forebrain, limbic areas, thalamic subnuclei and frontal cortex. Discharge rates, particularly tonic burst activity, correlate with aroused and positively rewarding states. This happens both during waking and REM sleep, suggesting that dopaminergic activation leads to central arousal associated with reward, but not necessarily to behavioural arousal and increased postural muscle tone. Unlike the histaminergic and noradrenergic neurons, there is much less variation in the firing rates of dopaminergic neurons over the 24-hour sleep–wake cycle, further indicating that dopamine plays a different role in sleep and waking compared with the other monoaminergic neurotransmitters. Dopamine reuptake blockers and dopamine releasers combine arousing and psychostimulant rewarding effects largely through activation of dopamine receptors in the ventral tegmental area. This probably accounts for the abuse potential of cocaine and amphetamine. These drugs can also cause profound insomnia. Although most dopamine reuptake inhibitors also inhibit the reuptake of noradrenalin, it is evident from studies with selective dopamine reuptake inhibitors and with dopamine receptor knockout mice that the wake-promoting effects of noradrenergic/dopaminergic compounds are to a large extent due to elevation of synaptic levels of dopamine.

In animals, dopamine D_1 agonists induce behavioural arousal. D_2-receptor agonists give rise to biphasic effects with low doses reducing wake time and augmenting SWS and REM sleep, while higher doses have opposite effects.

Dopaminergic Drug Effects

The complex sleep–wake effects of dopamine, dysregulation of dopaminergic systems in Parkinson's disease and other neuropsychiatric conditions, and the incomplete sub-type-selectivity of most dopaminergic drugs, all contribute to complex divergent and often biphasic effects of dopamine precursors and agonists on sleep and wakefulness. Dopaminergic medications can lead to sedation or sleep attacks in some patients while promoting psychomotor activity and causing insomnia in others. Anti-parkinsonian drugs also often cause abnormal dreams or nightmares although in a proportion of patients with impaired sleeping patterns related to dopamine deficiency, dopamine ago-nists can also improve sleep. In other patients, the activating effects of peak plasma concentrations of dopaminergic treatments can lead to sleep impairment, even at thera-peutic levels.

Reduction of dopamine as observed in patients with fluctuating Parkinson's disease is generally associated with excessive sleepiness. Similarly, inhibition of dopamine recep-tors by D_1- and D_2-receptor antagonists or reduction of dopaminergic tone by activa-tion of D_3 autoreceptors can induce somnolence. Central dopaminergic antagonists are mainly used to treat psychosis, although neuroleptics and atypical antipsychotics are also applied in anaesthesia and for neuropathic pain or dystonia. Peripheral dopaminer-gic antagonists are used to treat nausea and vomiting but they can also cause CNS effects if they penetrate the BBB sufficiently. This can be an issue in patients with CNS diseases or in susceptible individuals, particularly the elderly and children. Co-treat-ment with medications that disrupt the BBB or inhibit P-glycoprotein pump function may enhance these effects. The sedating effects of antipsychotic agents are not only due to inhibition of D_2 receptors, since most antipsychotics also have prominent inhibitory effects on other wake-related receptor types. These include $5HT_2$ receptors for atypical antipsychotics or H_1 receptors for most of the older neuroleptics.

Glutamate

Most of the thalamocortical projection relay neurons that stimulate the cortical mantle, after activation by both Ach and biogenic amines, have glutamate as their neurotrans-mitter. Subcortical glutamate levels in the nucleus accumbens are high during waking and low during SWS and REM sleep. Glutamate is such a widespread and important excitatory neurotransmitter that manipulations of its levels lack specific effects. Indeed, only few medications have been developed with an isolated or predominant effect on glutamatergic transmission largely due to the incidence of serious side effects. Direct or indirect inhibition of glutamatergic pathways, particularly subtypes of cationic gluta-mate receptors (NMDA, AMPA and kainate), will generally cause sedation and sleepi-ness. Most currently available antiglutamatergic drugs target the NMDA receptor although kainate and AMPA inhibitors ('ampanels') are slowly being introduced for conditions such as epilepsy and migraine.

Magnesium acts as a physiological inhibitor of glutamate-NMDA-cation channels by blocking the central pore of this pentameric peptide channel thus preventing intracellular passage of Na^+ or Ca^{2+} and neuronal excitation. For this reason, magnesium is used intravenously to treat seizures related to pre-eclampsia in pregnancy. Magnesium preparations are also used as antacids and have the potential to cause sedation and sleepiness.

Non-competitive glutamate NMDA antagonists are used for various indications and all are sedative. Memantine for dementia, amantadine for Parkinson's disease and influenza, riluzole for amyotrophic lateral sclerosis, acamprosate for alcohol addiction, ketamine and phencyclidine for anaesthesia and dextromethorphan in cough syrups can all cause drowsiness in clinical doses, albeit to variable degrees.

Although some anti-epileptic drugs such as levetiracetam and possibly lamotrigine inhibit glutamate release, in the former case by synaptic vesicle 2 inhibition, these compounds also seem to have other pharmacological effects on nerve conduction that are related to their sedative adverse effect profile. These other effects may explain why lamotrigine has stimulatory properties in about one third of patients, helping to reduce the side effects of sedative co-medication but also potentially causing sleep disturbance.

Sleep Regulators

Orexin

Activating orexin (hypocretin) producing neurons in the lateral hypothalamus project heavily to brainstem arousal nuclei and appear to play an important role in the stabilisation of the wakeful state through two G-protein coupled receptors (Ox_1 and OX_2). Orexin signalling is most active during the normal wake period and falls silent during the inactive period when orexin neurons are inhibited by the sleep-promoting centres of the lateral preoptic area, facilitating sleep. Orexin has been coined to be the neuropeptide that 'allows us to stay awake for dinner', and compounds that selectively target the hypocretin system are also being explored for alimentary and addictive disorders as well as sleep regulation.

Recently, the first orexin antagonist (suvorexant), which inactivates wakefulness through antagonism of both orexin receptor subtypes, was registered for the treatment of insomnia and several follow-up compounds are in development. Orexin antagonists appear not to be associated with the muscle relaxant, anxiolytic and amnestic properties that confound the use of benzodiazepines and non-benzodiazepine Z-hypnotics. There are two other salient advantages of orexin antagonists over benzodiazepines and Z-hypnotics. First, they appear to be devoid of tolerance and dependence allowing use in chronic insomnia and secondly, they appear not to interfere with the structure of sleep and promote more normal, physiological sleep. The most frequently reported side effect with suvorexant is morning somnolence, associated with its 12-hour half-life, while neurological symptoms such as hypnagogic hallucinations, sleep paralysis and cataplexy-like symptoms are only very occasionally (<0.5%) reported.

Melatonin

Melatonin is a pivotal regulator of circadian rhythms, including the sleep–wake cycle. Its production and release mainly occur during the early part of the dark cycle. Retinal fibres projecting to the suprachiasmatic nucleus of the hypothalamus play an important role in adjusting the clock mechanism. During the evening and early night, this 'physiological clock' stimulates the superior cervical ganglion which, in turn, activates melatonin production in the pineal gland through noradrenergic sympathetic nerve fibres. Melatonin$_{1a}$ receptors in the hypothalamus convey information about the light–dark cycle to other centres driving circadian physiological functions. Although melatonin itself penetrates the BBB only poorly and variably, it is widely used as a sleep-enabling 'food supplement'. Certain formulations with better characterised pharmacokinetic properties have been registered for medical use. Several melatonin agonists have been developed or are in various stages of assessment for insomnia. These include the antidepressant agomelatine (also a 5HT$_{2c}$ antagonist), which appears effective for comorbid insomnia in depression, ramelteon for the treatment of insomnia characterised by difficulty with sleep onset and tasimelteon for the treatment of non-24-hour sleep–wake disorder in the blind, specifically those born with conditions such as anophthalmia or micropthalmia.

Melatonin production is reduced by a number of different drugs including beta-blockers, corticosteroids, NSAIDs, cannabinoids and benzodiazepines, which at least partly explains why these drugs have the potential to disrupt normal sleeping patterns. Other medications can cause a phase shift in melatonin release, such as chronic levodopa treatment which causes a phase advance. Melatonin is metabolised through the cytochrome P450 system (mainly CYP1A2) and drugs that inhibit these liver enzymes can also prolong the activity of melatonin, particularly when production is at its peak early in the evening. These pharmacokinetic interactions can modulate the sleep effects of drugs that inhibit CYP1A2 such as caffeine, fluvoxamine and artemisinin. CYP1A2 inducers generally do not have a functionally significant impact on endogenous melatonin release, although many such inducers including barbiturates and smoking have prominent sleep effects of their own.

Opioid System

Opioids act at a variety of receptors, the main subtypes being mu, kappa, and delta. All three of these receptor subtypes appear to be involved in the analgesic effect of opioids, whereas the mu subtype plays a larger role, compared with the kappa subtype, in respiratory depression. Respiratory depression is one of the more serious adverse effects of opioids, particularly during sleep. Opioids act directly on the brainstem respiratory centres through mu and delta receptors and at chemoreceptors through mu receptors, depressing the regulation of respiratory rhythmicity. Individuals with pulmonary disease or obstructive sleep apnoea are known to be at greater risk for sustained hypoxaemia during sleep. Concomitant use of other sedatives, in particular hypnotics, increases the risk for potentially fatal respiratory depression. Although there is widespread belief that tolerance to the sedating effects of opioids develops with chronic use, there are no objective data to support this claim.

The limited PSG data available indicate that opioids decrease REM sleep and SWS. Subjective quality of sleep, however, is often improved in patients under opioid analgesics, but this is probably a secondary effect of improved pain control. The degree of sedation may depend on the specific drug, dosage, and duration of use, as well as on the severity of the underlying condition. In addition, the elderly appear particularly sensitive to opioids. Opioid mu antagonists used to treat overdosing and opioid or alcohol addiction can cause insomnia and other signs of acute drug abstinence.

Drugs Affecting Neuronal Conduction and Signal-effect Coupling

Neuronal conduction and electrochemical signalling are essential for all CNS activities at all stages of the sleep–wake cycle. It is not surprising therefore that drugs that affect neuronal conduction or the translation of the signal into a biological effect can also have an impact on wakefulness and sleep. Essentially, therefore, every agent that affects one of the numerous cell membrane conductance processes can influence sleep–wake regulation, depending on how much it penetrates the brain. The family of voltage-gated calcium (CaV) channels subserving a large spectrum of physiological functions are particularly important in this regard. N- and P/Q-type channels are the main subtypes of the calcium channel concentrated at nerve terminals, where they support the release of synaptic vesicles in synaptic transmission. L-type channels come in different varieties (CaV1.1–CaV1.4) and are involved in different physiological processes, ranging from excitation-contraction coupling to synaptic plasticity and retinal processing. R-type channels may be involved in neurotransmitter release and repetitive firing. T-type channels play a role in cardiac pacing, thalamocortical oscillations, hormone secretion and smooth muscle contraction. They also contribute to regulation of intracellular calcium levels. The involvement of T-type channels in thalamocortical oscillations suggests an interesting link to sleep rhythms and spike-wave discharges, especially since thalamocortical circuits play an important role in both sleep and epilepsy. These channels are inhibited by the anti-epileptics ethosuximide and valproate, drugs usually highly effective in absence epilepsy and often causing sedation. The effects of these drugs on sleep are less clear, however, with stabilisation of sleep phases in some studies and fragmentation in others.

The involvement of CaV channels in many different biological processes makes them interesting targets for physiological research and pharmacotherapy. L-type CaV channels, in particular, are unique substrates for a wide variety of treatments. However, the lack of tissue selectivity and functional homogeneity might be expected to produce significant undesired side effects that can be quite variable in character and intensity. L-type voltage-dependent calcium channel inhibitors such as verapamil and dihydropyridines such as nifedipine and nitrendipine are widely used to treat hypertension and cardiac insufficiency. These drugs regularly lead to insomnia and nervousness. The antihypertensive amlodipine, the bladder spasmolytic flavoxate, and both pregabalin and gabapentin, used for epilepsy and neuropathic pain, affect different types of L-type voltage-dependent calcium channels and are all known to be associated with sedation. The same side effect is reported for ziconotide, a N-type voltage-dependent calcium channel blocker recently registered for neuropathic pain. The drug flunarizine sometimes used for vertigo is a non-selective voltage-gated channel inhibitor potentially causing sleep impairment, although these effects are usually overshadowed by the sedative effects of its concomitant antihistaminergic properties. Similar effects are shown by the spasmolytic dantrolene, which blocks calcium release from cytoplasmic stores by inhibition of ryanodine.

Anti-epileptics

As a general rule, anti-epileptic drugs are developed to reduce neuronal conduction and signal transmission, preventing or interrupting the propagation of epileptic seizures. However, the underlying pharmacological mechanisms of action are often incompletely understood. A number of the most potent anti-epileptics block voltage-dependent sodium channels. Examples include carbamazepine, topiramate and zonisamide. Valproate and phenytoin inhibit (among others) CaV channels that are required for synaptic function. Levetiracetam and brivaracetam block neurotransmitter release by binding to a synaptic vesicle glycoprotein (SV2a). The impact of anti-epileptics on nerve conduction can lead to variable degrees of dose-dependent sedation. Many anti-epileptic drugs have prominent effects on sleep, although the evaluation of these effects in clinical populations of epileptic patients is complicated by arousals due to nocturnal seizures or abnormal interictal activity.

Neuropharmacology of Non-REM Sleep

While the activation of multiple neurotransmitter systems has been implicated in various aspects of wakefulness, the pharmacology of sleep induction has been dominated by a single neurotransmitter, namely, GABA (Figure 7.3). Despite an intensive search for other sleep-promoting substances, there has been limited success in the discovery of these so-called 'hypnogens'. It is evident that sleep is regulated not only by circadian factors but also by homeostatic control mechanisms that produce a 'sleep debt' with increasing time awake. It is likely that humoral factors are involved in this homeostatic control and purinergic receptors with adenosine responsivity may play an important role in this mechanism.

Gamma-Aminobutyric Acid

GABA is the primary inhibitory neurotransmitter in the CNS. Contrary to bioamine neurotransmitters, which are produced in a small number of highly specialised midbrain and brainstem nuclei, GABA-ergic neurons are widespread throughout the whole brain. Indeed, about 40% of central neurons contain GABA and 30% of synapses bind GABA. A small specific group of GABA-ergic cells in the ventrolateral preoptic area (VLPO) as well as in the adjacent basal forebrain (BF) and preoptic area (PO) appear to be crucial for the control and maintenance of non-REM sleep. Certainly, lesions in this region result in severe insomnia. Furthermore, neurons in these areas fire at higher rates during sleep than during waking and show high c-fos expression during sleep recovery after sleep deprivation. Basal forebrain sleep-promoting neurons project rostrally to the cortex alongside wake-promoting ACh-containing neurons. Their firing activity correlates positively with delta EEG activity and negatively with gamma EEG activity. VLPO GABA-ergic neurons also project caudally into the posterior lateral hypothalamus where they synapse onto orexinergic neurons. Further down they inhibit histamine-containing neurons in the tuberomamillary nucleus and brainstem noradrenergic and serotonergic neurons in the LCl and dorsal raphe nuclei. Sleep-active VLPO neurons, in turn, are under inhibitory control from noradrenaline, histamine and Ach systems. Accordingly, these neurons are inhibited during waking and are disinhibited when monoaminergic and cholinergic neurons decrease their discharge following the transition to drowsiness.

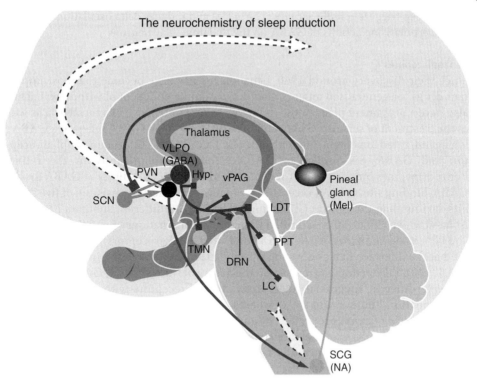

Figure 7.3 The light–dark cycle has an influence on sleep and wakefulness through the suprachiasmatic nucleus. This 'biological clock' controls the rhythmicity of melatonin release in the pineal gland through polysynaptic pathways. During light, the SCN suppresses the hypothalamic paraventricular nucleus through GABA-ergic projections. When night falls, the suprachiasmatic nucleus becomes less active and the paraventricular nucleus is disinhibited. This leads to melatonin production in the pineal gland, mediated by sympathetic (noradrenergic) nerve projections that originate in the superior cervical ganglion. Elevated melatonin levels (together with darkness and several neurochemical factors that are not shown in the figure) cause a disinhibition of the ventrolateral preoptic area of the anterior hypothalamus. This area is relatively inactive during wakefulness, but during sleep induction it exerts an inhibitory mainly GABA-ergic drive (ventrolateral preoptic area with connecting arrows) on all major arousing neurotransmitter systems. Brain regions: DRN, dorsal raphe nuclei; Hyp., hypothalamus; LC, locus coeruleus; LDT, laterodorsal tegmental nuclei; PPT, pedunculopontine tegmental nuclei; PVN, paraventricular nucleus; SCG, superior cervical ganglion; SCN, suprachiasmatic nucleus; TMN, tuberomammillary nucleus; VLPO, ventrolateral preoptic area; vPAG, ventral periaqueductal grey. Neurochemical: GABA, gamma-aminobutyric acid; Mel, melatonin; NA, noradrenaline.
Source: Courtesy of Dr Kari L. Franson.

Local GABA-ergic neurons in the brainstem reticular formation and LC also show increased activity during sleep. GABA-containing neurons in the caudal medullary reticular formation (RF), projecting to the spinal cord, are active during REM sleep together with glycine-containing neurons which directly inhibit spinal motor neurons. More fontally, GABA-ergic neurons in the thalamic reticularis nucleus inhibit thalamo-cortical relay neurons to dampen cortical activation. Their burst pattern of discharge during sleep triggers spindle activity (12–14 Hz) and induces delta oscillations through the hyperpolarising actions of GABA on the thalamic relay neurons.

Benzodiazepines

Since their discovery around 1960, benzodiazepines have become the most important drugs for generalised anxiety disorder, insomnia and alcohol withdrawal. They also have a prominent place in the induction and maintenance of anaesthesia as well as the treatment of seizures. There are three different main GABA receptors; $GABA_A$ is a ligand-gated ion channel for chloride (Cl^-), $GABA_B$ is a G-protein coupled receptor, and $GABA_C$, is similar to $GABA_A$, found predominantly in the retina. Benzodiazepines bind to $GABA_A$ receptors and increase the affinity of GABA for the GABA-binding site. $GABA_A$ receptors are heteropentameric, consisting of five subunits surrounding the central Cl^- channel. Thus far, 19 different subunits have been isolated which can occur in a limited number of combinations (6 α, 3 β and 3 γ units and 1 δ, ε, π and θ unit for $GABA_A$, and 3 ρ units for $GABA_C$ receptors). Benzodiazepines bind at the interface of α and γ subunits while GABA binds to the interface of the α and β subunit. Depending primarily on the nature of the α subunit, $GABA_A$ receptors subserve different functional roles. Activation of receptors with α_1 subunits produces sedation, amnesia and ataxia whereas α_2 subunits are associated with anxiolysis and muscle relaxant properties. α_3 and α_5 receptor activation also causes muscle relaxation and ataxia while seizure suppression is observed with all α subunits, particularly in combination. Currently, several subtype-selective $GABA_A$ agonists are in development for various indications with an improved side-effect profile. The benzodiazepines, however, show little difference in subunit selectivity, with the exception of α_4 and α_5 subunits which are insensitive to benzodiazepines. Their main therapeutic characteristics are due to differences in pharmacokinetic properties and dosage regimens. Long-acting low-level benzodiazepine dosing is used for generalised anxiety or seizure prevention, mainly in children, whereas fast-onset high-level concentrations are needed to treat status epilepticus or to induce anaesthesia. Non-benzodiazepine sleep-inducing agents such as zolpidem, zopiclone and zaleplon are characterised by a rapid absorption and a higher affinity for α_1 subunits, which are primarily associated with sedation.

It should be emphasised that benzodiazepines do not restore normal sleep. In contrast, they suppress deep sleep and REM-sleep stages while augmenting light stage 2 sleep. This reduced sleep quality along with persisting drug plasma levels of the longer-acting compounds may cause the 'hangover' effects that are frequently reported after use of benzodiazepines for insomnia. After a few weeks of daily treatment, most benzodiazepines also produce tolerance, associated with reduced efficacy and withdrawal symptoms after stopping. These withdrawal symptoms include insomnia and restlessness, which rapidly disappear after re-administration of the drug. This is an important cause for the dependency that many subjects experience after using benzodiazepines for more than 3 or 4 weeks. Very short-acting non-benzodiazepine drugs may show less propensity for drug dependency with once daily dosing. In general, however, most authorities recommend that prescriptions for GABA-ergic drugs for anxiety-related sleep disorders should be limited to a few weeks of uninterrupted use.

Barbiturates

Barbiturates allosterically enhance the binding of GABA to its receptor, thereby potently increasing and prolonging the effects of this neurotransmitter. Barbiturates also have other pharmacological effects such as reduced glutamatergic transmission that contribute to their strong CNS-suppressant properties.

Barbiturates are still used in anaesthesia and for the treatment or prevention of seizures, mainly as secondary treatment option. Their potency and long terminal half-life often cause prominent sedative adverse effects. Although patients seem to develop some tolerance to these side effects during prolonged treatment, much of this is due to behavioural adaptation to the long-lasting CNS depression caused by this class of drug.

Other GABA-ergic Drugs

Several GABA-ergic drugs with other pharmacological mechanisms have been developed. These include GABA-transferase inhibitors such as vigabatrin, now a rarely used anti-epileptic drug; GABA-release stimulators, a mechanism of action of the $GABA_B$-agonist baclofen used for dystonia and muscle spasticity; and GABA-reuptake inhibitors such as the antiepileptics tiagabine and stiripentol. In general, these drugs amplify the activity of endogenous GABA and hence cause fewer adverse effects. Nonetheless, all these GABA-ergic drugs cause dose-related sedation with less marked disturbance of sleep patterns. Ethanol is an allosteric enhancer of transmembrane receptors and many of its effects are mediated by enhancement of GABA-ergic signalling. In line with this effect, ethanol primarily causes sedation but also disturbs sleep maintenance.

GABA-A antagonists could theoretically play a role in the symptomatic treatment of a range of cognitive and movement disorders but, so far, their development has been limited by pro-convulsive side effects and agitation with insomnia.

Flumazenil is an inverse benzodiazepine receptor agonist that is used clinically to counteract benzodiazepine overdosing. Flumazenil can impair sleep at high doses but this may also reflect acute benzodiazepine withdrawal.

Adenosine

Adenosine is a degradation product of ATP, produced during cellular metabolic activity, the levels of which provides feedback on the cell's energy levels. Adenosine analogues are one of the few postsynaptic receptor agonists known to increase SWS. This may partly be mediated by adenosine A_1-induced decrease of neuronal firing and neurotransmitter release of both cholinergic basal forebrain cells and monoaminergic brainstem neurons. However, A_2-receptor-mediated stimulation of VLPO sleep-promoting neurons may also be involved. In the cortex and thalamus, adenosine has a hyperpolarising effect, switching these cells into a burst firing mode associated with SWS. Adenosine levels in the brain are higher during waking than during sleep and increase progressively with prolonged wakefulness, suggesting that adenosine might be a homeostatic sleep factor which builds up after prolonged wakefulness.

Adenosine itself is used as a class V anti-arrhythmic drug but does not penetrate the brain sufficiently to cause CNS effects. Phosphodiesterase (PDE) inhibitors decrease the inactivation of cyclic adenosine and guanosine monophosphates (cAMP and cGMP, respectively) and thereby prolong the active state of the cell. Caffeine, theophylline and other methylxanthines are both non-selective PDE inhibitors and adenosine A_1 receptor antagonists and thereby have a wake-promoting effect. PDE3 inhibitors such as enoximone and milrinone are used to treat cardiac failure by mimicking sympathetic stimulation. PDE4 inhibitors such as ibudilast and pentoxyfylline cause bronchodilation by a similar mechanism. PDE5 inhibitors including sildenafil and vardenafil are used to treat erectile dysfunction and pulmonary hypertension. Anagrelide reduces thrombocyte levels by PDE inhibition in platelets. The tissue selectivity of PDE subtypes is limited, and most of these drugs stimulate wakefulness and cause insomnia, depending on their BBB penetration. These stimulating properties have also led to the exploration of subtype-selective PDE inhibitors and adenosine antagonists as cognitive enhancers and CNS stimulants potentially for treating dementia, depression, and the negative symptoms of schizophrenia. So far, this approach seems to have been thwarted by the lack of brain selectivity for subtype selective PDE inhibitors and associated risks of insomnia, agitation and seizures.

Sleep Factors and Immune System Modulators

'Sleep factors' are homeostatic substances which, as proposed for adenosine, progressively build up with prolonged wake or physical activity. Most of these compounds have originally been isolated from brains of sleep-deprived animals. Apart from nitric oxide, uridine, oleamide and prostaglandin-D_2, most sleep factors have proved to be of peptidergic origin. The long list of these putative sleep factors include muramyl dipeptide, delta sleep inducing peptide, cortistatin, somatostatin, cholecystokinin, bombesin, insulin, neuropeptide S, prolactin, gallanin, grehlin, neuropeptide Y, growth hormone (GH), growth hormone releasing hormone (GHRH), melanin-concentrating hormone (MCH), tumour necrosis factor α (TNF-α) and interleukins (IL-1β). In most cases the physiological mechanisms that link these modulators to the sleep–wake cycle are still poorly characterised.

As evidenced by the dual role of orexin/hypocretin, sleep–wake regulation and feeding behaviour are closely linked, partly through the activation of the autonomic nervous system. Drugs that affect metabolic homeostasis also often have a significant impact on sleep or wakefulness. For instance, compounds that mimic aspects of food deprivation may cause insomnia. This may include lipid lowering drugs such as statins, anorectics and oral hypoglycaemics. Since stress also causes insomnia, most drugs that can be considered as stress hormones such as corticosteroids have similar properties. The sleep effects differ considerably among the various glucocorticoids, depending on their dose levels, CNS penetration and patient susceptibility. The effects of other hormones are also in line with their physiological effects. Thyroid hormones cause dose-dependent nervousness and insomnia as early signs of overstimulation. Oestrogen- or gonadotrophin antagonists can also produce insomnia in some patients, reminiscent of menopausal sleeping problems. Progestagens and oestrogens, however, usually do not have significant sleep–wake side effects.

Inflammatory processes have complex effects on sleep. In general, infections promote sleep as a consequence of stimulating the immunological defence systems. At the same time, serious infections cause considerable stress activation, tending to impair normal sleep. Infections change the interactions between the immune system and brain neurochemical systems involved in sleep–wake maintenance, particularly cytokine and serotonergic pathways. Considering the complicated role of the serotonergic system on sleep, it is perhaps understandable that many anti-inflammatory, immune-modulatory and antimicrobial drugs can variously cause insomnia, sedation or combinations of these side effects. This can also include some monoclonal antibodies and other proteins that are too large to penetrate into the CNS, but which have profound effects on interactive systems that connect the brain and the rest of the body.

Almost all antiviral medications can cause insomnia and abnormal dreaming occurs in a minority of patients. At the same time, several studies have shown that these drug-related side effects are aggravated by additional psychological stress. Most chinolone and some macrolide antibiotics have similar side effects. The majority of antimalarial drugs can also lead to moderate sedation. Cytostatics share many aspects of their mechanisms of action with antimicrobial drugs and about one third cause sedation, insomnia, or both at therapeutic doses, without a clear relationship to the underlying mechanism of action. About half of all cytostatic immunomodulators such as tyrosine kinase inhibitors, used to treat leukaemia, and some angiogenesis inhibitors can cause mild insomnia although, equally, a proportion of patients can become sedated. These effects may be partly due to an interaction with the underlying disease state or to associated factors, considering the large impact of cancer or severe infections on the sleep–wake cycle. Many cytostatic antihormones, particularly aromatase inhibitors used to treat breast cancer, reduce alertness or impair sleep. Reduction of normal hormone levels could also explain why the corticosteroid antagonist mitotane causes sedation in many patients with adrenal gland carcinoma, considering the well-known opposite effects of corticosteroids.

Some prostaglandin agonists, used for induction of childbirth or abortion, and most antagonists, namely NSAIDs and salicylates, can cause either limited sedation or insomnia and sometimes abnormal dreams, provided they act long enough and penetrate the CNS sufficiently. The same holds true for TNF-α inhibitors such as infliximab or adalimumab, although other disease modifying antirheumatic agents only seem to cause CNS effects at toxic drug levels. Most interferon preparations can produce mild insomnia, whether they are used to treat chronic viral infections (alpha, gamma) or multiple sclerosis (beta). For other immunological drug classes, the reports on either sedative or sleep impairing effects are less frequent or severe but hardly any class is completely devoid of such potential problems. The effects of most immunosuppressants or immunomodulators, therefore, can occasionally be added to the differential diagnosis of an impaired sleep–wake cycle in a susceptible patient. The highly complicated inflammation cascades are affected not only by anti-inflammatory drugs but also secondarily by other drug classes. Angiotensin converting enzyme (ACE) inhibitors, for instance, which secondarily increase bradykinin activity, can cause mild insomnia, sometimes related to coughing.

Key Points

- The circadian and functional changes during the sleep–wake cycle require coordinated changes of almost all pharmacological systems in the nervous system. Consequently, most CNS-active drugs can have a significant impact on sleep–wake regulation.
- Sedation and insomnia are determined by how the drug's primary or secondary pharmacological characteristics interact with sleep–wake regulation. The effects are modified both by drug levels in the CNS and by the sensitivity of the brain to the effects of medication.
- Centrally active anticholinergic drugs often cause sedation and memory disturbance. This is a relevant secondary pharmacological characteristic of many older compounds.
- Antihistaminergic [H1] drugs cause sleepiness in proportion to their brain penetration.
- Noradrenergic agonists (α1 agonists, release stimulators, reuptake inhibitors) often cause insomnia. Noradrenergic α_1 antagonists and presynaptic (auto-inhibitory) α_2 agonists usually cause sedation and promote sleep.
- Serotonergic drugs are used for different indications, and many show incomplete subtype selectivity. Such drugs can cause sedation (through 5HT1a receptors) or sedation (5HT2a), or both.
- Dopamine D_1 agonists induce behavioural arousal, whereas D_2-receptor agonists give rise to biphasic effects with low doses reducing wake time and augmenting SWS and REM sleep. Higher doses have opposite effects. D_2 antagonists induce some sedation, which for many antipsychotic drugs is also due to secondary antihistaminergic or -serotonergic effects.
- GABA is the primary inhibitory neurotransmitter in the CNS, and a small group of ventrolateral and basal GABA-ergic cells are involved in the control and maintenance of non-REM sleep. Benzodiazepines and barbiturates are GABA-ergic coactivators.
- Sleep factors such as adenosine build up with the amount of waking and physical activity. Phosphodiesterase inhibitors and adenosine A1 receptor antagonists such as caffeine and theophylline are activating and wake-promoting drugs.
- Sleep regulating hormones convey information about the light–dark cycle (melatonin) and coordinate the different neurophysiological systems involved in circadian rhythms (orexin). Recent improvements in hypnotic medication target these systems effectively. Beta-blockers reduce melatonin release and often cause abnormal dreams.
- The restorative function of sleep involves an intensive cross-talk with other fundamental homeostatic processes, such as immunologic, metabolic, endocrine and autonomic nervous systems. This complexity is reflected by the high frequency of sedation, sleepiness, insomnia and abnormal dreaming, during treatment with medications for infections, malignancies, and auto-immune, cardiovascular and other systemic conditions.

Appendix 7.A

Therapeutic class/Drugs	Primary mechanism [type II side effects]	Main (additional) indications	Sleep/wake disturbance	Severity[a]
Sedatives (insomnia/anxiety)				
Benzodiazepines (Chapter 5)	GABA-A agonism	Insomnia, anxiety disorders, sedation	Sleepiness, withdrawal insomnia	+++/– – –
z-hypnotics (Chapter 5)	GABA-A agonism	Insomnia	Sleepiness, withdrawal insomnia, abnormal dreams	++/–/~
Azapirones (buspirone,tandospirone)	Partial 5HT1a agonism partial 5HT5a agonism?	Anxiety disorders	Insomnia	++
Valerian	GABA-A agonism?	Insomnia, anxiety disorders	Sleepiness	+
Melatonin	MR1/2 agonism	Insomnia	Sleepiness, insomnia, abnormal dreams,	+/~/–
Sodium oxybate	GABA-B agonism?	Narcolepsy	Sleepiness, (withdrawal) insomnia, abnormal dreams	+++/– – – – /~ ~
Antipsychotics				
Chlorpromazine, perphenazine > fluphenazine, periciazine	D2 antagonism [H antagonism]		Sleepiness	+++
Chlorprotixene > zuclopentixol > flupentixol	D2 antagonism [H antagonism]		Sleepiness	+++
Clozapine	D2/5HT2 antagonism [H antagonism]		Sleepiness	+++
Olanzapine, quetiapine	D2/5HT2 antagonism [H antagonism]		Sleepiness	++
Haloperidol, bromoperidol, pipamperon, droperidol	D2 antagonism		Sedation	+
Amisulpride, sertindole, sulpiride	D2/5HT2 antagonism		Sedation	+
Risperidone, paliperidone, lurasidone	D2/5HT2 antagonism		Insomnia, sedation	–/+
Aripiperazole	Partial D2 agonism		Insomnia, sedatio[b]	–/+
Tiapride, pimozide, fluspirilene penfluridole	D2/5HT2 antagonism			

(Continued)

Appendix 7.A (Continued)

Therapeutic class/Drugs	Primary mechanism [type II side effects]	Main (additional) indications	Sleep/wake disturbance	Severity[a]
Antidepressants				
Agomelatine	5HT2c antagonism, MR1/2 agonism		Sedation, abnormal dreams	++/~
Amitriptyline, dosulepine, doxepine, nortriptyline	5HT/NA-reuptake inhibition [H antagonism]	Depression, anxiety disorders, neuro-pathic pain	Sedation, withdrawal insomnia, abnormal dreams	+++/--/~
Mianserine, mirtazapine	NA-release stimulation, 5HT1 stimulation [H antagonism]		Sleepiness	++
Trazodone	5HT-reuptake inhibition, NA-release stimulation, 5HT1 stimulation [H antagonism]		Sleepiness, insomnia	++/--
(es)citalopram, fluoxetine, paroxetine, sertraline	5HT-reuptake inhibition [5HT2 stimulation]	Depression, anxiety disorders	Sedation, (withdrawal) insomnia abnormal dreams, bruxism, yawning	++/--/~
Duloxetine*, venlafaxine, dapoxetine[†]	5HT/NA-reuptake inhibition	Depression, anxiety disorders, neuro-pathic pain*, premature ejaculation[†]	Sedation, (withdrawal) insomnia, abnormal dreams, bruxism, yawning	++/--/~
Fluvoxamine, paroxetine, sertraline	5HT-reuptake inhibition [5HT2 stimulation]	Depression, anxiety disorders, neuro-pathic pain	Sedation, (withdrawal) insomnia, yawning	++/--
Clomipramine, imipramine, desipramine	5HT/NA-reuptake inhibition [H antagonism]	Depression, anxiety disorders, neuro-pathic pain	Sedation, (withdrawal) insomnia	++/-
Moclobemide (A), selegiline (B), rasageline (B), tranylcypromine (A, B)	MAO-A/B inhibition		Insleep insomnia	--

Reboxetine, bupropion	NA(/D)-reuptake inhibition		Insomnia	--
Maprotiline	5HT/NA-reuptake inhibition		Sedation, abnormal dreams	+/~
Stimulants				
Atomoxetine	NA(/D)-reuptake inhibition	Attention deficit hyperactivity disorder	Insomnia, sleepiness[c]	---/++
Dexamphetamine	D/NA-release stimulation	Attention deficit hyperactivity disorder	Insomnia, sleepiness	---/++
Methylphenidate	D/NA-release stimulation	Attention deficit hyperactivity disorder	Insomnia, sleepiness	---/++
(ar)modafenil	D(/NA) agonism?	Narcolepsy	Insomnia, sleepiness, abnormal dreams	--/++/~
Epilepsy				
Barbiturates	GABA-A agonism	Epilepsy, anesthesia	Sleepiness	+++
Benzodiazepines	GABA-A agonism	Epilepsy, anesthesia	Sleepiness	+++
Chloralhydrate	GABA-A agonism	Epilepsy, anesthesia	Sleepiness	+++
Felbamate	GABA-A agonism		Insomnia, sedation	-/+
ethosuximide	calcium antagonism T-type VGCC		sedation, abnormal dreams	++/~~
Vigabatrin	GABA-transferase inhibition		Sedation	++
Carbamazepine[†], oxcarbazepine, phenytoin[‡], topiramate*, valproate*, zonisamide, rufinamide, lacosamine	Voltage-dependent Na inhibition	Neuropathic pain[†] (cardiac arrhythmia[‡]) (migraine prevention*)	Sedation	++(+)
Brivaracetam, levetiracetam	SV2A inhibition		Sedation	++
lamotrigine	Glutamate-release inhibition		Insomnia, sedation	-/+
Perampanel	Glutamate AMPA antagonism		Sedation	+++
Stiripentol, tiagabine	GABA-A agonism, GABA-reuptake inhibition		Sedation	+++
Retigabine	K-channel opener		Sedation	+++

(Continued)

Therapeutic class/Drugs	Primary mechanism [type II side effects]	Main (additional) indications	Sleep/wake disturbance	Severity[a]
gabapentin, pregabalin	calcium antagonism L-type VGCC	Epilepsy, neuropathic pain	Sedation	+++/--
Ziconotide	Calcium antagonism N-type VGCC	(neuropathic) pain (not epilepsy)	Sedation, insomnia	+++/--
Parkinson's disease				
Bromocriptine, ropinirole	Dopamine D2 agonism		Sedation (sleep attacks)	++(+)
tolcapone	COMT inhibition		Insomnia, abnormal dreams	--/+++/~~
Biperidene, dexetimide, trihexyphenidyl	M antagonism		Insomnia, sedation[b]	---/+++
Pergolide, pramipexole, rotigotine	Dopamine D2 agonism		Insomnia, sedation (sleep attacks)	--/+(+)/~~
Apomorphine	Dopamine D1/D2 agonism		Insomnia, sedation[b]	-/++
Entacapone	COMT inhibition		Insomnia, abnormal dreams	-/~~
Levodopa	Dopamine precursor		Insleep insomnia	-
selegiline	MAO-B inhibition		Insleep insomnia, sedation	--/++
Rasagiline	MAO-B inhibition		—	
Amantadine	Glutamate NMDA antagonism		Insomnia, sedation ('reduced concentration')	-/+
Multiple sclerosis				
Interferon beta-1a	Interferon	Relapse prevention	Insomnia	-
Interferon beta-1b	Interferon	Relapse prevention	—	
Glatiramer	Immunomodulation	Relapse prevention	Sedation, abnormal dreams	++/~
Fampridine	K-channel inhibition	Muscle weakness	Insomnia	-
Dementia, Huntington, amyotrophic lateral sclerosis (ALS)				
Riluzole	glutamate NMDA antagonism	ALS	Sedation	++
Memantine	glutamate NMDA antagonism	Alzheimer's disease, vascular dementia	Sedation	++
Donepezil, galantamine, rivastigmine	Cholinesterase inhibition	Alzheimer's disease	Insomnia, sedation	--/+
Tetrabenazine	Dopamine depletion	Huntington's chorea	Sedation, insomnia,	+++/--

Drug	Mechanism	Indication	Sleep effect	Rating
Migraine				
Almotriptan, frovatriptan, Naratriptan, rizatriptan, Sumatriptan, zolmitriptan	5HT1-antagonism	Migraine attack	Sleepiness	++
Eletriptan	5HT1-antagonism	Migraine attack	Sedation, insomnia	++/-
Methysergide	5HT2B-antagonism	Migraine attack	Sedation, insomnia	++/--
Flunarizine	Calcium inhibition VGCC [H-antagonism]	Migraine prevention (vertigo, allergy)	Insomnia, sedation	-/++
Pizotifene	5HT1/H-antagonism	Migraine prevention	Sleepiness[b]	+++
Muscle relaxants				
Baclofen	GABA-B-agonism		Sedation, sleepiness	+++
Dantrolene	Calcium inhibition, ryanodine antagonism		Sleepiness, insomnia	+/-
Hydroquinine	K-channel inhibition		—	
Tizanidine	Alpha2-agonism		Sleepiness, insomnia	+++/-
Succinylcholine	Nicotine agonism	Surgery	—	
(cis)atracurium, gallamine, mivacurium, pancuronium, rocuronium, vecuronium	Nicotine antagonism	Surgery, artificial respiration	—	
Neuromuscular disorders				
Distigmine, neostigmine, pyridostigmine	Cholinesterase inhibition	Myasthenia gravis	—	
Amifampridine (3,4-diaminopyridine)	K-channel inhibition	Lambert-Eaton myasthenic syndrome	Sleepiness, insomnia	+/-
Hypertension, vasodilation				
Acebutolol, betaxolol, bisoprolol, carvedilol, metoprolol*, nebivolol, oxprenolol, pindolol, *propranolol atenolol	Beta1 inhibition, lipophilic	(migraine prevention*)	Abnormal dreams	~
	Beta1 inhibition, hydrophilic		Insomnia	-
Celiprolol	Beta1 inhibition, hydrophilic		Insomnia, abnormal dreams	-/~
Esmolol, labetolol, sotalol	Beta1 inhibition, hydrophilic		—	

(Continued)

Appendix 7.A (Continued)

Therapeutic class/Drugs	Primary mechanism [type II side effects]	Main (additional) indications	Sleep/wake disturbance	Severity[a]
Carteolol, timolol	Beta1 inhibition	Intraocular hypertension	Abnormal dreams	~
Amlodipine, nicardipine, nifedipine, nitrendipine	Calcium antagonism L-type VGCC		Insomnia	–
isradipine, lercanidipine	Calcium antagonism L-type VGCC		Sedation	+
Other dihydropyridine Ca-antagonists	Calcium antagonism L-type VGCC		—	
Verapamil	calcium antagonism L-type VGCC		Insomnia/nervousness	– –
Diltiazem	Calcium antagonism L-type VGCC		Insomnia	–
Benazepril, captopril, enalapril, fosinopril, lisinopril, perindopril, quinapril, ramipril, zofenopril	ACE inhibition		Insomnia (partly related to cough)	–(–)
Acetazolamide	Carbonic anhydrase inhibition	Intraocular/intracranial hypertension	Sedation	++
Brimonidine	Alpha2 agonism	Intraocular hypertension	Insomnia	–
Moxonidine, rilmenidine	Imidazoline stimulation		Insomnia, sleepiness	–/+++
Telmisartan, valasartan,	AT1 antagonism		Insomnia	–
Losartan	AT1 antagonism		Sedation	+
Other AT1-antagonists	AT1 antagonism		—	
Isosorbide derivatives	NO donor		Sedation	+
Other nitrates	NO donor		Sedation[a]	+
Pentoxyphylline	Phosphodiesterase inhibition		—	
Doxazosine	Alpha1 inhibition	(urinary retention)	Sleepiness, abnormal dreams	++/~
Prazosine	Alpha1 inhibition		Sleepiness, abnormal dreams	+/~
Urapidil	Alpha1 inhibition		Insomnia	–

Drug	Mechanism	Indication	Sleep effect	
Phentolamine	Alpha1/2 inhibition			
Methyldopa	Alpha2 stimulation		Sleepiness, abnormal dreams	++/~
Clonidine	Alpha2 stimulation, imidazoline stimulation	(migraine prevention)	Insomnia, sleepiness	-/+++
Ketanserin	5HT2 antagonism [H1 antagonism]		Sleepiness	++
Hydralazine, minoxidil	Smooth muscle spasmolytic		—	
Ambrisentan, bosentan, macitentan, sitaxentan	Endothelin receptor antagonism		—	
Iloprost	Prostaglandin agonism		Sedation	++
Epoprostenol, treprostinil sildenafil	Prostaglandin agonism		—	
Sildenafil	Phosphodiesterase-5 inhibition	Primary pulmonary hypertension	Insomnia	— —
Sildenafil, vardenafil	Phosphodiesterase-5 inhibition	Erectile impotence	Insomnia	—
Avafenil	Phosphodiesterase-5 inhibition	Erectile impotence	Sedation (insomnia)	+/(—)
Tadalafil	Phosphodiesterase-5 inhibition	Erectile impotence		
Anti-arrhythmics				
Quinidine, disopyramide, procainamide	Na/K-channel inhibition	Class Ia Antiarrhythmics	—	
Lidocaine, mexiletine	Na-channel inhibition (fast dissociating)	Class Ia antiarrhythmics	—	
Flecainide, moricizine, Propafenone	Na-channel inhibition (slow dissociating)	Class Ic antiarrhythmics	—	
Dronedarone, ibutilide, dofetilide, sotalol	K-channel inhibition	Class III antiarrhythmics	—	
Amiodarone	K-channel inhibition	Class III antiarrhythmics	Insomnia, abnormal dreams	—/~~
Vernakalant	Na/K-channel inhibition	Classes I–III antiarrhythmics	Sedation	+
Adenosine, digoxin*	ATP inhibitor, parasympathicomimetic*	Class V antiarrhythmics	— (sedation)[a]	+
Isoprenaline	Beta1/2 agonism		Insomnia/ nervousness	
Atropine	M antagonism		—	

(Continued)

Therapeutic class/Drugs	Primary mechanism [type II side effects]	Main (additional) indications	Sleep/wake disturbance	Severity[a]
Hypotension, circulatory failure				
Ibopamine	Dopamine agonism, alpha-adrenergic agonism	Cardiac failure	Insomnia/ nervousness	–
Epinephrin	Alpha1/2-beta2 agonism		Insomnia/ nervousness	– –
Midodrine	Alpha1 agonism		Insomnia/ nervousness	–
Dobutamine, dopamine	Beta1 agonism		–	
Milrinon	Phosphodiesterase-3 inhibition	Cardiac failure	–	
Enoximon	Phosphodiesterase-3 inhibition	Cardiac failure	Insomnia	–
Fludrocortisone	Mineralocorticoid	Orthostasis, adrenal insufficiency	Insomnia	–
Ranolazine	Na-dependent Ca-channel inhibition	Cardiac failure	Insomnia, sedation	–/+
Caffeine	Phosphodiesterase inhibition	Orthostasis	Insomnia	–
Pentoxifylline	Phosphodiesterase inhibition	Intermittent claudication	Insomnia	–
Diuretics				
Spironolactone	Aldosterone receptor antagonist	K-sparing diuretics	Sedation	+++
Eplerenon	Aldosterone receptor antagonist	K-sparing diuretics	Insomnia	–
Amiloride	Tubular Na-channel blocker	K-sparing diuretics	Insomnia, sedation	–/+
Triamterene	Tubular Na-channel blocker	K-sparing diuretics	–	
	Thiazides		–	
	Osmotic Diuretics		–	
	Loop Diuretics		–	

Lipid lowering agents

Drug	Mechanism	Sleep effect	
Nicotinic acid	Lipolysis inhibition	Insomnia	–
Acipimox	Lipolysis inhibition	–	–
Fibrates (bezafibrate)	Lipoprotein lipase stimulation	Insomnia	–
Fibrates (ciprofibrate, gemfibrozil)	Lipoprotein lipase stimulation	Sedation	+
Atorvastatin, fluvastatin, pravastatin	HmGCoA inhibition	Insomnia	– –
Rosuvastatin, simvastatin	HmGCoA inhibition	–	
lomitapide	Microsomal transfer protein inhibition	Sedation	–

Blood coagulation

Drug	Mechanism	Sleep effect	
Carbasalate, acetylsalicylic acid	Prostaglandin synthetase inhibition	Sedation[a]	+
Abciximib, clopidogrel*, prasugrel, ticagrelor, dipyradimol*, eptifibatide, tirofiban	GPIIb/IIIa receptor inhibition/activation*	Platelet inhibition	
Dateparine, danaparoid, enoxaparine, fondaparinux, heparin, nadroparin, tinzaparin	(low molecular weight) heparins	–	
Warfarin, fenprocoumon	Coumarins	–	
apixaban, rivaroxaban	Factor Xa inhibitors ('-**xabans**')	–	
Argatroban, bivalirudine, dabigatran	thrombin inhibitors ('-**tr**(ob)ans)	–	
Alteplase, reteplase, streptokinase, tenecteplase, urokinase	thrombolytics	–	
	Coagulation factors	–	

Peptic disorders

Drug	Mechanism	Sleep effect	
Calcium/magnesium-carbonate, hydrocalcite, magnesiumoxide, -peroxide, -sulphate	Magnesium	Sedation[d,e]	+
Famotidine, nizatidine	H2 inhibition	Insomnia	–
Cimetidine, ranitidine	H2 inhibition	–	
Omeprazol	H^+/K^+ ATPase (proton pump) inhibition	Insomnia, sedation	– –/+ +

(*Continued*)

Appendix 7.A (Continued)

Therapeutic class/Drugs	Primary mechanism [type II side effects]	Main (additional) indications	Sleep/wake disturbance	Severity[a]
Rabeprazol	H⁺/K⁺ ATPase (proton pump) inhibition		Insomnia, sedation	−/+
Esomeprazol, lansoprazol	H⁺/K⁺ ATPase (proton pump) inhibition		Insomnia	−
Pantoprazol	H⁺/K⁺ ATPase (proton pump) inhibition		—	
Misoprostol	prostaglandin agonism	NSAID gastroprotection	Insomnia	(−)
Anti-emetics				
Cinnarizine	H antagonism		Insomnia, sedation	−/++
Cyclizine	H antagonism		Insomnia, sedation[f]	−/++
Meclozine	H antagonism		Sleepiness	++
Droperidol	D2 antagonism		Sedation	+
Domperidon	D2 antagonism		—	
Metoclopramine	D2/5HT3 antagonism		Sleepiness	++
Granisetron	5HT3 antagonism		Sedation	+
Ondansetron, tropisetron	5HT3 antagonism		—	
Aprepitant, fosaprepitant	NK1 inhibition		Insomnia, sleepiness	(−)/+
Scopolamine	M antagonism		Sleepiness	+++
Intestinal disorders				
Loperamide	Opioid	Diarrhoea	Sedation[c]	+
Chenodiol, ursodeoxycholate	Cholic acid derivatives		—	
	Contact laxatives		—	
	Osmotic laxatives		—	
	Fiber laxatives		—	
Antitussives				
Codeine	Opioid		Sleepiness	++
Noscapine	Opioid (?sigmoid)		Sedation	+
Dextromethorphan	Glutamate NMDA antagonism		Sleepiness	++

Pentoxyverine	Local anesthetic		—	
Acetylcysteine, Mercaptoethanesulphonate			—	
Allergies				
Alimemazine, promethazine	H1/M antagonism		Sleepiness	+++
Dimetindene, hydroxyzine	H1/M antagonism		Sleepiness	+++
Acrivastatine, fexofenadine, mizolastine, oxatomide, rupatadine	H1 antagonism		Sedation	+++
Hydroxizine	H1/M antagonism		Sedation	+
Cetirizine, ebastine,	H1 antagonism		Sedation	+
Oxomemazine	H1/M antagonism		Insomnia[g], sleepiness	−−/+++
Flunarizine	calcium inhibition VGCC [H antagonism]	(vertigo, migraine prevention)	Insomnia, sedation	−/++
Mebhydroline	H1/M antagonism		Insomnia, sedation	−/++
Clemastine	H1 antagonism		Insomnia[g], sedation	−−/+
Ketotifen	H1/M antagonism		(insomnia)[g], sedation	(−)/+
Desloratidine	H1 antagonism		(insomnia)[g], sedation	(−)/+
Loratadine	H1 antagonism		Insomnia/nervousness	−
Cromoglicate, nedocromil	chromium mast cell inhibition		-	
Anti-asthmatics				
Ephedrine	Alpha1/2 agonism		Insomnia/nervousness	−−−
Formoterol, salbutamol, salmeterol, terbutaline, phenoterol	Beta2 agonism		Insomnia/nervousness	−−
Indacaterol, olodaterol	Beta2 agonism		Insomnia/nervousness[d]	−
Theophylline	Phosphodiesterase inhibition		Insomnia/nervousness	−−
Ipratropium, tiotropium	Parasympathicolytic		-	
Montelukast	Leucotriene inhibitors		Insomnia	−
Omalizumab	FCeRI antagonist		Sedation	+
Bladder dysfunction				
Dariphenacine	M3 antagonism		Insomnia, sedation	−/+
Flavoxate	calcium antagonism L-type VGCC[h]		Sedation	+

(Continued)

Appendix 7.A (Continued)

Therapeutic class/Drugs	Primary mechanism [type II side effects]	Main (additional) indications	Sleep/wake disturbance	Severity[a]
Oxybutinine	Parasympathicolytic	Incontinence	Sedation	+
Fesoteridine	M antagonism[h]	Incontinence	Insomnia (sedation)	−−/(+)
Tolterodine, soliphenacine	M antagonism[h]	Incontinence	—	
mirabegron	Beta3 agonism	Incontinence	—	
Alfuzosine, terazosine	Alpha1 antagonism	Retention	Sedation	+
Tamsulosine, silodosine	Alpha1 antagonism	Retention	—	
Dutasteride, finasteride	5-alpha1-reductase inhibition	Retention	—	
Pregnancy, delivery				
Dinoprost, sulproston	Prostaglandin agonism	Delivery induction	Sedation	+
Carboprost	Prostaglandin agonism	Delivery induction	—	
Phenoterol	Beta2 agonism	Uterus spasmolytic	Insomnia/nervousness	−−−−
Atisoban	Oxytocin antagonist	Uterus spasmolytic	Insomnia	−
Anti-infectives: bacterial, protozoal, helminthine				
Benzathinebenzylpenicillin, pheneti-cillin, phenoxymethylpenicillin, flucloxacillin, amoxicillin, piperacillin	Penicillin		—	
Benzylpenicillin	Penicillin		Sedation	+
Nitrofurantoin			Sedation	+
Fusidic Acid			Sedation	+
	Aminoglycosides		—	
	Cephalosporins		—	
	Sulfonamides		—	
	Tetracyclins		—	
Norfloxacin	Chinolone		Insomnia, sedation	−/+(+)
Ciprofloxacin, levofloxacin, moxifloxacin, ofloxacin	Chinolone		Insomnia, abnormal dreams	−/~
Pipemidine	Chinolone		—	

Azithromycin, clarithromycin	Macrolide		Insomnia, abnormal dreams	-/~
Clindamycin, erythromycin, fidaxomicine, roxitromycin	Macrolide		—	—
Aztreonam, doripenem, imipenem, meropenem	Beta-lactam antibiotic			—
Ertapenem	Beta-lactam antibiotic		Insomnia	
Colistin, metronidazole, teicoplanin, vancomycin	(other antibiotics)		—	—
Daptomycin, linezolid	(other antibiotics)			
Dapsone		Lepra	Insomnia	—
Clofazimine		Lepra	Sedation	+
Artemotil, artemesinin, proguanil, pyrimethamine		Malaria	—	
Mefloquine		Malaria	Insomnia, sedation	--/++
Artemether, lumefantrine		Malaria	Insomnia, sedation	--/+
Atovaquon		Malaria, protozoa	Insomnia	-(-)
Pentamidine		Protozoa	—	
Metronidazole		Protozoa	Sleepiness	+(+)
Ethambutol, isoniazide, pyrazinamide, rifampicine, rifabutine		Tuberculosis	—	
Albendazole, ivermectine, mebendazole, niclosamide		Infestations		
Praziquantel		Infestations	Sleepiness	+(+)
Anti-infectives: viral				
Amantadine	[glutamate NMDA antagonism]	Influenza A (Parkinson's)	Insomnia, sedation ('reduced concentration')	-/+
Oseltamivir	Neuroaminidase inhibitor	Influenza A, B	insomnia	—
Zanamivir	Neuroaminidase inhibitor	Influenza A, B	—	
Peginterferon alpha 2a, 2b	Interferon	Hepatitis C	Insomnia, sedation, abnormal dreams	---/++/~~
Interferon alpha 2b	Interferon	Hepatitis B, C	Insomnia, sedation	---/++
Interferon alpha 2a	Interferon	Hepatitis B, C	Insomnia	—
Interferon gamma	Interferon	Hepatitis B	—	—
Telbivudine	DNA polymerase inhibition	Hepatitis B	—	

(Continued)

Appendix 7.A (Continued)

Therapeutic class/Drugs	Primary mechanism [type II side effects]	Main (additional) indications	Sleep/wake disturbance	Severity[a]
Boceprevir, simeprevir	Protease inhibition	Hepatitis C	Insomnia	– – –
Telaprevir	Protease inhibition	Hepatitis C	–	– –
Sofosbuvir	RNA polymerase inhibition	Hepatitis C	Insomnia	– –/~
Ganciclovir, valganciclovir	DNA polymerase inhibition		Insomnia/nervousness, abnormal dreams	– –/~
Valaciclovir	DNA polymerase inhibition		Insomnia/ nervousness, abnormal dreams	– –/~
Famcyclovir	DNA polymerase inhibition		Sedation	(+)
Adefovir, cidofovir, foscarnet	DNA polymerase inhibition		–	
Aciclovir	Nucleoside inhibition		Sedation	(+)
Entecavir	Nucleoside inhibition		Insomnia	– –
Peginterferon alpha 2a	Interferon		Insomnia	– – –
Ribavirin	RNA polymerase inhibition		Insomnia	– – –
Palivizumab	Fusion inhibition (RSV)		–	
Emtricitabine	Nucleoside inhibition	HIV	Insomnia, abnormal dreams	– –/~
Didanosine	Nucleoside inhibition	HIV	Insomnia	– –
Maraviroc	Fusion inhibition (CCR5)	HIV	Insomnia	– –
Enfuvirtide	Fusion inhibition (GP41)	HIV	Abnormal dreams	~~
Ritonavir	Protease inhibition	HIV	Insomnia, sedation	– –/++
Saquinavir	Protease inhibition	HIV	Insomnia, sedation	– –/+
Atazanavir, darunavir	Protease inhibition	HIV	Insomnia, abnormal dreams	– –/~
Amprenavir, lopinavir, tipranavir	Protease inhibition	HIV	Insomnia	– –
Fosamprenavir, indinavir, nelfinavir	Protease inhibition	HIV	–	
Lamivudine	Reverse transcriptase inhibition (nucleoside)	HIV	Insomnia	– –
Rilpivirine	Reverse transcriptase inhibition (non-nucleoside)	HIV	Insomnia, sedation	– – –/++
Etravirine	Reverse transcriptase inhibition (non-nucleoside)	HIV	Insomnia, sedation	– –/+
Efavirenz, zidovudine	Reverse transcriptase inhibition (non-nucleoside)	HIV	Insomnia	–

Drug	Class / mechanism	Indication	Sleep effect	
Abacavir, nevirapine, stavudine, tenofovir disoproxil	Reverse transcriptase inhibition (non-nucleoside)	HIV	—	—
Dolutegravir, raltegravir	integrase inhibition	HIV	Insomnia, abnormal dreams	-/~
Anti-infectives: mycotic				
Flucytosine			Sedation	+
Voriconazol			Insomnia	(−)
Posaconazol			Insomnia	− −
Amphotericin B, anidulafungine, capsofungine, fluconazole, itroconazole, ketoconazole, miconazole, nystatine, terbinafine			—	
Hormones, antihormones				
Testosterone, nadrolone	Androgen		Insomnia[a]	− −
Cyproterone	Androgen antagonism		—	
(ethinyl)estradiol, tibolone	Estrogens		—	
clomiphene	Estrogen antagonism		Insomnia	−
(medroxy)progesterone, desogestrel, dydrogesterone, etonogestrel, levonorgestrel, lynestrenol, norethisterone,uliprisal	Progestagens		—	
choriogonadotrophin 'relins' (uro)follitropin	GnRH		—	
	FSH			
	LH			
Lutropin	LH		Sleepiness	+++
Gonadorelin	LH-RH		—	
Danazole, gestrinone, cetrorelix, ganirelix, pegvisomant	anti GnRH		—	
Abarelix, buseriline	Anti GnRH		Insomnia	−
palifermine	Keratocyte growth factor	Mucositis	—	
Cabergoline	D2 antagonism	Prolactinoma	Sleepiness	+
Bromocriptine	D2 antagonism	Prolactinoma	Sleepiness	+
Quingolide	D2 antagonism	Prolactinoma	Insomnia, sedation	-/+
Somatropin	GH		—	
Mecasermine	IGF1		Sleep apnoea	

(Continued)

Therapeutic class/Drugs	Primary mechanism [type II side effects]	Main (additional) indications	Sleep/wake disturbance	Severity[a]
Somatostatin, 'reotides'	Somatostatin		—	
Tetracosactide	ACTH		—	
Desmopressin, terlipressin	AVP	Diabetes insipidus	—	
Diabetes mellitus				
	Insulin		—	
Exenatide	Incretin analogue		Sleepiness	++
Glibenclamide, gliclazide, glimepiride, tolbutamide	insulin secretagogue		—	
Metformin	Glucose-production inhibitor		—	
'Glitazones'	PPARgamma-agonist		—	
Repaglinide	insulin secretagogue (ATP-dependent K-channel inhibition)		—	
Sitagliptin, vildagliptine	Insulin degradation inhibition (DPP-4 inhibition)		—	
Diazoxide	Insulin secretion inhibition	Hypoglycaemia	Insomnia	−
Glucagon		Hypoglycaemia	—	
Thyroid disorders				
Carbimazol, iodide, propylthiouracil, thiamazol		Hyperthyroidism	—	
Thyroxines	Thyroid hormone		Insomnia/ nervousness[a]	− − −
Calcium regulators				
Parathyroid, teriparatide	Parathyroid hormone	Osteoporosis, Paget's	—	
Pamidronate	bisphosphonate	Osteoporosis, Paget's	Sleepiness	++
Alendronine, clodronine, etidronine, ibandronine, risedronine, tiludronine, zoledronine	Bisphosphonate		—	

Cinacalcet				—
Calcitonin		Osteoporosis, Paget's		—
Paracalcitol	Vitamin D			—
Bazedoxifene	Selective oestrogen receptor modulator	Osteoporosis	Sleepiness	++
Raloxifene	Selective oestrogen receptor modulator	Osteoporosis		—
Opioids				
Fentanyl, hydromorphone, buprenorphin	Opioid-mu agonist		Sleepiness	+++
Morphine	Opioid-mu agonist		Sleepiness, abnormal dreams	++/~
Alfentanil, codeine, dextromoramide, dextropropoxyphen, methadone, nicomorphine, piritramide, remifentanyl	Opioid-mu agonist		Sleepiness	++
Pentazocine, nalbuphine	Opioid-mu agonist partial opioid-mu agonist, M antagonist		Sedation, sleepiness	+++/++
Pethidine			Sleepiness	++
Sufentanyl	Opioid-mu agonist		Sedation	+
Oxycodon	Opioid-mu/kappa/delta agonist		Insomnia, sleepiness, abnormal dreams	−/++/~
Tapentadol	Opioid-mu agonist, NA-reuptake inhibitor		Insomnia, sleepiness, abnormal dreams	−/+++/~
Tramadol	Opioid-mu agonist		Insomnia, sedation	−/+
Analgesics				
'Salicylates'	Prostaglandin synthetase inhibition		Sedation	+
Mesalazine	Prostaglandin synthetase inhibition		Insomnia, sedation	−/+
Meloxicam, piroxicam	Prostaglandin synthetase inhibition		Sedation	+
Piroxicam	Prostaglandin synthetase inhibition		Insomnia, sedation	−/++

(*Continued*)

Appendix 7.A (Continued)

Therapeutic class/Drugs	Primary mechanism [type II side effects]	Main (additional) indications	Sleep/wake disturbance	Severity[a]
Aceclofenac, diclofenac	Prostaglandin synthetase inhibition		Insomnia, sedation, abnormal dreams	−/+/~
Naproxen, sulindac, tiaprophen	Prostaglandin synthetase inhibition		Insomnia, sedation	−/+(+)
Dexibuprofen, dexketoprofen, flurbiprofen, ibuprofen, indomethacin, ketoprofen, nabumetone,	Prostaglandin synthetase inhibition		Insomnia, sedation	−/+
Olsalazine, phenylobutazone, sulphasalazine	Prostaglandin synthetase inhibition		—	
Etoricoxib	Cyclo-oxygenase-2 inhibition		Insomnia, sedation	−/+
Celecoxib, parecoxib	Cyclo-oxygenase-2 inhibition		Insomnia	−−
Paracetamol	Cyclo-oxygenase-3 inhibition		—	
Corticosteroids				
Betamethasone, cortisone, dexamethasone, hydrocortisone, methylprednisolone, prednisolone, prednisone, triamcinolone	Glucocorticoid agonism		Insomnia	−−
Beclomethason, budesonide	Glucocorticoid agonism		Insomnia/nervousness[a]	−
Inflammation				
Methotrexate	Nucleoside inhibition	Autoimmune diseases	Sedation/CNS toxicity	+
Infliximab	TNF-alpha inhibition	Autoimmune diseases	insomnia, sedation	−/+
Adalimumab, golimumab	TNF-alpha inhibition	Disease modifying antirheumatic	Insomnia	−
Eternacept, certolizumab pegol	TNF-alpha inhibition	Disease modifying antirheumatic	—	
Leflunomide	DHODH inhibition	Disease modifying antirheumatic	—	

Abatacept	Fusion inhibition (T-cell)	Disease modifying antirheumatic	Insomnia	–
Anakinra	IL1α/ß inhibition	Disease modifying antirheumatic	—	
Tocilizumab	IL6 inhibition	Disease modifying antirheumatic	—	
Glucosamine	Glucosaminoglycan precursor	Osteoarthritis	—	
Aurothiomalate	Gold	Rheumatoid arthritis	Insomnia	–
Auranofin	Gold	Rheumatoid arthritis	—	
Hydroxychloroquine		Rheumatoid arthritis	—	
Rasburicase	Urate oxydase uricosuria	Gout	—	
Benzbromaron		Gout	—	
Febuxostat	Xanthine oxydase inhibition	Gout	Insomnia	–
Allopurinol	Xanthine oxydase inhibition	Gout	Sedation	(+)
Colchicine		Gout	—	
Pirfenidone	TGFß inhibition	Pulmonary fibrosis	Insomnia, sedation	–/+
Immunosuppression				
Muromonab	Anti CD3-lymphocyte antibody		Sedation	++
Daclizumab	Anti Tac-leucocyte antibody		Insomnia	– – –
Eculizumab	Anti complement C5 antibody	Paroxysmal nocturnal hemoglobinuria	Insomnia	– –
Mycophenolate (mofetil)	Inosinemonophosphate dehydrogenase inhibition		Insomnia	–(–)
Tacrolimus	Protein kinase inhibition		Insomnia	– –
Everolimus, sirolimus	Protein kinase inhibition		—	
Basiluximab	Anti CD20-leucocyte antibody		—	
Ciclosporine	Lymphokine inhibition		—	
Azathioprine	Nucleoside inhibition		—	

(Continued)

Therapeutic class/Drugs	Primary mechanism [type II side effects]	Main (additional) indications	Sleep/wake disturbance	Severity[a]
Macular degeneration				
Pegaptinib	VEGF antagonism	Angiogenesis inhibition	— Insomnia, abnormal dreams, nocturnal sweating	−/~
Aflibercept, axitinib, ranibizumab	VEGF antagonism	Angiogenesis inhibition	—	
Malignancies: cell cycle inhibitors				
Nelarabine	Nucleoside inhibition		Sedation/CNS toxicity	+++
Isophosphamide	Alkylating agent		Sedation/CNS toxicity[a]	++
Temozolomide	Alkylating agent		Sedation	++
Pixantrone	Alkylating agent		Sedation, insomnia	++/−
Bendamustine	Alkylating agent		Insomnia, sedation	−/+
Busulfan	Alkylating agent		Insomnia/nervousness	−
Procarbazine	Alkylating agent		Insomnia[b]	−
Chlorambucil, cyclophosphamide, dacarbazine*, lomustine, melfalan, thiotepa, treosulfan	Alkylating agent, Nucleoside inhibition*		—	
cladribine	Nucleoside inhibition		Insomnia/nervousness	−
Gemcutabine	DNA synthesis inhibition		Sedation	++
Hydroxycarbamide	DNA synthesis inhibition		Sedation	+
Capecitabine, oxilaplatin	DNA synthesis inhibition		Insomnia	−
Amsacrine, carboplatine, cisplatin, decitabine, mitomycine	DNA synthesis inhibition		—	
mitoxantrone	DNA/RNA synthesis inhibition		Sedation	++
Dactinomycin, daunorubicin, idarubicine	DNA/RNA synthesis inhibition		—	
Trabectedin	DNA degradation		Insomnia	−

Drug	Mechanism	Indication	CNS effect	
Arsenic trioxide, bleomycin dexrazoxane	DNA degradation topoisomerase II inhibition/ Chelating agent	Cardiotoxic antidote	— Sedation	++
Etoposide	Topoisomerase II inhibition		Sedation	+
Cytarabine	Nucleoside inhibition		Sedation/ CNS toxicity[a]	+
Fludarabine, fluorouracil, mercaptopurine, tegafur, thioguanine asparaginase	Nucleoside inhibition L-asparigine inhibition		— Sedation/ CNS toxicity	+
Bortezomib	Mitosis inhibition	Myeloma	Insomnia, sedation, abnormal dreams	--/+/~
Vincristine, vinflunine, eribulin docetaxel, doxorubicin, epirubicin, estramustine, paclitaxel, pemetrexed, teniposide, vinblastine, vinorelbine Irinotecan, topotecan	Mitosis inhibition Mitosis inhibition		insomnia —	—
Malignancies: growth factor inhibitors				
Mitotane	Corticosteroid antagonist	Adrenal carcinoma	Sedation	+++
Anastrazole	Aromatase inhibition	Breast carcinoma	Sedation	+
Aminogutethimide	Aromatase inhibition	Breast carcinoma	Insomnia, sedation	-/+++
Exemestane	Aromatase inhibition	Breast carcinoma	Insomnia	---
Flutamide	Androgen inhibition	Prostate carcinoma	Insomnia	—
Letrozole	Aromatase inhibition	Breast carcinoma	Insomnia/nervousness	—
Medroxyprogesterone	Progestagen	Breast carcinoma	Insomnia	—
Abiraterone, bicalutamide, Enzalutamide, nilutamide	Androgen inhibition	Prostate carcinoma		
Fluvestran, megestrol, tamoxifen	Oestrogen inhibition	Breast carcinoma	—	
Malignancies: specific growth inhibitors of cancer cells				
Anagrelide	Phosphodiesterase inhibition	Thrombocytosis	Insomnia/nervousness, Sedation	-/(+)
Sorafenib	Tyrosine kinase inhibition	Renal carcinoma	Sedation	++
Pazopanib	Tyrosine kinase inhibition	Renal carcinoma	Insomnia	—

(Continued)

Appendix 7.A (Continued)

Therapeutic class/Drugs	Primary mechanism [type II side effects]	Main (additional) indications	Sleep/wake disturbance	Severity[a]
Dasatinib, imatinib, nilotinib, ponatinib	Tyrosine kinase inhibition	Leukaemia	Insomnia	– –
Bosutinib, erlotinib, lapatinib, sunitinib	Tyrosine kinase inhibition	Leukaemia	–	
Afatinib, gefitinib	Tyrosine kinase inhibition	Lung carcinoma	–	
Vandetanib	Tyrosine kinase inhibition	Thyroid carcinoma	–	
Imatinib	Protein/tyrosine kinase inhibition	lymphoma, leukaemia	Insomnia, sedation	–/+
Regorafenib	Protein kinase inhibition	Colorectal carcinoma	–	
Temsirolimus	Protein kinase inhibition	Leukaemia	–	
Ruxolitinib	Protein kinase inhibition	Myeloproliferative Diseases	–	
Crizotinib	Protein kinase inhibition	Lung carcinoma	–	
Dabrafenib, vemurafenib	Protein kinase inhibition	Melanoma	–	
Bevacizumab	Anti VEGF antibody	Colorectal carcinoma	Sedation	+ +
Aflibercept, cetuximab, panitumumab	Anti EGFR antibody	Colorectal carcinoma	–	
Alemtuzumab	Anti CD52-leucocyte antibody	Leukaemia	Insomnia, sedation	–/++
Pertuzumab	Anti HER2 antibody	Breast carcinoma	Insomnia	– –
Trastuzumab	Anti HER2 antibody	Breast carcinoma	Insomnia/nervousness, sedation	–/++
Catumaxomab	Anti-Epithelial cell adhesion molecule antibody	Malignant ascites	Insomnia	–
Tretoine	Retinol derivative	Leukaemia	Insomnia/nervousness	– –
Rituximab, ibritumomab tiuxetan	Anti CD20-leucocyte antibody	Lymphoma	Insomnia/nervousness	– –
Vismodegib	Hedgehog pathway inhibitors	Basal cell carcinoma	–	
Ofatumumab	Anti CD20-leucocyte antibody	Lymphoma	–	
Brentuximab	Anti CD30-leucocyte antibody	Lymphoma	–	– –

Malignancies: immunomodulators

Lenalidomide	TNF-alpha/IL6 inhibition	Myeloma	Insomnia/nervousness, sedation	---/++
Thalidomide, pomalidomide	TNF-alpha/IL6 inhibition	Myeloma	—	
Mifamurtide	Specific monocyte stimulator	Osteosarcoma	Insomnia, sedation	-/+
Ipilimumab	Specific T-lymphocyte stimulating antibody	Melanoma	—	
Aldesleukin	Interleukin 2a, 2b	Renal carcinoma	Insomnia, sleepiness	--/+++
Interferon gamma	Interferon		—	
Antidotes, addictions, obesity				
Amifostine	Anti-alkylating agent	Radiotoxicity	Sedation	+
Flumazenil	Benzodiazepine Antagonist	Benzodiazepine overdose	—	
Naltrexon	Opioid-Mu Antagonist	Alcohol and opioid addiction	Insomnia/nervousness	---
Naloxone	Opioid-mu antagonist	Opioid overdose	—	
Acamprosate	glutamate NMDA antagonism	Alcohol addition	Insomnia, sedation ('impaired concentration')	--/+
Disulfiram	Aldehyde dehydrogenase inhibition	Alcohol addiction	Sedation	+
Nicotine, varenicline	Nicotinic agonist	Nicotine abuse	Insomnia/nervousness	---
Orlistat	Lipase inhibitor	Obesity	—	
Rimonabant	CB1 inhibition	Obesity	Insomnia	--
Sibutramine	5HT/NA-reuptake inhibition	Obesity	Insomnia	---

[a] Insomnia (−), sedation/sleepiness (+), abnormal dreams/nightmares (~):

−/+/~ mild/rare (0.1–1%);

−−/++/~~ moderate/frequent (1–10%);

−−−/+++/~~~ severe/very frequent (>10%).

[b] Increased sedative effects of CNS depressants.

[c] Children are more sensitive.

[d] At higher doses.

[e] During prolonged treatment.

[f] CNS stimulation at high doses.

[g] Insomnia particularly in children.

[h] High bladder affinity.

Further Reading

Espana, S.A. and Scammell, T.E. Sleep neurobiology for the clinician. Sleep 27; 811–820, 2005.

Imeri, L. and Opp, M.R. How (and why) the immune system makes us sleep. Nature Rev Neurosci 10; 199–210, 2009.

Kryger, M.H., Roth, T. and Dement, W.C. (Editors). Principles and Practice of Sleep Medicine, 5th edition. Elsevier Saunders, 2011.

Especially chapters by B.E. Jones and P.K. Schweitzer. Lee-Chong, T.L., Sateia, M.J. and Carskadon, M.A. (Editors). Sleep Medicine. Hanley & Belfus, 2002.

Especially Chapter 61 by T.J. Walter and J.A. Golish. Psychotropic and neurological medications, pp. 587–601. Nature 437(7063); 1253–1291, 2005 with a special Insight section on Sleep.

Especially C.B. Saper, T.E. Scammell and J. Lu. Hypothalamic regulation of sleep and circadian rhythms, pp. 1257–1264.

Part Two

Primary Sleep Disorders

8

Narcolepsy and Other Central Disorders of Hypersomnolence

Sebastiaan Overeem[1,2] and Paul Reading[3]

[1] Centre for Sleep Medicine 'Kempenhaeghe', Heeze, The Netherlands
[2] Eindhoven University of Technology, Eindhoven, The Netherlands
[3] Department of Neurology, James Cook University Hospital, Middlesbrough, UK

Introduction

Excessive daytime sleepiness can be a truly incapacitating symptom but is often not appreciated as such. Especially in the young, napping at inopportune times is often dismissed as laziness or as a consequence of 'overdoing it'. This is, in part, due to the fact that many of us think we understand symptoms of excessive sleepiness, having occasionally experienced particularly poor or reduced nocturnal sleep. On the other hand, patients themselves frequently have difficulty describing or articulating their situation, often mentioning terms such as 'fatigue' or 'lack of energy'. In such instances, it is crucial for doctors to ask the simple key question: 'do you fall asleep unintentionally during the day'?

When people have the opportunity to obtain nocturnal sleep of sufficient duration, unwanted daytime sleep episodes are invariably pathological, warranting further assessment [1]. Significant daytime sleepiness is most often caused by nocturnal sleep disorders, notably sleep-disordered breathing, although can be a symptom of chronic (neurological) disorders such as Parkinson's disease. What remains is a rather heterogeneous group of primary hypersomnias, or 'central disorders of hypersomnolence' according to the third edition of the International Classification of Sleep Disorders, ICSD-3 [2]. Narcolepsy is the prototypical disease in this category but alternative disorders are also included, including idiopathic hypersomnia and Kleine–Levin syndrome. Importantly, the category also describes 'insufficient sleep syndrome'. Although this is clearly not a 'central disorder' in a formal sense, it should always be considered in the differential diagnosis of chronic excessive sleepiness as it is often overlooked.

Sleep Disorders in Neurology: A Practical Approach, Second Edition.
Edited by Sebastiaan Overeem and Paul Reading.

Table 8.1 Hypersomnias of central origin, according to ICSD-3.

Narcolepsy type 1
Narcolepsy type 2
Idiopathic hypersomnia
Kleine–Levin syndrome
Hypersomnia due to a medical disorder[a]
Hypersomnia due to a medication or substance
Hypersomnia associated with a psychiatric disorder
Insufficient sleep syndrome

[a] Discussed in various chapters dealing with the primary disorder.

Diagnostic Categories

The point at which sleepiness becomes pathological is a grey area and not clearly defined in the literature. Originally, the term 'hypersomnia' was reserved for conditions in which there was an increase in the total amount of sleep over a 24-hour period [3]. However, that is not necessarily the case in disorders with daytime sleepiness as the core symptom. For example, because of disrupted overnight sleep, patients with narcolepsy often have only marginally increased total sleep times over 24 hours, despite multiple daytime sleep episodes [4]. For the symptom of unwanted daytime sleep periods without a clear increase in total sleep time, the term 'excessive daytime sleepiness' (EDS) has been coined. However, in clinical practice, EDS and hypersomnia are often used interchangeably and sometimes inappropriately. In ICSD-3, a more formal distinction is made, using the term 'hypersomnia' to denote a pathological condition or disease entity, and 'hypersomnolence' or EDS to describe a symptom.

Central disorders of hypersomnolence include a range of different disorders (Table 8.1). In this chapter, we will discuss the most important ones. General emphasis is put on narcolepsy, as the prototypical sleep disorder about which most is known. Idiopathic hypersomnia is another important category, albeit most likely forming a heterogeneous mix of pathologies as yet of unknown aetiology. Insufficient sleep syndrome is not a central hypersomnia, per se, but a highly important differential diagnosis for narcolepsy or idiopathic hypersomnia.

Kleine–Levin syndrome is a rare but fascinating recurrent hypersomnia with fairly specific diagnostic and therapeutic aspects [5].

Hypersomnia can also be caused by another medical (neurological) condition, and is classified in ICSD-3 as such. Important disorders associated with secondary hypersomnia include parkinsonian disorders, brain trauma, auto- immune or paraneoplastic disease and cerebrovascular disorders. These are covered in the chapters dealing with the primary disease.

General Aspects of Symptoms, Diagnosis and Management

The Sleepiness History

Obviously, an abnormal level of sleepiness is the core feature of the various hypersomnias of central origin. As discussed elsewhere in this book (e.g. Chapters 1 and 3), there often remains semantic confusion between symptoms such as hypersomnia, drowsiness,

Table 8.2 Topics to cover in the clinical interview.

Is there EDS? Separate from e.g. fatigue

Age at onset, circumstances at onset (trauma, etc.)

Pattern and severity of EDS. Continuous feeling of sleepiness, sleep 'attacks', circumstances, interference with daily life. Differences at weekends or on holidays? Duration of sleep episodes. Planned naps. Sleep episodes refreshing? Periodicity of symptoms

Automatic behaviour, memory complaints, concentration problems

Night-time sleep. Habitual sleep duration and sleep/wake timing. Sleep inertia. Signs of nocturnal sleep disorders

Associated symptoms, especially:

- **Cataplexy**: pattern of weakness, duration, triggers, etc.
- **Hypnagogic hallucinations**: frequency, content, impact
- **Sleep paralysis**: frequency, duration
- **Body weight/eating patterns**: weight increase, 'craving', night eating

Mood disturbances

Psychosocial aspects: social interactions, school, work, driving

---

sleepiness, and EDS. Therefore, a careful and focused history is paramount (Table 8.2, and Chapter 1). First, one has to establish if there is true abnormal sleepiness. Often, patients and carers report sleepiness as fatigue. The core feature of excessive sleepiness reflects the fact that people actually fall *asleep* during the day such that unintentional daytime naps are the single most distinguishing feature. The *pattern* of sleepiness should be thoroughly characterised (features to cover are listed in Table 8.2).

Automatic and often inappropriate behaviours may be a consequence of lapses in vigilance in the absence of overt sleep. Such phenomena are often reported in narcolepsy but are almost certainly present in other hypersomnias. Typical examples include reading back written text, only to find it either nonsensical, illegible or about a completely different subject. Rarer, but perhaps more specific instances include bizarre or inappropriate actions such as putting unusual objects in the fridge or washing machine.

Fully exploring the nature of the complaint of sleepiness often gives diagnostic clues which can then be further refined on the basis of associated symptoms.

Further Diagnostic Aspects

Questionnaires such as the Epworth Sleepiness Scale may confirm or even pick up hypersomnolence of central origin but a detailed or directed history remains the most important tool. As outlined previously, the pattern and nature of sleepiness may point to a specific diagnosis. Additional symptoms may have important diagnostic value, such as the presence of cataplexy or rapid eye movement (REM) sleep-related phenomena. Nocturnal polysomnography is used to rule out other primary sleep disorders as the main cause of the sleepiness. The flawed yet most established assessment tool for sleepiness remains the Multiple Sleep Latency Test (MSLT, see Chapter 3). It is used to confirm objectively a suspicion of hypersomnia and may also give clues to a specific diagnosis (e.g. multiple sleep-onset REM periods in narcolepsy). Sleep logs are useful in the diagnosis of insufficient sleep syndrome, and, when in doubt, actigraphy can be extremely valuable as an objective indicator of habitual sleep time. Other laboratory tests have only a limited place in the diagnosis of selected disorders but, importantly, include cerebrospinal fluid hypocretin-1 measurements for narcolepsy. Neuroimaging is indicated when a secondary or symptomatic hypersomnia is suspected.

Management Principles

In most central hypersomnias, the goal is to improve daytime functioning of a patient. The disabling effects of EDS should not be underestimated and focused effort on improving sleepiness is invariably appropriate. However, one should not expect to completely eliminate symptoms of excessive sleepiness and this should clearly be communicated with the patient.

Behavioural advice forms the starting point for the treatment of all central disorders of hypersomnolence [6,7]. It is important for patients to try and keep a sleep–wake schedule that is as regular as possible. Often, scheduled daytime naps may be of benefit, particularly for narcolepsy [8]. Some may well be restored by two or three naps per day, each lasting 10–20 minutes or so. Longer naps may suppress the sleep drive later and interfere with nocturnal sleep onset, however. Anecdotally, some patients benefit from avoiding carbohydrate-rich food which reportedly exacerbates post-prandial sleepiness, preferring a high-protein diet.

In general, behavioural approaches are rarely sufficient for satisfactory symptom control and pharmacotherapy is appropriate [6,7]. The various stimulant medications available for narcolepsy are discussed in Chapter 6. The current 'mainstay' drugs are modafinil and amphetamine-like agents such as methylphenidate or dexamphetamine. Pitolisant, a wake-promoting drug that enhances central histamine levels has recently been introduced and may well become established as an effective treatment to improve alertness with few side effects [9]. In general, the treatment guidelines for narcolepsy can be applied to all hypersomnias with a presumed central cause and a pragmatic approach is recommended, given the lack of formal treatment protocols.

Narcolepsy

Epidemiology

Prevalence figures for narcolepsy differ between countries, with estimates ranging from 0.02 to 0.18% for Western populations [10]. Men and women are affected equally. In most patients, symptoms present in adolescence, between 15 years of age and 25 years of age although, importantly, studies have shown that the time between first symptoms and final diagnosis is often more than 7 years [11]. Furthermore, when looking back, patients often report having had symptoms at an earlier age, but mild enough not to raise the suspicion of a disease process. Sometimes, narcolepsy can develop at a particularly young age, even before 10 years old [12]. Recently, reports of young-onset narcolepsy have markedly increased, perhaps suggesting that age-at-onset estimates were previously too high.

Core symptoms

Classical narcolepsy, now designated Narcolepsy type 1, is predominantly characterised by two core symptoms: EDS and cataplexy [13]. Other elements of the often quoted and somewhat outdated 'tetrad' of symptoms are hallucinations around sleep–wake transitions and sleep paralysis. Importantly, fragmented night-time sleep is nowadays regarded as a core symptom and, not infrequently, may be the most bothersome aspect to patients. It is also increasingly recognised that the narcolepsy phenotype is broad, including symptoms such as metabolic disturbances potentially fuelling obesity, eating disorders, depression and anxiety [14–16]. Memory and cognitive complaints, especially in attentional domains, are extremely common. Based on specific findings from ancillary sleep studies, a form of narcolepsy without cataplexy is recognised, Narcolepsy type 2, although this is likely to be a heterogeneous disorder, almost certainly overlapping with idiopathic hypersomnia [17].

Sleepiness

The sleepiness in narcolepsy is typically characterised by relatively short and refreshing sleep episodes. In between sleeps, patients may have seemingly normal vigilance, but lapses are common. The sleepiness may be truly imperative but usually patients can postpone sleep for a while by engaging in physical activity, for example. Sudden 'sleep attacks' without any recognised prior warning of sleep are certainly possible but are relatively rare. Although the patterns described are typical, exceptions do occur. For example, prolonged daytime sleep episodes are described and some may report virtually continuous feeling of sleepiness with superimposed lapses into frank sleep.

Cataplexy

Cataplexy is the most specific symptom of narcolepsy and in combination with EDS virtually pathognomonic for Narcolepsy type 1 [18]. In its typical form, cataplexy manifests as attacks of bilateral muscle weakness with preserved consciousness, triggered by an emotional stimulus. Cataplexy can affect all skeletal muscles except those subserving respiration and eye movements. Attacks can be complete, causing the patient to slump to the ground, or partial. Preferential sites for partial cataplexy include the face, neck or legs. Symptoms, therefore, include dropping of the jaw and/or speech arrest/slurring, head drooping, and buckling of the knees. Although attacks start relatively abruptly, they usually progress over a few seconds at least, enabling the patient to break any fall and avoid significant injury. The duration of cataplexy is generally short with most episodes lasting a matter of seconds. Attacks longer than a minute or two should prompt the suspicion of disorders other than cataplexy although can sometimes be caused by an accumulation of several attacks when the trigger is continuously present. The most common trigger for cataplexy is mirth, or the expression of mirth, namely laughter. However, many other emotions can trigger cataplexy, including surprise, anger, frustration, and elation. Because a subjective feeling of weakness in the knees when laughing is quite prevalent in the normal population [19], the additional presence of other triggers makes a diagnosis of cataplexy more specific. Generally, a degree of mental relaxation is necessary for patients to experience cataplexy such that it is rarely encountered in the consultation room and attempts to provoke episodes are usually fruitless. When a cataplexy attack is witnessed, it can be useful to assess limb muscle tone and, if a tendon hammer is available, try to elicit deep tendon reflexes. Cataplexy, even when only partial, is invariably accompanied by transient areflexia.

Associated Symptoms

Hypnagogic hallucinations are realistic dream-like experiences around sleep onset whereas the term 'hypnopompic' is used if they occur from awakening. The experiences can be extremely realistic and, not infrequently, patients need to check retrospectively whether an imagined event happened for real or not. This feeling of reality is reinforced by the fact that the dream-like experience often incorporates the actual sleeping environment. Hypnagogic hallucinations are typically 'multimodal', combining visual, auditory and tactile modalities.

Sleep paralysis can occur during arousals from sleep or, typically for narcolepsy, at sleep onset. The patient is conscious but unable to move voluntarily. In contrast to cataplexy, there is no defined trigger and attacks can be prolonged, sometimes lasting up to 10 minutes. It is important to realise that sleep paralysis may occur with a low frequency in the normal population, especially in the context of sleep deprivation.

Narcolepsy is often associated with a clear increase in body mass index with sudden weight gain often around the onset of the other core symptoms. Many also report dysregulation of appetite control with night-time eating behaviours and 'carbohydrate craving' [15].

Concentration difficulties and memory problems are almost universal although formal testing generally yields normal results. This implies any cognitive symptoms are most likely due to (micro-)sleep episodes or deterioration in vigilance levels when sustained levels of concentration are required for task performance.

Diagnostic Procedures and Considerations

The ICSD-3 criteria for Narcolepsy type 1 reflect the current established knowledge that this disorder is caused by a deficiency in hypothalamic hypocretin-1 signalling [20]. Narcolepsy type 1 can be diagnosed when there is a combination of daily and persisting EDS, combined with clear-cut cataplexy and a sleep latency less than8 minutes on the MSLT with at least two sleep onset REM periods (SOREMPs). Based on recent epidemiological studies, a SOREMP is also deemed to have occurred if detected on the polysomnogram preceding the MSLT. Patients with sleepiness and very low or absent hypocretin-1 levels in the cerebrospinal fluid are also classified as Narcolepsy type 1, regardless of whether there is cataplexy or whether the MSLT criteria are strictly fulfilled. So, in clinical practice, the single most important diagnostic clue is the presence of typical cataplexy. Given the implications of the diagnosis, a polysomnogram followed by an MSLT is nearly always undertaken to help confirm Narcolepsy type 1. In Figure 8.1, typical results are shown in a patient with narcolepsy. Although hypocretin-1 measurements are now part of the diagnostic armamentarium, the logistical issues around a lumbar puncture may limit availability to specialist centres. However, in several instances, hypocretin-1 measurements are specifically indicated and of value. Such indications include the presence of comorbid sleep disorders such as sleep-disordered breathing (making the MSLT difficult to interpret), medication use that cannot easily be discontinued such as antidepressants, diagnosis in young children where there are no normative MSLT data, or a 'negative' MSLT when narcolepsy is strongly suspected clinically.

More than 90% of patients with clear-cut cataplexy carry the HLA subtype DQB1*0602. However, the same holds true for 25–30% of the general Caucasian population. Moreover, in cases of diagnostic doubt such as when cataplexy is atypical, the HLA association is much less secure. Therefore, while HLA typing can be used to 'complete' the diagnostic picture and define a homogenous patient population, it should not be used as a primary diagnostic tool and is not listed in ICSD-3 as such.

The criteria for Narcolepsy type 2 are more elaborate and less straightforward. A positive diagnosis requires the combination of persisting daytime EDS, a sleep latency less than 8 minutes at the MSLT, and at least two SOREMPs, again one of which can be

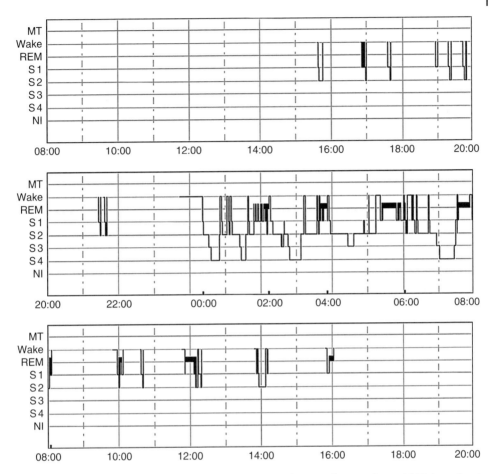

Figure 8.1 Typical narcolepsy findings on a polysomnographic recording starting at 16:00 throughout the night, followed by a MSLT. Several spontaneous sleep episodes can be seen in the afternoon and early evening. There is a fragmented sleep pattern, with several awakenings throughout the night. During all episodes of the MSLT stage 2 is reached, with a mean sleep latency of 4 minutes. In addition, there are three sleep-onset REM periods (during episodes 1, 2 and 4). Finally, a spontaneous nap occurred between MSLT episodes 1 and 2.

derived from the preceding polysomnogram. By definition, cataplexy should be clearly absent but, if it develops later, the patient should be reclassified as having Narcolepsy type 1. Further criteria state that hypocretin-1 is either not measured or found to be within the normal range. Importantly, the symptoms or MSLT findings should not be better explained by another disorder, most notably insufficient sleep.

Management

Behavioural Therapy and Lifestyle Adjustments

Patients should be counselled with respect to sleep hygiene, its timing and the importance of sufficient night-time sleep. In narcolepsy, short daytime naps can be both helpful and restorative in a significant proportion of patients such that they are actively encouraged in combination with pharmacotherapy. It is often useful to have the help of other healthcare workers such as psychologists or nurses, particularly for children. A social worker can also provide useful guidance for choices in school or work but also with respect to activities of daily life and (social) relationships.

Pharmacotherapy

Pharmacotherapy for sleepiness should be tailored towards the individual patient. For most patients, modafinil is a first-line agent, especially as it provides a background level of increased alertness and has relatively few side effects. If it is not tolerated or better control is needed, traditional psychostimulants can be used instead or in addition to modafinil. These drugs are generally short-acting and can be used 'on demand' for dips in alertness. Pitolisant is another alternative with a novel histaminergic mode of action which has become available recently. Chapter 6 provides details on these stimulants, as well as other options.

Although cataplexy and hypnagogic hallucinations may improve if general daytime wakefulness in increased, if troublesome, they are usually treated separately, typically with antidepressant medications that generally suppress REM sleep [7,13]. Although controlled or comparative data are severely lacking, the most widely used drugs are either tricyclic antidepressants or combined serotonin/norepinephrine reuptake inhibitors such as venlafaxine. In mild cases, these are often efficacious in relatively low doses (e.g. 10 mg clomipramine or 75 mg venlafaxine), which helps to limit the occurrence of significant side effects. Anecdotally, selective serotonin reuptake inhibitors are used to good effect but often need to be dosed somewhat higher.

Subsequent to a large body of good quality randomised trial evidence, sodium oxybate (gamma-hydroxybutyrate) has grown into a first line treatment choice for cataplexy in many countries [21]. It is a potent hypnotic with a short half-life, usually taken in two doses through the night. Besides improving night-time sleep quality, probably by enhancing the slow wave component, sodium oxybate is also very efficacious for cataplexy. The precise mechanism is unknown and the anticataplectic effects appear to build over a few weeks. Treatment with sodium oxybate should only be instituted by physicians familiar with the drug and the issues around its prescription.

The disturbed nocturnal sleep in narcolepsy can sometimes be its most challenging or disturbing aspect. Classical hypnotics have limited clinical effects and tolerance is common. Moreover, they tend to produce unrefreshing sleep in contrast to sodium oxybate which generally improves the perceived quality of sleep in the majority of subjects.

Idiopathic Hypersomnia

Epidemiology

There have been no formal prevalence studies for idiopathic hypersomnia, especially for the clinical subtypes with and without long sleep time. Studies are hampered by the fact that the only available diagnostic test (the MSLT, see Chapter 3) is neither particularly sensitive nor specific.

Core Symptoms

Idiopathic hypersomnia (IH) is characterised primarily by excessive sleepiness but without the ancillary symptoms and diagnostic features that point either to Narcolepsy type 1 or 2. ICSD-3 lists one diagnostic category for IH, albeit many acknowledge that two clinical subtypes can be recognised in practice [2]. Indeed, one may encounter IH patients with a normal amount of nocturnal sleep and relatively short, refreshing daytime sleep episodes [22] whereas other patients may have considerably increased total amounts of sleep over 24 hours and a particularly long nocturnal sleep episode (usually of more than 10 hours) [3]. These patients do not feel refreshed in the morning, have significant difficulty waking up, and are strikingly less vigilant for some time after awakening, reflecting so-called 'sleep inertia'.

Diagnostics

ICSD-3 requires that a set of criteria are all met to make a positive IH diagnosis. There should be daily excessive sleepiness for at least 3 months, cataplexy should be absent, and the MSLT or polysomnogram should not show more than one SOREMP. Furthermore, the MSLT should demonstrate a mean sleep latency of less than 8 minutes. When measured with 24-hour polysomnography or wrist actigraphy, the total 24-hour sleep time is more than 11 hours and, typically, 12–14 hours. As with Narcolepsy type 2, it is important to specifically exclude insufficient sleep syndrome, even if it requires an empirical trial of sleep extension. Clearly, other potential diagnoses explaining excessive sleepiness should also be actively ruled out.

Although not part of the formal diagnostic criteria, severe and prolonged sleep inertia in the morning is supportive of an IH diagnosis, as are prolonged and unrefreshing daytime sleep episodes together with frequent acts of automatic behaviour. In the absence of insufficient sleep as an explanation, a high sleep efficiency (>90%) on polysomnography is also supportive of the diagnosis.

Management

Theoretically, an agent to reduce the theoretical excessive sleep drive in IH would be a potential first-line therapy although no consistent treatment data are available for such an approach. Instead, IH is generally treated symptomatically with daytime stimulants in the absence of specific or controlled data from therapeutic trials. Several authors have indicated that IH with excessive sleep time is relatively resistant to traditional stimulants or modafinil such that higher doses than usual are often required and specialist advice is appropriate. Anecdotally, drugs taken before nocturnal sleep either to enhance sleep quality (sodium oxybate) or to potentially lighten sleep (modafinil) have sometimes been useful, particularly in the difficult situation of severe sleep inertia.

Kleine–Levin Syndrome

Epidemiology

Kleine–Levin syndrome is generally considered as extremely rare with a recent prevalence study estimating a prevalence of 3.2 per million [23]. However, previously published case series may have been biased towards 'full blown' or classical cases comprising intermittent hypersomnia, cognitive disturbances, megaphagia *and* hypersexuality. It seems likely that mild or atypical forms of the condition characterised simply by periodic hypersomnolence are more prevalent. It is likely such patients are not routinely encountered in clinical practice.

Core Symptoms

The Kleine–Levin syndrome is characterised by a pattern of intermittent sleep-related and behavioural symptoms in subjects who appear entirely normal between symptomatic episodes [5,24]. The core feature is periodic hypersomnia with prolonged episodes of sleep or profound stupor that may dramatically reduce useful wakefulness during a symptomatic day. The duration of episodes varies between a few days to several weeks. The symptom-free interval between episodes is also variable, from 1 or 2 months up to a year.

Besides recurrent hypersomnia, a positive diagnosis requires there to be additional behavioural or cognitive symptoms [5,24]. Although often cited as the most pathognomonic features, megaphagia and hypersexuality are relatively rare and probably overemphasised. However, almost all patients report feelings of derealisation with dream-like altered perceptions of the physical environment, often described as like being 'in a bubble'. Irritability, confusion, hallucinations or inappropriate child-like behaviour are all commonly reported.

Diagnostics

The diagnosis of Kleine–Levin syndrome is essentially based on a characteristic clinical picture. Between symptomatic episodes, the sleep–wake cycle is within normal limits. The MSLT may be abnormal during an episode, but it is often difficult to perform due to confusion or lack of collaboration from the patient. Electroencephalography studies often show non-specific general slowing of background cortical activity indicative of a mild encephalopathy. For a positive diagnosis to be made, ICSD-3 requires that the patient has experienced at least two recurrent episodes with excessive sleepiness and increased total sleep duration, between 2 days and 5 weeks. In addition, episodes need to occur either more than once a year or at least every 18 months. There is normal alertness, behaviour and cognitive function in between episodes. At least one of the following should also be present besides excessive sleepiness during an episode: cognitive dysfunction, altered perception, eating disorder (either hyperphagia or anorexia), or disinhibited behaviour such as hypersexuality. Finally, the hypersomnolence and associated symptoms are not better explained by another disorder or intermittent use of drugs or medications.

Management

In our experience, it is of the utmost importance to provide guidance to patients and close care-givers, especially given the limited availability of effective symptomatic treatments. Not infrequently, patients feel shame or embarrassment for their behaviour during episodes. Kleine–Levin syndrome episodes pose a particular burden on parents of younger patients during episodes who invariably require 24-hour supervision. A supportive home environment is essential as is provision of information to school and/or work about the disorder, its symptoms and typical course. Occasionally triggering factors such as sleep deprivation can be identified and active behavioural approaches to prevent them are worthwhile.

During episodes, any attempts to treat EDS with stimulant drugs are largely unsuccessful with limited responses even at relatively high doses. Moreover, stimulants do not seem to improve any associated cognitive or behavioural problems. Many compounds have been tried as a prophylactic approach to decrease the frequency of episodes, typically anticonvulsant or anti-migraine agents. However, lithium is the only drug that has been used with moderate success and is therefore regarded by most to be the medication of choice when treatment is considered appropriate [25]. Given the rarity of the disorder and the uncertainties over treatments, it is advisable to concentrate the care for Kleine–Levin syndrome patients in centres with previous experience.

Insufficient Sleep Syndrome

Epidemiology

In the absence of formal prevalence studies, there is a clinical impression that adolescents are more susceptible, probably due to a combination of high sleep need and social pressure to delay the sleep phase.

Symptomatology

Insufficient sleep syndrome remains an important differential diagnostic possibility, especially in younger people with EDS [26,27]. However, habitual self-imposed sleep restriction can be difficult to recognise, especially in those long-sleeping subjects who constitutionally require more nocturnal sleep than average. Relative sleep deprivation is a likely possibility when there is a reported tendency to extend the sleep periods during weekends or vacations. If daytime sleepiness disappears when the sleep period is extended during holidays, for example, insufficient sleep is the most likely diagnosis. Chronic sleep deprivation associated with insufficient sleep may also result in other symptoms such as irritability, attention or concentration problems, restlessness or dysphoria. These symptoms may sometimes be more obvious than daytime sleepiness, potentially creating diagnostic confusion, especially in adolescents.

Diagnostics

When insufficient sleep syndrome is suspected, it can usually be confirmed using a patient-completed sleep diary completed over 2 weeks at least. However, it is highly recommended to measure the habitual sleep–wake cycle objectively using actigraphy for a similar period. ICSD-3 requires several criteria to be met: a daily complaint of hypersomnolence or, in the case of prepubertal children, behavioural abnormalities that are attributable to sleepiness; a sleep time that is shorter than expected for age, based on patient history, sleep logs or actigraphy; a curtailed sleep pattern that is present for at least 3 months; a need for alarm clocks; resolution of symptoms with sleep extension; and, finally, that symptoms are not better explained by another disorder.

Management

If insufficient sleep is diagnosed, patients should simply extend their time in bed gradually until symptoms resolve. Pharmacological wake-promoting treatment should be avoided and, if necessary, help from a behavioural sleep therapist obtained. It is often necessary to adjust a subject's mind-set towards an appropriate time of sleep length. Support with lifestyle changes in social or professional settings may be needed in order for the subject to adhere to the advised sleep times.

Key Points

- It is important to distinguish (excessive) daytime sleepiness from fatigue.
- A careful and directed clinical history is the most important diagnostic tool.
- Always bear in mind the possibility of insufficient sleep syndrome, especially in young people with EDS.
- Behavioural treatments are not to be overlooked, emphasising regular sleep/wake timing and, if possible, beneficial planned daytime naps.
- There should be a low threshold for medical treatment, given the disabling consequences of EDS in many patients.

References

1 Guilleminault C, Brooks SN. Excessive daytime sleepiness: a challenge for the practising neurologist. *Brain* 2001;124(Pt 8):1482–91.

2 American Academy of Sleep MedicineMedicine AAoS International Classification of Sleep Disorders, 3rd edn. Darien, IL: American Academy of Sleep Medicine, 2014.

3 Billiard M, Dauvilliers Y. Idiopathic hypersomnia. *Sleep Medicine Reviews* 2001;5(5):349–58.

4 Broughton R, Dunham W, Newman J, et al. Ambulatory 24 hour sleep-wake monitoring in narcolepsy-cataplexy compared to matched controls. *Electroencephalography and Clinical Neurophysiology* 1988;70(6):473–81.

5 Arnulf I, Rico TJ, Mignot E. Diagnosis, disease course, and management of patients with Kleine-Levin syndrome. *The Lancet Neurology* 2012;11(10):918–28.

6 Morgenthaler TI, Kapur VK, Brown T, et al. Practice parameters for the treatment of narcolepsy and other hypersomnias of central origin. *Sleep* 2007;30(12):1705–11.

7 Billiard M, Bassetti C, Dauvilliers Y, et al. EFNS guidelines on management of narcolepsy. *European Journal of Neurology* 2006;13(10):1035–48.

8 Mullington J, Broughton R. Scheduled naps in the management of daytime sleepiness in narcolepsy-cataplexy. *Sleep* 1993;16(5):444–56.

9 Szakacs Z, Dauvilliers Y, Mikhaylov V, et al. Safety and efficacy of pitolisant on cataplexy in patients with narcolepsy: a randomised, double-blind, placebo-controlled trial. *The Lancet Neurology* 2017;16(3):200–7.

10 Longstreth WT, Jr, Koepsell TD, Ton TG, et al. The epidemiology of narcolepsy. *Sleep* 2007;30(1):13–26.

11 Morrish E, King MA, Smith IE, Shneerson JM. Factors associated with a delay in the diagnosis of narcolepsy. *Sleep Medicine* 2004;5(1):37–41.

12 Rocca FL, Pizza F, Ricci E, Plazzi G. Narcolepsy during childhood: an update. *Neuropediatrics* 2015;46(3):181–98.

13 Kornum BR, Knudsen S, Ollila HM, et al. Narcolepsy. *Nature Reviews Disease Primers* 2017;3:16100.

14 Kok SW, Overeem S, Visscher TL, et al. Hypocretin deficiency in narcoleptic humans is associated with abdominal obesity. *Obesity Research* 2003;11(9):1147–54.

15 Fortuyn HA, Swinkels S, Buitelaar J, et al. High prevalence of eating disorders in narcolepsy with cataplexy: a case-control study. *Sleep* 2008;31(3):335–41.

16 Fortuyn HA, Lappenschaar MA, Furer JW, et al. Anxiety and mood disorders in narcolepsy: a case-control study. *General Hospospital Psychiatry* 2010;32(1):49–56.

17 Baumann CR, Mignot E, Lammers GJ, et al. Challenges in diagnosing narcolepsy without cataplexy: a consensus statement. *Sleep* 2014;37(6):1035–42.

18 Pillen S, Pizza F, Dhondt K, et al. Cataplexy and its mimics: clinical recognition and management. *Current Treatment Options in Neurology* 2017;19(6):23.

19 Overeem S, Lammers GJ, van Dijk JG. Weak with laughter. *Lancet* 1999;354(9181):838.

20 Mignot E, Lammers GJ, Ripley B, et al. The role of cerebrospinal fluid hypocretin measurement in the diagnosis of narcolepsy and other hypersomnias. *Archives of Neurology* 2002;59(10):1553–62.

21 Group TUSXMS. A randomized, double blind, placebo-controlled multicenter trial comparing the effects of three doses of orally administered sodium oxybate with placebo for the treatment of narcolepsy. *Sleep* 2002;25(1):42–9.

22 Bassetti C, Aldrich MS. Idiopathic hypersomnia. A series of 42 patients. *Brain* 1997;120(Pt 8):1423–35.

23 Habra O, Heinzer R, Haba-Rubio J, Rossetti AO. Prevalence and mimics of Kleine-Levin syndrome: a survey in French-speaking Switzerland. *Journal of Clinical Sleep Medicine* 2016;12(8):1083–7.

24 Lavault S, Golmard JL, Groos E, et al. Kleine-Levin syndrome in 120 patients: differential diagnosis and long episodes. *Annals of Neurology* 2015;77(3):529–40.

25 Leu-Semenescu S, Le Corvec T, Groos E, et al. Lithium therapy in Kleine-Levin syndrome: an open-label, controlled study in 130 patients. *Neurology* 2015;85(19):1655–62.

26 Dauvilliers Y. Differential diagnosis in hypersomnia. *Current Neurology and Neuroscience Reports* 2006;6(2):156–62.

27 Komada Y, Inoue Y, Hayashida K, et al. Clinical significance and correlates of behaviorally induced insufficient sleep syndrome. *Sleep Medicine* 2008;9(8):851–6.

9

Insomnia

Ingrid Verbeek and Angelique Pijpers

Centre for Sleep Medicine 'Kempenhaeghe', Heeze, The Netherlands

Introduction

In essence, insomnia can be defined as dissatisfaction with sleep quantity or quality resulting in daytime impairment, despite adequate opportunity and circumstances for sleep. Patients can present with difficulties initiating sleep, maintaining sleep, or early morning awakenings with an inability to return to sleep. These symptoms can occur together and often vary over time. Insomnia is considered a chronic condition when present for at least three times per week for a period of least 3 months. The sleep/wake difficulties should not be better explained by another (primary) sleep disorder [1]. The third edition of the International Classification of Sleep Disorders (ICSD-3) distinguishes three categories of insomnia: acute; chronic; and 'other'. Chronic insomnia disorder is the most relevant in practice, and will be the focus in this chapter. The diagnostic criteria for chronic insomnia are listed in Table 9.1 [1].

Insomnia should be considered a significant public health problem with a high prevalence. Indeed, about one third of adults report occasional sleep problems (transient insomnia symptoms) and approximately 6–10% meet the diagnostic criteria for insomnia disorder [2,3]. Insomnia has an important negative impact both on psychological well-being and quality of life. Moreover, insomnia is a risk factor for the development of major depression and, when associated with an objective sleep duration of less than 6 hours, is associated with serious health conditions [4,5].

Insomnia in Neurology

Insomnia often exists in conjunction with other medical or psychiatric disorders, including neurological diseases [6]. In practice, when insomnia is a prominent and/or persistent complaint, it is strongly advisable to consider a separate insomnia diagnosis and treat it accordingly. The main reason to do so is the typical reciprocal or bidirectional relationship between the sleep complaint and the comorbid condition

Sleep Disorders in Neurology: A Practical Approach, Second Edition.
Edited by Sebastiaan Overeem and Paul Reading.
© 2018 John Wiley & Sons Ltd. Published 2018 by John Wiley & Sons Ltd.

Table 9.1 ICSD-3 criteria for chronic insomnia disorder.

a) The patient reports, or the patient's parent or caregiver observes, one or more of the following:
   1) Difficulty initiating sleep.
   2) Difficulty maintaining sleep.
   3) Waking up earlier than desired.
   4) Resistance to going to bed on appropriate schedule.
   5) Difficulty sleeping without parent or caregiver intervention.

b) The patient reports, or the patient's parent or caregiver observes, one or more of the following related to the night-time sleep difficulty:
   1) Fatigue or malaise
   2) Attention, concentration, or memory impairment
   3) Impaired social, familial, occupational or academic performance
   4) Mood disturbance or irritability
   5) Daytime sleepiness
   6) Behavioural problems (e.g. hyperactivity, impulsivity, aggression)
   7) Reduced motivation, energy or initiative
   8) Proneness for errors or accidents
   9) Concerns about or dissatisfaction with sleep

c) The reported sleep–wake complaints cannot be explained purely by inadequate opportunity (i.e. enough time is allotted for sleep) or inadequate circumstances (i.e. the environment is safe, dark, quiet, and comfortable) for sleep

d) The sleep disturbance and associated daytime symptoms occur at least three times per week

e) The sleep disturbance and associated daytime symptoms have been present for at least 3 months

f) The sleep–wake difficulty is not better explained by another sleep disorder

(medical or psychological). As a consequence, if the sleep component is left untreated, it can adversely affect the co-morbid condition. Moreover, insomnia can persist when the co-morbid condition is adequately treated. Actively treating the insomnia disorder may therefore improve not only sleep quality but positively influence the co-morbid condition. Finally, possible direct consequences of insomnia such as mood disturbances, anxiety, increased pain perception may, in turn, also worsen insomnia [7–9].

Although no systematic reviews on the prevalence of insomnia disorder co-morbid with neurological disorders have been performed, it is safe to assume the numbers are high. For instance, prevalence rates of chronic insomnia of more than 50% have been reported in various diverse disorders including multiple sclerosis, stroke and traumatic brain injury [10–12].

Clinical Pathophysiology

The pathophysiology of chronic insomnia is not completely understood, but can be conceptualised in a clinically useful way using the '3-P' model of Spielman and Glovinsky [13]. This model describes how a relatively stable predisposition, combined with varying

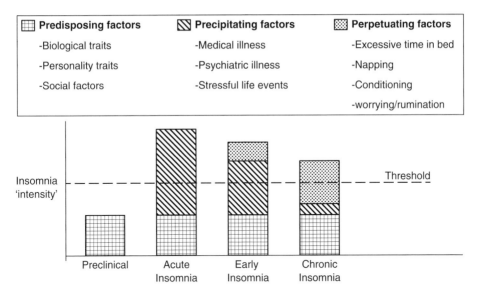

▦ **Predisposing factors**	◺ **Precipitating factors**	▨ **Perpetuating factors**
-Biological traits	-Medical illness	-Excessive time in bed
-Personality traits	-Psychiatric illness	-Napping
-Social factors	-Stressful life events	-Conditioning
		-worrying/rumination

Figure 9.1 The '3-P' model of insomnia. Predisposing, precipitating and perpetuating factors co-contribute to the development of chronic insomnia. *Source:* Adapted from Ref. [13].

precipitants and perpetuating factors interact in the development of chronic insomnia (Figure 9.1). Predisposing factors include (epi)genetic mechanisms [14], personality traits such as perfectionism and need for control, and social factors such as living in an unsafe or unsuitable environment. On this background, a medical or psychiatric illness or stressful life event may then lead to acute insomnia. Gradually, the influence of these precipitating factors reduces and perpetuating factors start to play a more dominant role. For example, to cope with the insomnia, patients may develop dysfunctional habits such as spending excessive time in bed or napping during the day. Moreover, negative conditioning and dysfunctional thinking towards sleep, the bed and the bedroom may develop. For example, worrying may lead to insomnia but, consequently, insomnia leads to more time to worry causing a patient to get trapped in a vicious circle of insomnia (Figure 9.2).

There are several other models explaining the development of insomnia. The neuro-cognitive model is an extension of the 3-P model and suggests that patients with insomnia suffer from an attenuation of normal so-called 'mesograde' amnesia of sleep because of increases in cortical arousal. According to the psychobiological inhibition model, however, chronic insomnia is less a hyperarousal disorder but characterised by the failure to inhibit wakefulness. The cage exchange model suggests that insomnia represents a hybrid state; one that is, from a neurobiological perspective, part wake and part sleep. Simultaneously, there are higher than normal levels of central nervous system activation and failure to inhibit processes normally associated with wakefulness.

Whatever model is used to conceptualise the underlying mechanisms, stress responses, attention bias, conditioning and altered neurobiology all play a role in promoting the trajectory from acute to chronic insomnia [15].

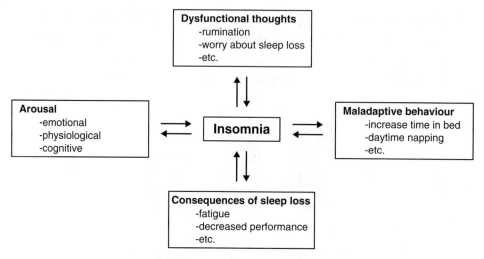

Figure 9.2 The vicious circle of chronic insomnia. *Source:* Adapted from Ref. [2].

Assessment of the Insomniac

History

As stated, insomnia complaints deserve an evaluation in their own right [15,16]. As a starting point, this encompasses a complete sleep history, including attention to the presence of other sleep disorders, such as sleep-related breathing disorders and restless legs syndrome (RLS). In case of sleep difficulties associated with other medical or psychiatric conditions, it is important to tease out how one influences the other. Other aspects of the interview are outlined in Table 9.2.

There can sometimes be 'mismatches' between the view of the patient and the healthcare professional regarding both the sleep complaint and its treatment. When evaluating a complaint of insomnia, it is important to realise that there is no solid definition of 'good' or 'poor' sleep, so the evaluation is largely based on an individual's subjective sleep experience. It is also important to note that sleep duration and sleep timing show sizeable inter-individual differences and vary considerably with age. Moreover, there is a significant night-to-night variability.

In general, average sleep onset latencies and periods of wakefulness after sleep onset lasting longer than 20–30 minutes are deemed clinically significant whereas waking at least 30 minutes prior to the desired rising time is considered an early morning awakening.

Patients often tend to emphasise any daytime symptoms over their night-time sleep difficulties [17]. In addition to those mentioned in the diagnostic criteria (Table 9.1), somatic symptoms such as gastro-intestinal complaints, general malaise and headaches can even be a presenting symptom of insomnia. Of importance, although daytime sleepiness can be reported, only a minority of insomniacs actually fall asleep during the day unintentionally.

Screening for psychopathology is important, because of the intricate relationship between insomnia and (new onset) psychiatric disorders, most notably depression, anxiety and substance misuse [18]. When the presence of a mood or anxiety disorder is suspected, referral to a psychologist or psychiatrist for further evaluation should be considered.

Table 9.2 The insomnia history.

Primary complaint
Onset; sudden or gradually, age, precipitating event(s)
Type; difficulties initiating sleep, maintaining sleep, early morning awakening, mixed
Course; severity, changing types
Frequency; every night, specific nights or circumstances, continuous or episodic, seasonal influence
Previous treatments and responses
Improving and exacerbating factors
Assess daytime consequences
Fatigue/sleepiness, mood/cognition, performance, quality of life
Pre-sleep conditions
Sleep environment
Lifestyle; social, occupational histories, exercise, travel
Current sleep–wake hygiene and attitude towards sleep
Sleep–wake schedule
Sleep onset latency, wake after sleep onset, total sleep time. Napping, weekday and weekend pattern. Preferably in a sleep–wake diary
Nocturnal symptoms of other sleep disorders
Sleep-related breathing disorders, movement disorders, parasomnias, etc.
Prior medical and psychiatric history
Specifically ask for treatments pain, discomfort, nocturia or other external factors that may interfere with sleep. Past and present life events
Screening for current psychopathology
Depression, anxiety disorder, chronic fatigue syndrome, attention deficit disorder, substance abuse, personality disorder
Intoxications
Alcohol, caffeine, smoking, drugs
Medications

Special attention should be given to the use of drugs and medications, as these can have a significant negative impact on sleep quality (see also Chapter 7). It is clear that alcohol is probably one of the most used substances for insomniacs to self-medicate. Alcohol can initially facilitate sleep onset but this effect is abolished after a few days. Importantly, alcohol disrupts normal sleep architecture and reduces sleep stability in the second half of the night [19].

As many people receive informal advice from people around them, it is very useful to explore what patients have already tried themselves to conquer their sleep difficulties. Typical techniques include medication, herbal cures, and behavioural adjustments. Documentation of the effects such interventions have had, if any, combined with the expectations of the patient should be made.

The sleep diary

Besides the history, the most valuable tool for the assessment of sleep is the sleep diary, in which subjective sleep is tracked during several nights (see for example http:// yoursleep.aasmnet.org/pdf/sleepdiary.pdf). A diary gives a very useful overview of the overall sleep pattern, including aspects such as sleep–wake scheduling, time spent in bed, work-to-weekend differences, as well as subjective sleep latencies and duration. Activities before bedtime, alcohol, caffeine and medication use can also be tracked. It is important to instruct the patient to fill the log retrospectively in the morning, based on subjective estimations and to avoid becoming obsessed with clock watching.

One can use several questionnaires to assess insomnia severity and sleep quality. For example, the Insomnia Severity Index and the Pittsburgh Sleep Quality Index [20,21] may be useful to evaluate the past 2–4 weeks for sleep difficulties, the interference with daytime function as well as the degree of concern about the insomnia.

Polysomnography

Polysomnography is not needed to diagnose insomnia disorder. However, it can be useful in selected patients to identify other sleep disorders if they are suspected to be related to the insomnia complaints. In addition, when sleep state misperception is suspected, polysomnography can be used to show the mismatch between self-perceived and recorded total sleep time. This helps to reassure the patient that some sleep is obtained and explains the mechanism how repeated awakenings can lead to the sensation of continued wakefulness.

Management of Insomnia

As stated, even when insomnia appears in the context of another (co-morbid) disorder, it should typically be treated on its own. Cognitive behavioural therapy for insomnia (CBTi), benzodiazepine receptor agonists and non-benzodiazepine 'z' drugs are all supported by best empirical evidence [15,22]. Most experts currently agree that CBTi is the evidence-based first-choice treatment for chronic insomnia.

Non-pharmacological Therapies for Chronic Insomnia Disorder

Although probably more time consuming than pharmacotherapy, CBTi can produce sleep improvements that are sustained over time. Moreover, the therapy is appropriate and accepted even in the presence of co-morbid neurological conditions [23–25]. Meta-analyses [26,27] and systematic reviews [28–30] show that CBTi has moderate to large effects for sleep onset latency (range 0.41–1.05) and sleep quality (0.94–1.14), and small to moderate effects for total sleep time and the number and duration of awakenings. Importantly, 70–80% of patients achieve a therapeutic response, and about 40% even achieve clinical remission [31].

CBTi is a brief, sleep-focused, multimodal intervention, encompassing 4–6 weekly or biweekly sessions [28–31]. The pillars of treatment are:

- Monitoring of subjective sleep.
- Psycho-education about sleep including the changes of sleep during the life span, the development of chronic insomnia, the vicious circle of insomnia and basic sleep hygiene principles.
- Behavioural techniques (sleep restriction and stimulus control) to change dysfunctional sleep habits, and reverse negative-conditioning.

- Relaxation strategies and exercises, not only just before sleep, but during the waking day.
- Changing dysfunctional beliefs and attitudes about sleep.

CBTi starts with psycho-education about sleep, and the rationale of common and well-known sleep hygiene advises (Table 9.3). The goal is to create optimal circumstances for sleep and to set a realistic goal for treatment. It is often surprising for patients to learn that not all of us need 8 hours of sleep. Looking at sleep in the context of the 24-hour period is also new to most patients.

The goal of sleep restriction is to temporary reduce bedtime in order to enhance sleep [32]. The time spent in bed is typically shortened to the subjective total sleep time currently reported, though never below 5 hours. Time in bed is gradually increased when sleep efficiency rises above 80–85%. It is important to guide the patient how to cope with fatigue in the first week and how to fill the extra time. Sleep restriction should be used cautiously in patients who are prone to seizures or bipolar disorder, as well as occupational drivers or people with potentially hazardous occupations.

Stimulus control aims to strengthen the association between the bed and sleep [33]. Patients are instructed to go to bed only when feeling sleepy, to get out of bed when unable to sleep after 15–30 minutes, and repeat these steps as often as needed. It is also important to get out of bed at the same time each morning, irrespective of the amount of time slept. Both sleep restriction and stimulus control are very powerful in decreasing sleep onset latency and the amount of wake after sleep onset. At first, total sleep time may decrease, but in the second half of the therapeutic process it usually increases.

Relaxation techniques are also taught to the patient. Subsequently, the focus of therapy shifts towards identifying dysfunctional beliefs and attitudes towards sleep and to confront and challenge their validity and replace them with more adaptive and rational substitutes (cognitive restructuring). Finally, patients are made aware of the changes that are happening allowing evaluation of whether the goals are achieved. Importantly, strategies are discussed to deal with relapses.

Edinger et al. performed an elegant 'dose response' study on the effect of CBTi [34], in which both the patient and therapist were initially blinded for the number of treatment sessions. The data showed that psycho-education about sleep and sleep hygiene advice can, by itself, have a significant impact. Physicians could therefore consider starting with these aspects of therapy (Table 9.3) and evaluate the response, before referring for full CBTi.

CBTi can be delivered in several ways, varying from self-help approaches, online therapy, group therapy or individual therapy. Unfortunately, CBTi is time consuming and not readily available in all clinical settings. However, before converting to pharmacological therapy for insomnia complaints, it would be wise to consider referral to a sleep centre that has experienced CBTi therapists available. Although we feel that patients with neurological disorders can also benefit from online or group therapy, the underlying condition may make individual CBTi sometimes more advisable.

Several other, less well established, non-pharmacological treatment approaches have been advocated for insomnia, including acceptance-based therapy (ACT) and mindfulness [35] or the appliance of bright light therapy in the morning in the case of sleep-onset insomnia, or late afternoon in the setting of early morning awakenings.

Table 9.3 Tips, strategies and psycho-education to improve sleep hygiene.

The following instructions can be discussed with and given to the patient

Before bedtime

- *Take time for a break during the day.* If we are hyper aroused the whole day we cannot expect to just push our 'off' button and soundly go to sleep
- *Relax before going to sleep, taking time to wind down.* This can be very personal and achieved in many ways (going for a walk, taking a shower or bath, watching TV, having a conversation). Avoid strenuous exercise in the last 4–6 hours before bedtime
- *Electronic devices.* It is recommended to turn off all electronic devices 'with a screen' at least 30 minutes before bedtime, due to emittance of blue light and possible (hyper)arousal
- *Take a power nap during the day.* A power nap with a maximum duration of 30 minutes outside the bed before 15:00 may be helpful, unless it worsens sleep difficulties during the night
- *Prevent worrying in bed.* Take time for a 'worry moment' during the day or early evening to prevent worrying in bed
- *Avoid caffeine except in the morning.* Caffeine stimulates our brain and therefore interferes with sleep. It can be used to reduce tiredness in the morning. When having trouble falling asleep limit the daily intake of coffee and caffeinated beverages. It can also be present in (dark) chocolate and some medications
- *Nicotine.* This also stimulates our brain. When quitting smoking, due to withdrawal, sleep can initially become worse
- *Reduce the amount of alcohol and avoid it within 4–6 hours of bedtime.* Alcohol might temporarily help you fall asleep faster at first, but it also causes frequent awakenings during the night and potential nightmares
- *Food.* Limit eating close to bedtime to a light snack and avoid upsetting your stomach

In bed

- *Create a good sleeping environment.* A comfortable bed in a dark, quiet room, with a comfortable temperature
- *Try to keep a regular sleep schedule, even on the weekend or during holidays.* Irregular sleep–wake schedules offset the biological clock. Especially rising time gives a clear signal to our biological clock
- *Reduce time in bed to a maximum of 8 hours.* Average sleep time is about 7–8 hours. It takes time to fall asleep and it is normal to have a few awakenings during the night. When you are a biological short sleeper, 8 hours can be too long.
- *Reserve the bed for sleeping, having sex or recovering from illness.* Sleep is a behaviour which can be 'unlearned' when there are too many waking activities in bed. Only go to bed when sleepy and get up when you are restless and cannot fall asleep within 20–30 minutes (depending on age). Go to another room and relax. Go back to bed when sleepy.
- *Try to distract yourself from worrying.* Individuals who remain more cognitively aroused in the pre-sleep period experience more sleep difficulties than those who are able to control their pre-sleep arousal (listen to music, reading, focus on pleasant thoughts).
- *Do not watch the time.* Excessive arousal alters time estimation, which in turn affects the perception of sleep–wakefulness. Wake time will be overestimated when looking at the clock all the time.

In the morning

- *Start the day with sufficient light.* Bright light in the morning helps to establish a regular sleep rhythm and is a clear 'timing messenger' for our biological clock.

Pharmacotherapy for Chronic Insomnia Disorder

When CBTi is not available or ineffective, pharmacological treatment for insomnia could be considered [36]. Importantly, pharmacological treatment for insomnia should be tailored to the patients' needs and presence of co-morbid conditions, together with treatment of any underlying disorder(s) and optimal sleep–wake hygiene. We recommend using an explicit shared decision-making approach when considering pharmacological treatment for insomnia. Expectations, benefits, risks and costs should be thoroughly discussed before initiating therapy. A detailed description of the available pharmacological options is provided in Chapter 5.

Although (non) benzodiazepine receptor agonists are clinically proven to be effective for chronic insomnia, there are clear drawbacks for prescribing such medications over prolonged periods of time, especially in the presence of co-morbid neurological conditions. These include impaired daytime functioning (sedation, sleepiness, cognitive impairment), suppressed ventilation during sleep, increased risk of falls, tolerance, dependence, addiction and rebound insomnia with discontinuation.

To date, supporting evidence for other pharmacological treatments of chronic insomnia in patients with neurological disorders remains scarce and of limited methodological quality. Depending on the country, these agents might be specifically approved to treat insomnia, or regarded as off-label use. Examples include melatonin receptor agonists, selective histamine H1 receptor antagonists (e.g. doxepin, one of few agents indicated for sleep maintenance difficulties), sedating antidepressants (e.g. amitriptyline or mirtazapine, even though these may potentially worsen RLS), antipsychotics (e.g. quetiapine, risperidone, in the absence of known risk–benefit profile), anticonvulsants (gabapentin and pregabalin, anecdotally effective in our personal experience), and the new hypocretin receptor antagonists (e.g. suvorexant, currently not widely available).

In some patients, a useful strategy is to start with pharmacological treatment and CBTi simultaneously, tapering the medication when behavioural therapy has commenced [31].

Key Points

- Insomnia frequently occurs together with neurological disorders.
- If insomnia is present, ideally, it should be assessed and treated separately.
- Recognition of insomnia is important as effective treatment options are available which improve quality of life.
- Best first-line treatment for insomnia is generally considered to be cognitive behavioural therapy.
- Often, psycho-education about sleep and advice regarding sleep hygiene can make a useful impact.

References

1 American Academy of Sleep Medicine, International Classification of Sleep Disorders, 3rd edn. Darien, IL: American Academy of Sleep Medicine, 2004.

2 Morin, C.M., Insomnia: Psychological Assessment and Management. New York, NY: Guilford Press, 1993.

3 Roth, T., Jaeger, S., Jin, R., et al., Sleep problems, comorbid mental disorders, and role functioning in the national comorbidity survey replication. *Biol Psychiatry*, 2006. 60(12): 1364–71.

4 Riemann, D., Baglioni, C., Spiegelhalder, K., [Lack of sleep and insomnia. Impact on somatic and mental health]. *Bundesgesundheitsblatt Gesundheitsforschung Gesundheitsschutz*, 2011. 54(12): 1296–302.

5 Baglioni, C., Battagliese, G., Feige, B., et al., Insomnia as a predictor of depression: a meta-analytic evaluation of longitudinal epidemiological studies. *J Affect Disord*, 2011. 135(1–3): 10–19.

6 Morin, C.M., Benca, R., Chronic insomnia. *Lancet*, 2012. 379(9821): 1129–41.

7 Amtmann, D., Askew, R.L., Kim, J., et al., Pain affects depression through anxiety, fatigue, and sleep in multiple sclerosis. *Rehabil Psychol*, 2015. 60(1): 81–90.

8 Naylor, C., Parsonage, M., McDaid, D., et al. Long-term conditions and mental health. The cost of co-morbidities. King's Fund and Centre for Mental Health, 2012.

9 Smith, M.T.,Haythornthwaite, J.A., How do sleep disturbance and chronic pain inter-relate? Insights from the longitudinal and cognitive-behavioral clinical trials literature. *Sleep Med Rev*, 2004. 8(2): 119–32.

10 Viana, P., Rodrigues, P., Fernandes, C., et al., InMS: Chronic insomnia disorder in multiple sclerosis – a Portuguese multicentre study on prevalence, subtypes, associated factors and impact on quality of life. *Mul Scler Relat Disord*, 2013. 4(5): 477–83.

11 Hermann, D.M., Bassetti, C.L., Role of sleep-disordered breathing and sleep-wake disturbances for stroke and stroke recovery. *Neurology*, 2016. 87(13): 1407–16.

12 Baumann, C.R., Sleep and Traumatic Brain Injury. *Sleep Medicine Clinics* 2016. 11(1): 19–23.

13 Spielman, A.J., Glovinsky, P., The varied nature of insomnia, in Case Studies in Insomnia, P.J. Hauri (ed.). New York: Plenum Press, 1991, pp. 1–15.

14 Palagini, L., Biber, K., Riemann, D., The genetics of insomnia – evidence for epigenetic mechanisms? *Sleep Med Rev*, 2014. 18(3): 225–35.

15 Schutte-Rodin, S., Broch, L., Buysse, D., et al., Clinical guideline for the evaluation and management of chronic insomnia in adults. *J Clin Sleep Med*, 2008. 4(5): 487–504.

16 Leibowitz, S., Batson, A., Difficulty falling or staying asleep. *Sleep Medicine Clinics* 2014. 9(4): 463–79.

17 Araujo, T., Jarrin, D.C., Leanza, Y., et al., Qualitative studies of insomnia: Current state of knowledge in the field. *Sleep Med Rev*, 2017. 31: 58–69.

18 Breslau, N., Roth, T., Rosenthal, L., et al., Sleep disturbance and psychiatric disorders: a longitudinal epidemiological study of young adults. *Biol Psychiatry*, 1996. 39(6): 411–8.

19 Roehrs, T., Roth, T., Sleep, sleepiness, sleep disorders and alcohol use and abuse. *Sleep Med Rev*, 2001. 5(4): 287–97.

20 Morin, C.M., Belleville G., Bélanger, L., et al., The Insomnia Severity Index: psychometric indicators to detect insomnia cases and evaluate treatment response. *Sleep*, 2011. 34(5): 601–8.

21 Buysse, D.J., Reynolds, C.F., 3rd, Monk, T.H., et al., The Pittsburgh Sleep Quality Index: a new instrument for psychiatric practice and research. *Psychiatry Res*, 1989. 28(2): 193–213.

22 Mayer, G., Jennum, P., Riemann, D., Dauvilliers,Y., Insomnia in central neurologic diseases – occurrence and management. *Sleep Med Rev*, 2011. 15(6): 369–78.

23 Clancy, M., Drerup, M., Sullivan, A.B., Outcomes of cognitive-behavioral treatment for insomnia on insomnia, depression, and fatigue for individuals with multiple sclerosis: a case series. *Int J MS Care*, 2015. 17(6):261–7.

24 Ouellet, M.C., Morin, C.M., Efficacy of cognitive-behavioral therapy for insomnia associated with traumatic brain injury: A single-case experimental design. *Arch Phys Med Rehabil*, 2007. 88(12): 1581–92.

25 Geiger-Brown, J.M., Rogers, V.E., Liu, W., et al., Cognitive behavioral therapy in persons with comorbid insomnia: A meta-analysis. *Sleep Med Rev*, 2015. 23: 54–67.

26 Morin, C.M., Culbert, J.P., Schwartz, S.M., Nonpharmacological interventions for insomnia: a meta-analysis of treatment efficacy. *Am J Psychiatry*, 1994. 151(8): 1172–80.

27 Murtagh, D.R., Greenwood, K.M., Identifying effective psychological treatments for insomnia: a meta-analysis. *J Consult Clin Psychol*, 1995. 63(1): 79–89.

28 Morin, C.M., Bootzin, R.R., Buysse, D.J., et al., Psychological and behavioral treatment of insomnia: update of the recent evidence (1998–2004). *Sleep*, 2006. 29(11): 1398–414.

29 Morgenthaler, T., Kramer, M., ALessi, C., et al., Practice parameters for the psychological and behavioral treatment of insomnia: an update. An american academy of sleep medicine report. *Sleep*, 2006. 29(11): 1415–9.

30 Riemann, D.., Perlis, M.L., The treatments of chronic insomnia: a review of benzodiazepine receptor agonists and psychological and behavioral therapies. *Sleep Med Rev*, 2009. 13(3): 205–14.

31 Morin, C.M., Vallières, A., Guay, B., et al., Cognitive behavioral therapy, singly and combined with medication, for persistent insomnia: a randomized controlled trial. *JAMA*, 2009. 301(19): 2005–15.

32 Spielman, A.J., Saskin, P., Thorpy, M.J., Treatment of chronic insomnia by restriction of time in bed. *Sleep*, 1987. 10(1): 45–56.

33 Riedel, B., Lichstein, K., Peterson, B.A., et al., A comparison of the efficacy of stimulus control for medicated and unmedicated insomniacs. *Behav Modif*, 1998. 22(1): 3–28.

34 Edinger, J.D., Wohlgemuth, W.K., Radtke, R.A., et al., Dose-response effects of cognitive-behavioral insomnia therapy: a randomized clinical trial. *Sleep*, 2007. 30(2): 203–12.

35 Ong, J.C., Manber, R., Segal, Z., et al., A randomized controlled trial of mindfulness meditation for chronic insomnia. *Sleep*, 2014. 37(9): 1553–63.

36 Riemann, D., Baglioni, C., Bassetti, C., et al., European guideline for the diagnosis and treatment of insomnia. *J Sleep Res*, 2017. 26(6): 675–700.

10

Sleep-related Breathing Disorders

Timothy G. Quinnell

Respiratory Support and Sleep Centre, Royal Papworth Hospital, Cambridgeshire, UK

Sleep-disordered Breathing

Sleep-disordered breathing (SDB) generally refers to two separate but occasionally related entities, namely, obstructive and central sleep apnoea (OSA and CSA, respectively). Both can cause debilitating symptoms with reduced alertness and excessive daytime sleepiness (EDS) as the most recognised consequences. The impairments in quality of life and daytime functioning are the main reason for therapeutic intervention. The strong association of SDB with cardiovascular disease and diabetes adds to its clinical importance, although the complexities of these relationships are still being explored.

Hypoventilation during sleep complicates many respiratory and neurological disorders, potentially leading to life-threatening ventilatory failure. While it can overlap with both OSA and CSA, its investigation and management are complex and beyond the scope of this chapter (see Chapter 17).

Obstructive Sleep Apnoea

Definition and Pathophysiology

OSA is defined by repeated pauses in breathing (apnoeas) due to upper airway occlusion, usually in the oropharynx. It is precipitated by sleep-related muscle relaxation and positional changes which alter airway dimensions and increase collapsibility. Furthermore, the normal protective reflex increase in upper airway dilator muscle activity during inspiration fails in OSA, resulting in intermittent pharyngeal collapse. If occlusion is partial then airflow is only diminished, causing so-called 'hypopnoeas'. Respiratory events are often associated with oxygen desaturation but, arguably, the increased work of breathing is probably the main arousal mechanism that disturbs sleep continuity. With arousal there is sympathetic activation and a return of pharyngeal dilator activity, so that airflow improves and sleep usually resumes. When sleep disruption from frequent nocturnal arousals leads to EDS then OSA syndrome (OSAS) is said to exist (Figures 10.1–10.3) [1].

Sleep Disorders in Neurology: A Practical Approach, Second Edition.
Edited by Sebastiaan Overeem and Paul Reading.
© 2018 John Wiley & Sons Ltd. Published 2018 by John Wiley & Sons Ltd.

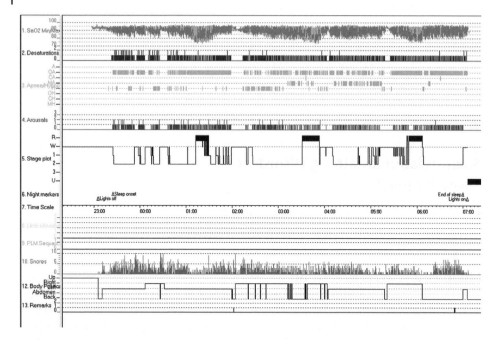

Figure 10.1 Polysomnogram overview showing severe obstructive sleep apnoea. Note: Respiratory events are associated with microarousals and oxygen desaturations. Sleep is fragmented and there are frequent body position changes.

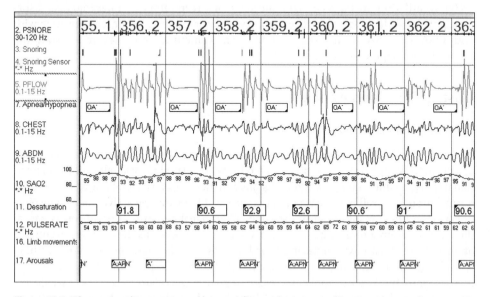

Figure 10.2 Obstructive sleep apnoeas. Absent airflow with attenuated but ongoing respiratory movement indicating continuing effort.

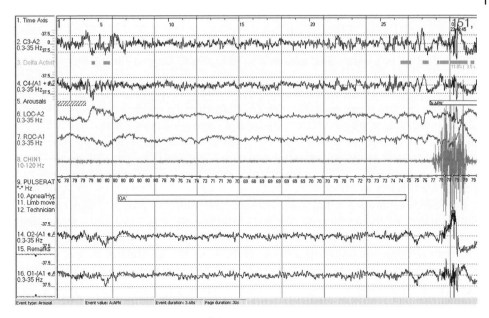

Figure 10.3 Microarousal at termination of obstructive apnoea.

Epidemiology and Risk Factors

OSAS affects 2–7% of the adult population [2] with males approximately twice as likely to develop the condition [3,4]. It is common in middle age [3] and prevalence may increase further with increasing age [5]. Obesity is a major risk factor for OSAS, particularly when distributed around the neck and upper body [6,7]. Causality is supported by longitudinal evidence of fluctuating disease severity in association with weight change [4,8]. Other lifestyle risk factors include smoking and alcohol use. Medical conditions having a probable causal association through physical craniofacial effects include hypothyroidism, polycystic ovary syndrome and acromegaly. Congenital syndromes including Down's, Marfan's and Turner's are also strongly associated [2,6].

Consequences of OSA

OSA is causally linked with hypertension [9]. There is a 2.5-fold associated increase in cardiovascular risk [10] with a reported 6% increase in stroke risk per unit increase in Apnoea–Hypopnoea Index (AHI/hour) [11]. This association has biologically plausible mechanisms which include hypertension, oxidative stress linked to oxygen desaturation and sympathetic overdrive. The beneficial cardiovascular effects of OSA treatment have been well described [12]. However confounding factors such as coexistent metabolic syndrome mean that causation and the impact of OSA treatment on cardiovascular disease are still being explored. Other effects of OSAS include a two to three times higher road traffic accident risk [13], such that it is notifiable to the driving authorities in most countries. Health-related quality of life (HRQoL) is impaired [14], while healthcare usage is almost doubled in OSAS [15].

Diagnosis

Clinical Features

Figure 10.4 gives a schematic overview of the diagnostic and therapeutic pathway. Although sleep studies are required to diagnose OSA, whether to perform them depends on the index of clinical suspicion. The evaluation of EDS requires focused history taking but can be supported by questionnaires. The ubiquitous Epworth Sleepiness Scale (ESS) [16] is susceptible to placebo effects, misinterpretation and manipulation but is helpful in monitoring real-life response to OSAS treatment. Although daytime sleepiness can also be objectively measured with electroencephalography (EEG)-based nap tests, these are more useful in non-respiratory sleepiness disorders [17] and have limited utility in OSAS (see Chapter 3).

Excessive sleepiness is often not the main presenting symptom in OSAS as many individuals come to attention due to nocturnal choking or simply finding sleep unrefreshing. Less specific symptoms include morning headaches, nocturia, reduced libido, emotional lability, and impaired memory and concentration. The bed partner, if available, is a key historian and often the main driver for seeking medical help, with snoring, apnoeas and other nocturnal OSA effects causing anxiety and sleep disruption. Sometimes OSA comes to medical attention when patients either have an accident or declining performance at work leads to occupational health referral. Not infrequently it

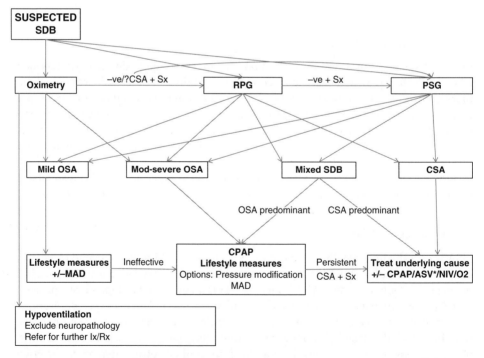

Figure 10.4 Diagnostic and treatment pathway for sleep-disordered breathing. ASV, adaptive servo ventilation (*contraindicated in left ventricular systolic failure); CPAP, continuous positive airway pressure; CSA, central sleep apnoea; MAD, mandibular advancement device; NIV, non-invasive ventilation; OSA, obstructive sleep apnoea; O2, oxygen; PSG, polysomnography; RPG, respiratory polygraphy; SDB, sleep-disordered breathing; Sx, symptoms; −ve, negative result.

is observed during unrelated hospital stays. Occasionally severe OSA, in association with nocturnal hypoventilation, presents with ventilatory failure.

Physical examination is not always discriminatory for OSA but elevated body mass index (BMI) with central obesity involving neck and upper body is typical. Oropharyngeal crowding is also seen but more extensive evaluation of physical features, including oropharyngeal scoring tools, does not usefully improve diagnostic precision. In the author's opinion the prevalence and treatability of OSAS, and the simplicity of basic sleep studies, mean there should be a low threshold for investigating anyone with suggestive symptoms.

Sleep Studies

There are several levels of OSA investigation, spanning a range of complexity and cost. Nocturnal pulse oximetry is a useful first line test given it is portable, user-friendly and most commonly used in patients' homes without supervision. It provides an hourly oxygen desaturation index (ODI/hour; ≥4% index most used) as a surrogate marker of important respiratory events. Other relevant parameters include mean and minimum oxygen saturation, and percentage of time spent below 90%. Although oxygen desaturations are key to confirming or excluding OSA and gauging severity, the other values can alert to coexistent nocturnal hypoventilation, for example due to obesity, lung disease, or a neuromuscular disorder, which may require further investigation and influence management.

The key pitfall of oximetry is its variable sensitivity and specificity [18]. Factors affecting this include patient physiology, duration and nature of obstructive events, and sleep stage. Precision varies between oximeters, partly due to differences in device set-up. Optimal sampling frequency and signal averaging balance sensitivity and artifact control. Although different oximeters with similar settings may still give discordant results, clinically important differences are less likely and severe disease is rarely missed. It is important to remember that abnormal oximetry does not always mean an obstructive aetiology. The pattern of desaturation can help distinguish OSA, CSA and hypoventilation but this is more discriminatory if done in conjunction with clinical features. Even then, oximetry analysis is still something of an art and best undertaken by experienced practitioners, as with more complex investigations.

A trial of treatment may help clarify the nature of hypoxic dips, but CSA and hypoventilation sometimes also respond to OSA therapy. Although the immediate clinical outcome can be positive, misdiagnosis means that underlying diseases could be overlooked, with potentially serious consequences. False negative oximetry is also not uncommon. This is more likely to occur when respiratory events are associated with only minor or no oxygen desaturation, due to arousal occurring before frank hypoxia develops. If there is uncertainty as to the nature of nocturnal hypoxia and/or symptoms are compelling for SDB but oximetry is negative, more sophisticated sleep studies should be performed.

Respiratory polygraphy (RPG) and full polysomnography (PSG) provide an apnoea-hypopnoea index (AHI/hour). Pulse oximetry is combined with oronasal temperature and pressure monitors that measure airflow together with thoracic and abdominal movement gauges marking respiratory effort. Resulting breath by breath analysis helps distinguish obstructive from central SDB. Full PSG incorporates limited EEG, electro-oculography (EOG) and submentalis electromyography (EMG), which allow precise scoring and staging of wake, sleep and micro-arousals.

The AHI is considered a more sensitive and specific index of SDB. The American Academy of Sleep Medicine (AASM) arbitrarily defines mild OSA as an AHI of 5–15 events per hour; moderate OSA as 15–30 events per hour; and severe OSA as an AHI of greater than 30 events per hour [19]. Respiratory events must last at least 10 seconds and apnoeas involve complete cessation of airflow. Hypopnoeas are variously defined by different classification systems. Common is a degree of airflow amplitude reduction, which must be accompanied by either significant oxygen desaturation or EEG micro-arousals on PSG. Both types of events are characterised by evidence of continuing respiratory effort from the thoracic and abdominal bands. The multiple scoring systems for hypopnoea introduce heterogeneity into what is otherwise a relatively precise index. They can give a significantly different AHI for the same individual, sometimes large enough to influence clinical management. Until a single standardised hypopnoea definition is established, it is important to factor in these potential discrepancies when interpreting sleep studies from other units [20].

Respiratory polygraphy is sometimes used as the entry-level investigation but can also miss significant OSA. Again, this is more common if an arousal prevents frank hypoxia, as desaturation is required to score hypopnoea in the absence of EEG recording. Another caveat is automated computer scoring (ACS) which should not be relied on in isolation. Despite inter-scorer variability, manual scoring is considered by most to be the gold standard and variability is manageable with training and audit [21].

Overdiagnosis or overestimation of the severity of OSA is of less concern than the erroneous exclusion of clinically significant SDB. Treatments for OSA can be intrusive but adverse effects are rarely severe. Early review after starting treatment should identify ineffective intervention, triggering diagnostic review. Ideally, however, PSG should be available when there is diagnostic uncertainty.

Management

Treatment choice depends on sleep study findings, symptom severity, and patient preference, and usually requires specialist input. Definitive intervention should not exclude lifestyle modification, with its wider potential benefits. Although the extent of EDS in OSAS varies greatly, only moderately correlating with the AHI, it remains the main treatment indication given uncertainty over the impact OSA control has on cardiovascular endpoints. Therefore, OSAS is alternatively classified according to EDS severity and treatment effects are measured by symptom response as much as sleep study results.

Lifestyle Measures

Weight reduction can improve OSA to the extent that other treatment can be deferred or discontinued. Sleep hygiene advice, smoking cessation, alcohol reduction and position management in supine preponderant OSA may be sufficient. Lifestyle measures are useful across the disease spectrum but are particularly relevant in milder OSAS, where other interventions may be inappropriate or poorly tolerated [22].

Continuous Positive Airway Pressure therapy

Continuous positive airway pressure (CPAP) therapy is the cornerstone of OSAS treatment. It is applied using a nasal or face mask, connected via tubing to an electric pump. The resulting pneumatic splint prevents pharyngeal collapse.

CPAP greatly reduces obstructive respiratory events and improves daytime sleepiness, cognitive function and quality of life. There are proven beneficial effects on blood pressure and possible secondary improvements in other cardiovascular endpoints [12,14,22]. CPAP therapy also improves driving simulator performance and road traffic accident risk [23]. The clinical and cost effectiveness of CPAP in moderate to severe OSAS is reflected in clinical guidelines recommending it as first-line treatment [14,22].

Traditionally CPAP pressure settings have been determined using attended inpatient sleep studies. Predictive formulae, incorporating OSA and patient parameters are a simpler but less precise outpatient alternative. Auto-titrating CPAP (auto-CPAP) is increasingly popular as a means of determining pressure requirements without hospital admission. It tracks patients' breathing, adjusting pressure to control apnoeas while minimising pressure delivery to optimise tolerance. Although auto-CPAP can be used long term, it is usually more economical to use titration periods to guide subsequent fixed CPAP prescription.

The intrusive nature of CPAP can undermine its effectiveness. Not everyone accepts treatment and published adherence figures range from around 29 to 85% [24]. Masks continue to be refined and developed in attempts to improve CPAP tolerance. Other innovations include pressure modification using so-called 'bi-level' devices, auto-CPAP or expiratory pressure relief as well as circuit humidification. Although helpful in overcoming an individual's CPAP intolerance, none of these reliably improve adherence [25]. In the author's opinion it would seem reasonable to start with standard fixed CPAP and mask, with recourse to more sophisticated solutions if needed.

As important to optimising adherence is patient education and support, especially early in treatment. Various structured approaches continue to be tried, but techniques are diverse and the quality of evidence is too low to guide patient selection or choice of intervention [24]. Unfortunately, while CPAP implementation without support may succeed in many patients with OSAS and is rewarding to patients and clinicians alike, a significant proportion will fail on treatment without appropriate back-up.

The role of CPAP in the management of mild OSAS is less clear-cut. Clinical and cost effectiveness are more marginal [14] and compliance may be worse. Guidelines recommend CPAP be tried when significant symptoms fail to respond to lifestyle measures 'and any other relevant treatment options' [22]. In practice the different means of grading OSAS severity should allow flexibility such that if a patient with mild OSA is significantly sleepy, a CPAP trial can be justified. It is important to initiate CPAP well and support closely, while considering other factors that might be responsible for a patients' symptoms. A failed trial of CPAP should represent a step in a diagnostic and therapeutic process rather than simply treatment failure.

Mandibular Advancement Devices

Mandibular advancement devices (MADs) offer an alternative to CPAP. Worn intra-orally, they hold the mandible and tongue forward to maintain upper airway patency. Although MADs do not perform as well as CPAP objectively, both treatments improve subjective sleepiness and other health outcomes similarly, possibly due to better MAD tolerance [14]. Numerous types are available, covering a range of sophistication and cost in terms of device design and provision. Titratable MADs with specialist dental input are increasingly favoured but their superiority remains unproven, and simpler devices may work just as well for many patients.

Factors which may favour a MAD include milder, supine preponderant OSA and lower BMI. It is important to check that the patient is able to open their mouth sufficiently to accommodate a MAD and that there is some degree of jaw protrusion possible. Gums and teeth must be healthy and dentition needs to be adequate. If there are any concerns about oral health or marginal dentition but a MAD is the preferred option, then referral to a dentist with OSA expertise should be considered as a bespoke device may still be possible.

With existing evidence, CPAP is the first option in moderate to severe OSAS, defined by sleep study indices and/or degree of EDS. With milder OSA, conservative measures may be all that is necessary or acceptable. Mandibular devices potentially bridge the gap with a role in mildly symptomatic OSA but also more severe disease according to patient preference. In cases where fitness to drive is of concern, the usual clinician preference is for CPAP although a MAD need not be ruled out [14].

Other Treatments

Various surgical techniques have been developed to try to treat OSAS. Most aim to prevent pharyngeal occlusion by increasing upper airway dimensions or reducing collapsibility. Although several short-term studies have been reported, diverse techniques, inconsistent effects and a lack of longer term data mean that conclusive evidence of effectiveness is still lacking [26]. Hypoglossal nerve stimulation is a novel treatment which may have a role in selected patients with moderate to severe OSA when other treatments have failed. Upper airway dilator muscles (primarily the genioglossus) are activated by an implanted electrical stimulator. Evidence of effectiveness is accumulating but device specific [27], and access to this treatment is currently limited. Tracheostomy is highly effective as an extreme treatment but complications and side effects make it controversial.

Pharmacotherapy continues to be explored in OSAS. Several drugs have been investigated, attempting to exploit various pharmacological mechanisms to reduce respiratory events and/or improve symptoms. Despite some positive results from individual trials, effectiveness is unproven [28].

Central Sleep Apnoea

CSA is a term that covers a group of disorders that involve repeated, sometimes cyclical, central apnoeas and hypopnoeas. Pathophysiology of CSA is complex and aetiologies are diverse but a common thread is temporary loss or diminution of central respiratory effort. CSA is probably more common than realised and may be asymptomatic since, unlike with OSA, apnoea termination does not always produce an arousal from sleep. However, awareness of CSA is important because it is another cause of repetitive oxygen desaturations, potentially causing symptoms itself and possibly reflecting significant underlying cardiovascular, neurological or renal disease.

The categories of pathological CSA seen in adults include: Cheyne–Stokes Breathing CSA (CSB-CSA); CSA due to medical conditions excluding Cheyne–Stokes; drug-induced CSA; and primary idiopathic CSA. CSA can coexist with OSA, especially in heart failure and neuromuscular disorders. So-called 'complex sleep apnoea' describes persistent or emergent CSA after initiation of CPAP therapy. Physiological CSAs have no pathological association, usually occur at sleep–wake transition and are self-limiting. High altitude periodic breathing and primary CSA of infancy will not be covered here [29–31].

Aetiology and Pathophysiology

Transitions from wake to sleep and between the various sleep states lead to changes in the apnoea threshold for arterial carbon dioxide ($PaCO_2$). Central apnoeas are far less likely to occur in wake when the threshold is lowest and cortically driven respiration is protective. Although $PaCO_2$ also rises during sleep, various factors can bring it closer to the apnoea threshold, including hypoxia. Carbon dioxide is then more likely to drop below the apnoea threshold and breathing stops. Ventilation restarts when a $PaCO_2$ rise above the threshold is detected in the medulla [29,30].

Pathological CSA occurs when there is either ventilatory instability or central respiratory depression. The automatic control of ventilation during sleep relies on feedback loops, making it vulnerable to instability. Loop gain describes the response of a system to feedback with high loop gain representing a response that is fast and strong and low loop gain with one that is slow and weak. Loop gain is subdivided into controller and plant gain. Controller gain describes the strength of a system's response to feedback, in this case a medullary chemo-response to rising $PaCO_2$. Plant gain describes how efficiently change is achieved, in this case $PaCO_2$ reduction. If chemoreceptors respond too readily to relatively minor $PaCO_2$ changes, and/or plant gain is too high, then there is greater chance of $PaCO_2$ being driven below the apnoea threshold. A repetitive cycle of hyperventilation and apnoea will develop if loop gain is too high (>1) and is more likely if other factors such as heart failure increase respiratory drive [29,30].

Delayed detection of $PaCO_2$ fluctuations also predispose to CSA. Blood levels first change at the pulmonary capillaries and if medullary transit is prolonged due to cardiac failure then chemoreceptors are continually playing catch-up. The delay produces a late response to a $PaCO_2$ rise. The peak ventilatory response will be greater but also occur after $PaCO_2$ has begun to fall. Ventilatory overshoot follows and $PaCO_2$ falls below the apnoea threshold, triggering an apnoea before the cycle repeats. This underlies the crescendo–decrescendo pattern of ventilation-apnoeas seen in CSB-CSA of heart failure and other types of periodic breathing (Figure 10.5) [29,30].

Depression of the medullary ventilatory centres also causes CSA and is usually distinct from the above in being associated with hypercapnia. Brainstem disorders including infection, stroke, tumour and neurodegeneration are predisposing factors. Central apnoeas after stroke can persist or resolve with time. Congenital central hypoventilation syndrome is a rare but serious condition which usually manifests shortly after birth as CSA or ventilatory failure during sleep, and a similar condition can present de novo in adulthood. Opioids can unpredictably cause CSA through inhibition of medullary mu-opioid receptors in sensitive individuals. This is sometimes associated with OSA, possibly due to hypoglossal inhibition [29,30].

Mixed SDB occurs in other scenarios. Physiological apnoeas occurring during sleep–wake transitions can be increased by OSA-induced sleep fragmentation. In cardiac failure, OSA and CSA sometimes appear unrelated, beyond OSA and ischaemic heart

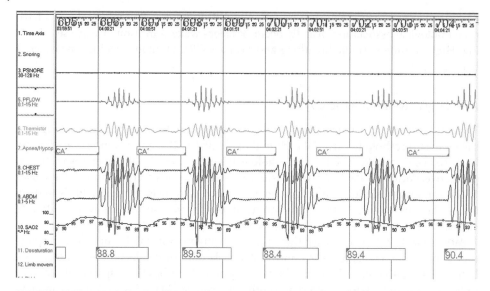

Figure 10.5 Cheyne–Stokes Breathing central sleep apnoea. Note: Crescendo–decrescendo ventilation alternating with apnoeas. Airflow cessation (PFLOW and Thermistor) is associated with absent chest and abdominal deflection, indicating loss of central respiratory drive.

disease sharing risk factors. However, OSA may be exacerbated by upper airway oedema or be a factor in cardiac dysfunction complicated by CSA. Central respiratory depression can cause OSA if both genioglossal and diaphragmatic activity are reduced. Depending on the extent and pattern of deactivation and reactivation, obstructive, central or mixed apnoeas occur. CSA that occurs in predominantly obstructive sleep-disordered breathing can persist or only emerge when CPAP is commenced. This complex sleep apnoea commonly resolves without intervention [29,30].

Epidemiology

Primary CSA is an uncommon diagnosis of exclusion, representing less than 5% of sleep clinic patients assessed for SDB [29]. Cheyne–Stokes respiration is found in one third of patients with left ventricular systolic dysfunction when it is associated with a poorer prognosis [29,30]. Opioid-induced CSA has been reported in up to 50% of patients taking opioids [29].

Diagnosis

Clinical Features

Sleepiness is not always present in CSA but the bed partner may describe apnoeas. If closer questioning yields crescendo–decrescendo breathing or absence of snoring then CSA needs to be considered. Alternatively, patients may wake up breathless during the hyperventilation phase of CSB-CSA, which could be mistaken for paroxysmal nocturnal dyspnoea. History and examination should explore for features of underlying conditions and concomitant opioids.

Sleep Studies

Investigation of CSA is best undertaken by a specialist. Oximetry is reasonably sensitive, depending on device and set-up, but characteristic features are not reliable enough to differentiate from OSA, particularly as mixed SDB is common [30]. One way to deal with symptomatic oximetry-positive SDB of uncertain nature is with a CPAP trial, and subsequent RPG or PSG if desaturations persist. Although CPAP sometimes controls CSA, and OSA control in mixed SDB may be all that is necessary to improve symptoms, such an approach is best confined to cases where predominant OSA is most likely or when sophisticated sleep studies are a scarce resource. If predominant CSA is suspected then in the author's opinion it is better to perform RPG or PSG before starting treatment, as CPAP can sometimes worsen CSA or trigger it in genuine OSA, causing further confusion.

Central apnoeas are defined similarly to obstructive events [19]. However, they are accompanied by cessation of respiratory effort, with absent deflection in chest and abdominal gauges. Arousal and oxygen desaturation may be associated but, while giving an indication of whether SDB is causing sleep disruption, these are not mandatory criteria [19]. Hypopnoeas are more difficult to characterise and unlike OSA are not formally recognised in the most widely used scoring system [19]. Both obstructive and central hypopnoeas are associated with reduced respiratory excursion: the former because reduced airflow lessens chest displacement and the latter because respiratory effort is genuinely reduced. Oesophageal manometry can differentiate by showing inspiratory pressure drop in OSA, but this technique is invasive and not routinely used. Severity criteria for CSA are at least as arbitrary as for OSA due to the variety of pathophysiology and uncertainty regarding the role of treatment. It is reasonable to adhere to the same arbitrary cut-offs as OSA but to place particular importance on symptoms when considering management options.

Management

The role of intervention is less clear in CSA and again requires specialist input. Apnoeas can be incidental and may spontaneously improve. Active treatments do not reliably improve the AHI, sleep architecture or daytime symptoms. Furthermore, long-term health benefits are unproven. The decision to treat should be based on symptoms, typically EDS, and the likelihood of CSA being the cause (Figure 10.4) [29,32].

The best chance of improving symptomatic CSA may be through addressing the underlying cause. Heart failure treatment should be optimised and opioid-induced CSA should respond to weaning of medication. Nocturnal dialysis may improve CSB-CSA associated with renal failure [29].

When a treatable cause cannot be identified then direct treatment of CSA can be tried. Oxygen may be considered when hypoxia is thought to be one of the factors underlying respiratory instability or sleep fragmentation. However, the potential for precipitating significant hypercapnia, particularly in central hypoventilation, means oxygen should only be initiated by those with specialist expertise and monitoring facilities [29,32].

CPAP can improve CSA although is less effective than for OSA. It can improve cardiac function but long-term benefits are unproven. Bi-level non-invasive ventilation has been studied less but is probably similarly effective to CPAP. However, it is more expensive and can worsen CSA if over ventilation increases respiratory instability [29,32]. Adaptive servo-ventilation (ASV) is also expensive but may be the most effective at stabilising CSB-CSA. By titrating inspiratory pressure according to the patient's own ventilation, ASV stabilises CSB and maintains airway patency to control any coexistent OSA. ASV used to be considered reasonable to try in CPAP failures [32]. However trial data showing a mortality disadvantage for this modality when used in patients with left ventricular systolic heart failure [33] cast doubt on the safety and utility of ASV, at least in that patient group.

Finally, acetazolamide and theophylline are respiratory stimulants which have been shown to ameliorate CSA although their use remains controversial, largely due to insufficient evidence [29,32].

Conclusions

OSA and CSA are both common and can cause significant symptoms, often in association with serious medical disorders. In specialist hands they are relatively straightforward to diagnose. For both types of apnoea, the main indication for treatment is symptom control although the safety profile of the key interventions means the threshold for starting treatment need not be high. Treatment is highly effective at controlling respiratory events and symptoms of OSA but less reliable in CSA. The long-term impact of intervention on associated disorders such as cardiovascular disease and diabetes remains unclear.

Key Points

- Sleep-disordered breathing is defined by recurrent pauses in breathing during sleep either due to upper airway obstruction (OSA) or reduced ventilatory drive (CSA).
- OSA is a very common cause of sleep disruption fuelling significant daytime sleepiness and impaired function.
- Patients with a high suspicion of having OSA may be diagnosed using home oximetry or polygraphy; in other cases full PSG is warranted.
- It is possible but unproven that successful OSA treatment has major long-term benefits on cardiovascular and possibly neurological health.
- CSA is a heterogeneous phenomenon and a complex area that benefits from expert management together with treatment of potential underlying factors such as cardiac failure.

References

1 Douglas NJ, Polo O. Pathogenesis of obstructive sleep apnoea/hypopnoea syndrome. *Lancet* 1994;344:653–5.
2 Punjabi NM. The epidemiology of adult obstructive sleep apnea. *Proc Am Thorac Soc* 2008;5:136–43.
3 Young T, Palta M, Dempsey J, *et al.* The occurrence of sleep disordered breathing among middle-aged adults. *N Engl J Med* 1993;328:1230–5.

4 Newman AB, Foster G, Givelber R, *et al*. Progression and regression of sleep-disordered breathing with changes in weight: the Sleep Heart Health Study. *Arch Intern Med* 2005;165:2408–13.

5 Ancoli-Israel S, Kripke DF, Klauber MR, *et al*. Sleep disordered breathing in community-dwelling elderly. *Sleep* 1991;14:486–95.

6 Al Lawati NM, Patel SR, Ayas NT. Epidemiology, risk factors, and consequences of obstructive sleep apnea and short sleep duration. *Prog Cardiovasc Dis* 2009;51:285–93.

7 Young T, Shahar E, Nieto FJ, *et al*. Predictors of sleep-disordered breathing in community-dwelling adults: the Sleep Heart Health Study. *Arch Intern Med* 2002;162:893–900.

8 Peppard PE, Young T, Palta M, *et al*. Longitudinal study of moderate weight change and sleep-disordered breathing. *JAMA* 2000;284:3015–21.

9 Stradling JR, Pepperell JC, Davies RJ. Sleep apnoea and hypertension: proof at last? *Thorax* 2001;56(Suppl. 2): ii45–9.

10 Dong JY, Zhang YH, Qin LQ. Obstructive sleep apnea and cardiovascular risk: metaanalysis of prospective cohort studies. *Atherosclerosis* 2013;229:489–95.

11 Redline S, Yenokyan G, Gottlieb DJ, *et al*. Obstructive sleep apnea-hypopnea and incident stroke: the sleep heart health study. *Am J Respir Crit Care Med* 2010;182:269–77.

12 Bradley TD, Floras JS. Obstructive sleep apnoea and its cardiovascular consequences. *Lancet* 2009;373:82–93.

13 Ellen RL, Marshall SC, Palayew M, *et al*. Systematic review of motor vehicle crash risk in persons with sleep apnea. *J Clin Sleep Med* 2006;2:193–200.

14 McDaid C, Griffin S, Weatherly H, *et al*. Continuous positive airway pressure devices for the treatment of obstructive sleep apnoea hypopnoea syndrome: a systematic review and economic analysis. *Health Technol Assess* 2009;13:iii–iv, xi–xiv, 1–119, 43–274.

15 Tarasiuk A, Greenberg-Dotan S, Simon-Tuval T, *et al*. The effect of obstructive sleep apnea on morbidity and health care utilization of middle-aged and older adults. *J Am Geriatr Soc* 2008;56:247–54.

16 Johns MW. A new method for measuring daytime sleepiness: the Epworth sleepiness scale. *Sleep* 1991;14:540–5.

17 Arand D, Bonnet M, Hurwitz T, *et al*. The clinical use of the MSLT and MWT. *Sleep* 2005;28:123–44.

18 Netzer N, Eliasson AH, Netzer C, *et al*. Overnight pulse oximetry for sleep disordered breathing in adults: a review. *Chest* 2001;120:625–33.

19 Iber C, Ancoli-Isreal S, Chesson A, *et al*. The American Academy of Sleep Medicine Manual for the Scoring of Sleep and Associated Events: Rules, Terminology and Technical Specifications, 1st edn. Westchester, IL: American Academy of Sleep Medicine, 2007.

20 Ruehland WR, Rochford PD, O'Donoghue FJ, *et al*. The new AASM criteria for scoring hypopneas: impact on the apnea hypopnea index. *Sleep* 2009;32:150–7.

21 Masa JF, Corral J, Pereira R, *et al*. Effectiveness of sequential automatic-manual home respiratory polygraphy scoring. *Eur Respir J* 2013;41:879–87.

22 National Institute for Health and Care Excellence (NICE). Continuous positive airway pressure for the treatment of obstructive sleep apnoea/hypopnoea syndrome. *TA* 139. 2008. https://www.nice.org.uk/guidance/ta139. Accessed 24 January 2018.

23 George CF. Reduction in motor vehicle collisions following treatment of sleep apnoea with nasal CPAP. *Thorax* 2001;56:508–12.

24 Wozniak DR, Lasserson TJ, Smith I. Educational, supportive and behavioural interventions to improve usage of continuous positive airway pressure machines in obstructive sleep apnoea. *Cochrane Database Syst Rev* 2014;1(Art. No.: CD007736). doi: 10.1002/14651858.CD007736.pub2.

25 Smith I, Lasserson TJ. Pressure modification for improving usage of continuous positive airway pressure machines in adults with obstructive sleep apnoea. *Cochrane Database Syst Rev* 2009;4(Art. No.: CD003531). doi: 10.1002/14651858.CD003531.pub3.

26 Sundaram S, Bridgman SA, Lim J, Lasserson TJ. Surgery for obstructive sleep apnoea. *Cochrane Database Syst Rev* 2005;4(Art. No.: CD001004). doi: 10.1002/14651858. CD001004.pub2.

27 Strollo P, Soose R, Maurer J, et al. Upper-airway stimulation for obstructive sleep apnoea. *N Engl J Med* 2014;370:139–49.

28 Mason M, Welsh EJ, Smith I. Drug therapy for obstructive sleep apnoea in adults. *Cochrane Database Syst Rev* 2013;5(Art. No.: CD003002). doi: 10.1002/14651858. CD003002.pub3.

29 Eckert DJ, Jordan AS, Merchia P, *et al.* Central sleep apnea: pathophysiology and treatment. *Chest* 2007;131:595–607.

30 Javaheri S. Central sleep apnea. *Clin Chest Med* 2010;31:235–48.

31 Series F, Kimoff RJ, Morrison D, *et al.* Prospective evaluation of nocturnal oximetry for detection of sleep-related breathing disturbances in patients with chronic heart failure. *Chest* 2005;127:1507–14.

32 Aurora RN, Chowdhuri S, Ramar K, *et al.* The treatment of central sleep apnea syndromes in adults: practice parameters with an evidence-based literature review and meta-analyses. *Sleep* 2012;35:17–40.

33 Cowrie M, Woehrle H, Wegscheider K, et al. Adaptive-servo ventilation for central sleep apnoea in systolic heart failure. *N Engl J Med* 2015;373:1095–105.

11

Circadian Rhythm Sleep Disorders

Kirstie N. Anderson

Regional Sleep Service, Newcastle upon Tyne Hospital NHS Foundation Trust, Newcastle upon Tyne, UK

> *Just to satisfy my curiosity I have gone through files of the British Medical Journal and could not find a single case reported of anybody being hurt by loss of sleep.*
>
> Thomas Edison

Introduction

Virtually all life on the planet has evolved to accommodate the 24-hour cycle of the earth's rotation around the sun giving a regular cycle of light and dark. Circadian rhythms (from the Latin, circa 'about' and dies 'a day') describe the regular, near 24-hour cycles that influence nearly all aspects of animal and plant physiology.

At a molecular level, in virtually all animal species, 12–14 highly conserved circadian clock gene proteins oscillate by means of an autoregulatory feedback loop, generating self-sustained timing systems that are highly regulated with a period of about 24 hours [1]. Biological clocks within all cells drive or alter our sleep patterns, alertness, cognition, mood, and virtually every other aspect of our physiology and behaviour.

In humans, a cellular pacemaker in the hypothalamus called the suprachiasmatic nucleus (SCN) acts as the master timekeeper for the body, synchronising all the individual cellular clocks. Lesions of the SCN in animals abolish circadian rhythms whilst isolated preparations of SCN neurons reveal they can an act as a self-sustaining oscillator with near daily rhythms for weeks in complete isolation. However, the intrinsic period of the SCN oscillator is *not* exactly 24 hours. For most human subjects it runs at just over 24 hours and will drift out of phase with the solar day unless synchronised or 'entrained' by sensory inputs, the most important of which is light.

We now know through the pioneering work of Russell Foster and others that we are 'hard wired' to light stimulation via a direct retino-hypothalamic link from the 1–2% of melanopsin-secreting, non-rod and non-cone photoganglion cells in the retina that respond to light intensity [2]. Environmental light spans nine orders of magnitude from starlight to the dawning sun (400 lux) to the overhead sun at midday (up to 100 000 lux).

Sleep Disorders in Neurology: A Practical Approach, Second Edition.
Edited by Sebastiaan Overeem and Paul Reading.
© 2018 John Wiley & Sons Ltd. Published 2018 by John Wiley & Sons Ltd.

The average office light level rarely goes above 400 lux although the eye is such an efficient camera that this does not affect visual acuity. Therefore, we rarely think about the effect of long periods of indoor light levels upon our circadian rhythm and sleep.

Michel Siffre, the self-styled father of chronobiology, performed one of the key experiments on himself in a cave in 1962 when he simply recorded his sleep–wake cycles in the complete absence of sunlight for 63 days. Without any time or light cues, he was still able to maintain a rhythm of approximately 24.5 hours for about 4 weeks and in fact reported 'some of the best sleep of my life'. However, after this time there was complete desynchronisation with sleep–wake cycles that were entirely irregular ranging from 18 to 48 hours. Many others have replicated the experiments in more comfortable laboratory conditions using so-called 'forced desynchrony protocols' [3].

Although light remains the most important 'zeitgeber' or timekeeper, melatonin secreted by the pineal gland also directly affects the SCN. Suppressed by light and absent or minimal during the day, melatonin secretion commences around 14 hours following the natural time of awakening and acts to stabilise the nocturnal sleep period. The timing of melatonin secretion and the core body temperature serve as useful proxy measures of the intrinsic circadian system.

There is natural genetic variation that accounts for an individual chronotype – whether we are morning 'larks', evening 'night owls' or, like the majority of us, set somewhere in the middle. Validated questionnaires to determine chronotype are used more in research than routine clinical practice [4].

For optimal sleep, the actual sleep time should match the timing of the circadian rhythm of sleep and wake propensity. However, in the last 250 years, the industrial revolution, availability of 24-hour electric light and, most recently, the digital revolution have not just reduced total sleep time but have eroded day–night patterns, making abnormal circadian rhythms a universal and pervasive part of modern living.

Changes in Circadian Rhythm with Age

Development of circadian sleep phase preference of either 'eveningness' versus 'morningness' develops between 6 years of age and 12 years of age. There is then a natural tendency for a delay in the onset of sleep by about 1–2 hours and an increase in total sleep time during later adolescence. At the other end of life, the sleep phase tends to advance with older adults waking earlier. Melatonin production itself declines significantly and the circadian rhythm weakens alongside the homeostatic drive to sleep. Generally, older adults deal with shifts in circadian rhythm such as those induced by jet lag less well than their younger counterparts [5].

Circadian Rhythm Sleep–Wake Disorders

Published criteria within the most recent International Classification of Sleep Disorders (ICSD-3) as well as the Diagnostic and Statistical Manual of Mental Disorders (DSM V) define six distinct circadian rhythm sleep–wake disorders (CRSWDs) [6,7]: delayed sleep–wake phase disorder; advanced sleep–wake phase disorder; irregular sleep–wake rhythm disorder; non-24 hour sleep–wake rhythm disorder (free running or non-entrained disorder); shift work disorder; and jet lag disorder.

In the context of a sleep medicine clinic, delayed sleep phase, shift work disorder, and irregular sleep–wake cycle disorder (often alongside other physical or mental health problems) are the most likely to be seen. By definition, all of the conditions have to be associated with functional impairment and distress. For example, a baker who happily gets up at 03:30 and goes to bed at 18:30 may be 'out of sync' with the rest of the world but he does not harbour a true circadian rhythm disorder.

History and Investigations

Even within dedicated sleep clinics, CRSWDs can often remain unrecognised for some time. Questions within the history can be focused more upon snoring, vivid dreams and night-time events rather than the actual timing of the sleep period over days and weeks. A CRSWD should be considered within the differential diagnosis of all patients presenting with either sleepiness or sleeplessness. One of the fundamental features of circadian rhythm disorders is that sleep quantity is often entirely normal over the 24-hour period. The sleep quality can also be good but simply the timing of the sleep period is abnormal. Therefore, questions that focus upon the patterns of sleep and wake over time are necessary and the diagnostic value of simple sleep diaries over 2 weeks usually far outweighs that of scales such as the Epworth sleepiness score.

Useful and targeted questions within the clinic to screen for CRSWD include:

- *Take me through your typical 24-hour day.* The specific patterns and rotas for any shift work, time out of the house, light exposure during the day should all be included. Ask about any difference between weekends and weekdays.
- *If you are allowed to sleep when you feel the need to, do you sleep well?* Insomniacs will usually say 'no' but those with circadian problems can often describe long periods of sleep.
- *Do you go out of the house at least once a day?* One could argue that for those with any chronic mental or physical health problem, if they then remain within standard room lighting (averaging 100–400 lux, equivalent to environmental twilight) then they will acquire circadian rhythm disruption that will contribute to their other symptoms.

Sleep Diaries

A well completed sleep diary can be all that is required alongside a characteristic history to make a diagnosis of a CRSWD. The diary should not only encompass the night alone, but can show environmental zeitgebers such as food, exercise as well as caffeine and alcohol consumption.

The latest ICSD diagnostic criteria specify a minimum assessment period of 7 days but state that 14 days is better to encompass both free days and work/school days. Diaries in clinical practice need to span at least one full weekend if the patient works in a conventional job but often longer is needed to detect those who 'free run', have irregular sleep–wake cycles or those who work variable shifts. Ideally, a subject should provide 2 weeks of a sleep diary, completed before attending the sleep clinic appointment. Of course, not all subjects can efficiently complete diaries. Actigraphy may provide more useful information in those at the extremes of age or those who have significant cognitive impairment and/or mental health issues.

Actigraphy

The technique of accelerometry has been used for over 25 years to generate physical activity data that can be used as a surrogate marker of sleep–wake cycles [8]. Simple, well tolerated and ideal for recording sleep–wake patterns over time, there are now a number of medical devices available. Increasingly, non-medical devices or commercial accelerometers are also being used as health 'apps' with printouts brought in to clinics by patients. Examples include the 'fit-bit' or 'jawbone'. Few of these non-medical devices have been clinically validated against the arguable gold standard of polysomnography.

These devices are usually wrist worn and can supplement diary data with practice parameters developed by the American Academy for Sleep Medicine [9]. Non-compliance is very easy to detect and of course the role of physical activity as a key zeitgeber can also be monitored. The lack of validated norms across different populations has possibly limited the use of these devices in clinical practice. A typical recording of a normal 2 weeks is shown in Figure 11.1 in which the sleep–wake cycle is clearly seen alongside periods of daytime exercise.

Polysomnography

This is rarely indicated unless evaluating other potential causes for sleep-related complaints. Examples might include restless legs syndrome driving a delay in sleep phase or a shift worker who has also developed obstructive sleep apnoea syndrome.

Delayed Sleep Phase Syndrome

This disorder has been estimated to account for up to 10% of those presenting with insomnia complaints to a sleep medicine clinic. Delayed sleep phase syndrome (DSPS) is characterised by habitual sleep–wake times that are at least 2 hours later than conventional or socially acceptable patterns and often delayed by 3–6 hours. If subjects are allowed to sleep to their preferred schedule, sleep is typically of normal duration.

It is a condition recognised much more commonly in the adolescent population and can be viewed as a pathological exaggeration of the normal delay in the circadian rhythm that peaks in males at age 21 and females at age 19 during the final changes post-puberty [5,10].

Social factors such as reduced parental influence and omnipresent light sources from laptops and smart phones in the bedroom may contribute to this disorder. It typically starts in late teenage years although mean presenting age is around 20 years old. Prevalence amongst adolescents when defined according to ICSD criteria has ranged between 1.9% and 3.3% with a much lower prevalence in surveys across populations of all ages of 0.15–0.17% [11].

Up to 40% of subjects have a family history and some appear to show an autosomal dominant trait with either polymorphisms in clock genes (hPer3, Clock) or HLA associations in small case series [12,13]. Typical patients will have 'evening' chronotypes and will show a delayed phase in all the circadian markers including melatonin and temperature, parameters not routinely evaluated in clinical practice. Interestingly, there is

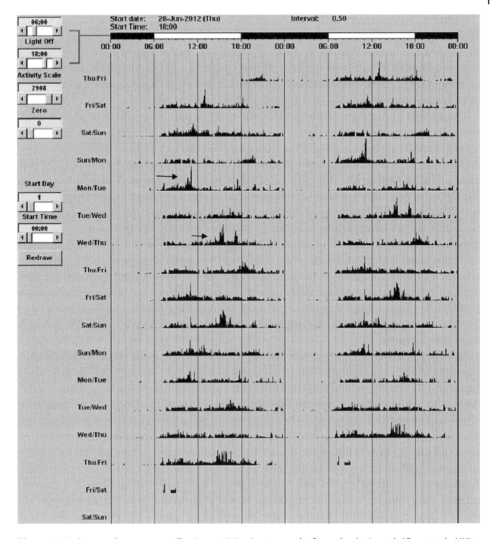

Figure 11.1 A normal actogram collecting at 0.5-minute epochs from the Actiwatch (Camntech, UK) plotted over a 48-hour timescale to show a regular day–night pattern in a 61-year-old female. Arrows denote periods of intense exercise (horse riding) which occurred regularly.

also recent evidence that the circadian period length itself (so-called 'Tau') is longer than that of normal sleepers, predisposing them to 'drift' from day to day and possibly accounting for the tendency in some to relapse after treatment [14]. Extreme difficulty with waking for school or college can lead to truancy and behavioural difficulties along-side descriptions of sleep drunkenness and confusion if subjects are forcibly woken too early. There is increasing recognition of the association between DSPS and mental health problems, especially depression. However, it may also be the case that the sleep restriction invariably caused by DSPS contributes directly to mental health issues and behavioural difficulties such as an attention deficit hyperactivity disorder (ADHD) phenotype [15,16].

Diagnosis can be made with well completed sleep diaries, preferably for 2–3 weeks, and actigraphy can be particularly useful if diaries are unclear or for younger subjects. Treatment can be satisfying and rapidly effective, often after patients have tried routine hypnotics or behavioural techniques and sleep hygiene without success. However, often treatment strategies seem to be more effective for those who have acquired a DSPS later in life rather than those with abnormal sleep timing from early on.

The American Academy of Sleep Medicine practice parameters have produced treatment guidelines recommending precisely timed melatonin administration before bed alongside morning light exposure but then point out the lack of consensus in important details such as actual timing and melatonin dose in the published studies [7,17]. Small case series and three placebo controlled trials have demonstrated benefit but noted variability of dose and assessment measures. Many chronobiology experts highlight the benefits of careful assessment of dim light melatonin onset (DLMO) to enable perfect timing of the melatonin dose [18] but in regular clinical practice few have access to these tests. Giving melatonin at a dose of 1–2 mg, 6 hours before a consistent sleep diary recorded sleep onset can be effective, especially alongside exposure to a light box at around 8 a.m. in the morning (at least 2500 lux and at least 1 hour in most studies). There are often practical difficulties encouraging compliance in the use of light boxes and a simple explanation of just how many more lux come from the cloudiest November day at 9 a.m. compared with the brightest light in the house may be helpful to patients and their parents.

So-called 'chronotherapy' can be helpful for some. This might start with a 2-week schedule where subjects initially fix their bed and wake time at their ideal delayed sleep phase (e.g. bed at 4 a.m. and rise time at 1 p.m.), and then delay time in bed (and wake) further by 2 hours every 2 days to take them right around the clock to the desired or conventional bed and wake time. The author has found it very effective in selected cases but published data only come from case control studies. It is undeniably disruptive and needs all aspects of schedule to be moved so can only practically be undertaken outside of work or school during holiday periods. After completion of a cycle of chronotherapy, subsequent use of melatonin and bright light to hold patterns in place can prevent relapse. How long to continue melatonin is not clear given that, without treatment, many come to clinic with chronic histories over many years [19]. However, for those with short histories or a clear societal trigger and a rapid response to therapy, it is worth trying melatonin withdrawal at least once after 3–6 months of therapy. This may be more relevant in health care systems where melatonin is a prescribed drug with associated restrictions compared with those in which it is available over the counter in health food retailers. There have been no trials using modified release preparations of melatonin to treat DSPS, although anecdotally some have also reported success.

Advanced Sleep Phase Syndrome

Advanced sleep phase syndrome (ASPS) can be viewed as the polar opposite to DSPS, where sleep comes too early in the evening and patients wake early with subsequent difficulty maintaining sleep. Rarely, younger familial cases have been described with identifiable mutations in key clock genes [20]. However, although prevalence figures are hard to establish, possibly 1% of those over 65 can be considered to have a form of ASPS.

Sleep diaries typically show relatively little difficulty with sleep early in the night or possible evening napping before bed but then waking often from 3 to 4 a.m. onwards. Typically, many of these subjects will undergo investigations such as polysomnography to exclude co-morbid sleep disorders which are invariably more frequent in an older population. Within the differential diagnosis, obstructive sleep apnoea is typically worse in the second half of the night and depression must also be carefully screened for. It is also a consideration in older patients who present with insomnia but simply cannot tolerate the sleep restriction component of therapy. Furthermore, decreased mobility, poor eyesight and daytime napping may all contribute or exacerbate symptoms.

There is level 2 evidence for the effectiveness of Bright Light Therapy given between 18:00 hours and 20:00 hours in the evening, using lux levels over 2500. Melatonin when used should be given in the morning but again doses and clear schedules have not been established and many simply use evening light alone. This seems better tolerated in an older age group who may be able to sit more easily at this time of day [21].

Shift Work Disorder

Cultural changes in work patterns have been so great over the last century that it often seems hard for doctors and patients alike to consider this aspect of modern life as a potential sleep disorder. An estimated 20% of the western world now work some form of shift pattern that will encroach into the usual or natural time for sleep. Also included are prolonged work shifts that will contribute to fatigue and sleepiness. Overall, the prevalence of clinically significant sleep disturbance and excessive daytime sleepiness is estimated to be 2–5% of the general population with this rising to between 10% and 38% within rotating or night shift workers [22]. Innate circadian preference will influence the ability to tolerate different shifts with morning 'larks' clearly struggling more with nights or evenings than 'owls'.

In practice, shift work often produces both sleep restriction and a circadian rhythm disorder. The current ICSD criteria define shift work disorder as more than 3 months of insomnia and/or excessive sleepiness, accompanied by a reduction of total sleep time, which is associated with a recurring work schedule that overlaps the usual time for sleep. The reduction in measured total sleep time over 24 hours is often striking with many studies showing a mean loss of between 1 hour and 4 hours.

An extensive body of research suggests that this causes both immediate difficulties with concentration, attention and mood as well as longer term problems with mental and physical health as well as quality of life [23]. When compared with those who work regular hours, shift workers have been shown in various studies to have impaired glucose tolerance, increased cardiovascular risk, lower mood, increased reflux, a greater cancer risk and more mental health problems such as depression and substance abuse. Worryingly, many studies have also demonstrated the impact upon decision making and rate of errors in those within health care [24,25].

People with co-morbid medical, psychiatric, and other sleep disorders such as sleep apnoea and those with a more prolonged sleep need may be at particular risk. Social pressures tend to lead to workers switching straight back to daytime schedules on holidays or days off so reducing the likelihood of spontaneous circadian adjustment. The social support for shift workers and the availability of a comfortable, dark sleeping environment can often play a major part in either helping or contributing to symptoms. Those who suffer most tend to be those working night shifts, early morning shifts, and rotating shifts. Predictably most of us will struggle to work and function at our best between 04:00 hours and 06:00 hours in the morning. Almost certainly, increasing age exacerbates the problem given that sleep homeostasis and the robustness of circadian rhythms diminish with age.

The diagnosis should be straightforward in those with a clear history for ongoing shift work and completed diaries but the variability of work patterns can produce a complex history. In practice, many can tolerate shifts without symptoms in youth but gradually develop intolerance over time so may not attribute their fatigue, somatic symptoms and new onset sleepiness to their longstanding evening or occasional night shifts. Polysomnography may well be indicated for co-morbid sleep disorders such as sleep apnoea and specific questioning for associated sleep disruptors in shift workers such as gastro-oesophageal reflux is indicated. In clinical practice there is little evidence that morningness/eveningness questionnaires or measurement of circadian phase markers are useful in diagnosis or predicting who will have greatest trouble working shifts.

Clearly the ideal treatment is to avoid shift work! There are often financial and social considerations making this impossible but it may be important for a sleep specialist to at least support the employee in finding the best shift pattern for long-term health benefit and work efficiency. Aiming for fixed pattern shifts, avoiding back-to-back night to day shifts and trying to align the individual's innate preference to their work pattern is important where possible. Sleep hygiene and an explanation of the role of light and stimulants during the day can help to some extent [26].

Beyond educational input, the timing of light exposure, the use of stimulants or planned naps all have moderate evidence but some are more practical to apply than others. Planned naps prior to the start of a night shift or during a long shift where possible have been shown to improve alertness. Modafinil 200 mg at the start of a shift (licensed for use in shift work in some countries) and caffeine (250 mg and 400 mg) have both shown benefit in increasing alertness and improving psychomotor performance during a night shift. Hypnotics and melatonin have been shown to improve the duration and quality of daytime sleep following night shifts but not to clearly improve alertness during the next shift. There is no convincing evidence to favour melatonin at present and the optimal dose remains debated.

Bright light (2350–12 000 lux in trials) given early in the shift can be shown to improve alertness and performance but for practical purposes a future goal may involve the use of smart lighting at intensities that truly mimic daylight selectively applied across the entire workplace. There is increasing commercial interest in these devices across hospitals and other workplaces that require night shift workers but evidence for improved well being and productivity are lacking at present.

Jet Lag Disorder – 'East is a Beast, West is Best'.

Rarely seen in a sleep clinic but much debated in the lay press, jet lag refers to the transient misalignment of the intrinsic circadian rhythm to the external environment resulting from flying distances spanning greater than two time zones. Typically, symptoms develop over the course of 1–2 days. The circadian system has an innate ability to realign to local time, adapting to delays or advances of 1–2 hours per day. This should mean that, for most, jet lag causes transient symptoms of night time sleep disturbance and daytime fatigue, often with gastrointestinal disturbance and malaise. Travelling west generally has less impact because the intrinsic circadian rhythm is slightly greater than 24 hours making it easier to delay rather than advance one's circadian rhythm.

However, long haul flights often come alongside many other sleep disruptors or 'toxins' that are independent of circadian rhythm. Many of us arrive at the airport sleep deprived, having overused alcohol and/or caffeine and having failed to sleep upright. Long queues in passport control and customs also contribute significantly to sleep–wake disturbance at the destination.

Timed light exposure has a clear evidence base with schedules that the organised traveller can strategically plan depending on destination time zone [27].

Melatonin at variable doses has also been studied and shown to effectively improve sleep in a number of trials, mainly for eastward travel and with variable schedules and dose regimes [7]. However, there is greatest adherence to the simplest dosing schedule of 0.5–5 mg close to the local bedtime for 3–4 days upon arrival. It should be noted that Zopiclone and Zolpidem have an equal effect, so it may well be that a substantial effect is coming from the hypnotic action rather than true phase shifting effect per se.

Free Running Circadian Rhythm Disorder

This rare condition is characterised as a gradual drift of the major sleep period by 1–2 hours every day with a circadian system that appears not entrained by the normal external zeitgebers. If scheduled sleep–wake times are attempted, patients report insomnia and excessive daytime sleepiness. Some subjects with DSPS appear to have an overlap disorder in which they occasionally move into a free running pattern. Indeed, this has been reported in some individuals with DSPS undergoing chronotherapy.

Until recently, the majority of cases have been described in the blind, particularly those blind from birth who are never exposed to photic entrainment [28]. An estimated 50% of those blind from birth have a free running circadian rhythm with at least 70% having chronic sleep disturbance.

This is one condition that may clearly be missed by only 2 weeks of sleep diaries and certainly by 1 week. Often 4 weeks are required alongside actigraphy to confirm the diagnosis. Objective markers such as melatonin levels may be easier to interpret.

In the cases reported in sighted individuals, there is a recognised increase in psychiatric and neurodegenerative conditions [29]. Up to a quarter will have mental health problems, typically post-dating the sleep disturbance. An important recent study carefully controlling for social zeitgebers such as employment status in schizophrenia patients compared with controls found high rates of circadian rhythm disorders including free running patterns and irregular sleep–wake schedules. The findings suggested that the circadian rhythm disturbance may be an integral part of the schizophrenic illness itself [30]. Given that complaints of sleep disturbance in severe mental health problems are very common but often attributed to medication or lifestyle factors, this condition may well be under recognised in this group and represents a potential avenue for treatment. There is some preliminary evidence that stabilising the sleep–wake cycle may be beneficial even in those with severe and enduring psychosis [31] and there are now several ongoing randomised controlled treatment trials in schizophrenia and bipolar disorder.

Irregular Sleep–Wake Rhythm Disorder

This phenomenon is characterised by multiple episodes of sleep night and day, usually 2–4 hours at a time with no fixed temporal pattern. This seems more common in those with a variety of severe neurodegenerative disorders [32] or in children with neurodevelopmental delay. Total sleep time over 24 hours may be relatively normal for age but is usually taken in three or more periods of sleep taken at entirely unpredictable times. They key feature distinguishing irregular sleep–wake rhythm disorder from other disorders is the lack of a prolonged sleep period and the random distribution of sleep. Certain chromosomal abnormalities are associated with particularly disruptive circadian rhythm abnormalities. These include Angelman's syndrome, Williams syndrome and Smith–Magenis syndrome, often with significant disruptive impact upon carers.

In those with Alzheimer's disease the specific phenomenon of 'sundowning' – marked agitation and wandering that occurs in the evening – may reflect a subtype of an irregular sleep–wake pattern [33]. The problem of night time sleep disturbance in dementia is cited as one of the commonest reasons for institutionalisation where the loss of many zeitgebers and lack of natural light may contribute further to an already irregular sleep–wake cycle.

Trials of various combinations of melatonin, bright light, exercise and behavioural therapies have all shown relatively modest benefits with no one modality clearly acting as the best zeitgeber. The difficulty of treating this problem probably reflects a degenerate or dysfunctional SCN that is less amenable to entrainment.

It is probably important to emphasise that there may be those with a very irregular sleep–wake cycles as measured by actigraphy who do not have any subjective sleep complaints. This is often apparent in large scale studies in normal populations where there is an association between disrupted sleep and dementia but also considerable variability within the range of normal ageing. The highly abnormal actogram shown in Figure 11.2 represents a patient who completed normal sleep diaries, had no discernible sleep–wake pattern on actigraphy and denied sleep–wake disturbance.

Conclusion

Broken or disrupted body clocks potentially have profound effects on physical and mental health. Many of us either spend long periods exposed to constant and relatively low levels of light or work far beyond the comfort of our natural chronotype. It is very likely that circadian rhythm disorders are significantly under recognised even within specialist sleep clinics.

Treatment can be effective and satisfying but the lack of any controlled trial data or consensus on therapy needs to be addressed in future research. The increasing recognition of circadian rhythm disruption within severe and enduring mental health problems should prompt attempts to better align a subject's clock with the sleep homeostat.

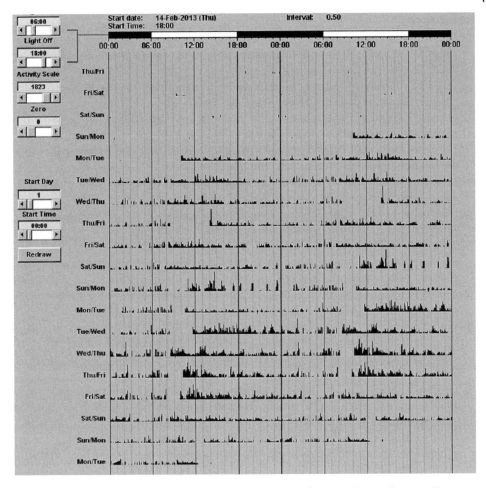

Figure 11.2 An actogram in a patient with a 3-year history of Parkinson's disease who was still working and driving with few subjective sleep complaints. Sleep diaries were completed showing consolidated blocks of sleep during the night only.

Key Points

- Sleep diaries should be a routine part of the assessment of all those with complaints of insomnia and/or daytime sleepiness. Actigraphy adds more information if history or diary keeping is unreliable for any reason and is particularly useful for free running circadian rhythm disorder.
- Think of delayed sleep phase syndrome in an adolescent 'insomniac'.
- Significant circadian rhythm disorders are likely to be common but under-recognised in those with significant mental health problems and may represent a fundamental part of disease biology.
- Our brains have evolved not to work at night, particularly as we age. The significant sleep restriction alongside circadian rhythm disturbance make shift work disorder an often underdiagnosed but troublesome sleep disorder in those over 40 years of age.

References

1 Fisher SP, Foster RG, Peirson SN. The circadian control of sleep. *Handb Exp Pharmacol* 2013; 217: 157–83.

2 Hughes S, Hankins MW, Foster RG, Peirson SN. Melanopsin phototransduction: slowly emerging from the dark. *Prog Brain Res* 2012; 199: 19–40.

3 Czeisler CA, Duffy JF, Shanahan TL, et al. Stability, precision, and near-24-hour period of the human circadian pacemaker. *Science* 1999; 284: 2177–81.

4 Horne JA, Ostberg O. A self-assessment questionnaire to determine morningness-eveningness in human circadian rhythms. *Int J Chronobiol* 1976; 4: 97–110.

5 Yoon IY, Kripke DF, Elliott JA, et al. Age-related changes of circadian rhythms and sleep-wake cycles. *J Am Geriatr Soc* 2003; 51: 1085–91.

6 International Classification of Sleep Disorders 3: Diagnostic and Coding Manual. American Sleep Disorders Association, Rochester, MN, 2014 (epub).

7 Morgenthaler TI, Lee-Chiong T, Alessi C, et al. Practice parameters for the clinical evaluation and treatment of circadian rhythm sleep disorders: An American Academy of Sleep Medicine report. *Sleep* 2007; 30: 1445–59.

8 Ancoli-Israel S, Cole R, Alessi C, et al. The role of actigraphy in the study of sleep and circadian rhythms. *Sleep* 2003; 26: 342–92.

9 Littner M, Kushida CA, Anderson WM, et al. Standards of Practice Committee of the American Academy of Sleep Medicine. Practice parameters for the role of actigraphy in the study of sleep and circadian rhythms: an update for 2002. *Sleep* 2003; 26: 337–41.

10 Gruber R, Sheshko D. Circadian sleep disorders in children and adolescents. In Ivanenko A (ed.), Sleep and Psychiatric Disorders in Children and Adolescents. Informa Healthcare USA, New York, 2008; 61–78.

11 Sivertsen B, Pallesen S, Stormark KM, et al. Delayed sleep phase syndrome in adolescents: prevalence and correlates in a large population based study. *BMC Public Health* 2013; 13: 1163.

12 Archer SN, Carpen JD, Gibson M, et al. Polymorphism in the PER3 promoter associates with diurnal preference and delayed sleep phase disorder. *Sleep* 2010; 33: 695–701.

13 Ancoli-Israel S, Schnierow B, Kelsoe J, Fink R. A pedigree of one family with delayed sleep phase syndrome. *Chronobiol Int* 2001; 18: 831–41.

14 Micic G, de Bruyn A, Lovato N, et al. The endogenous circadian temperature period length (tau) in delayed sleep phase disorder compared to good sleepers. *Sleep Res* 2013; 22: 617–24.

15 Dagan Y, Stein D, Steinbock M, et al. Frequency of delayed sleep phase syndrome among hospitalized adolescent psychiatric patients. *Psychosom Res* 1998; 45: 15–20.

16 Gruber R, Fontil L, Bergmame L, et al. Contributions of circadian tendencies and behavioural problems to sleep onset problems of children with ADHD. *BMC Psychiatry* 2012; 12: 212.

17 MacMahon KM, Broomfield NM, Espie CA. A systematic review of the effectiveness of oral melatonin for adults (18 to 65 years) with delayed sleep phase syndrome and adults (18 to 65 years) with primary insomnia. *Curr Psychiatry Rev* 2005; 1: 103–13.

18 Bijlenga D, Van Someren EJW, Gruber R, et al. Body temperature, activity, and melatonin profiles in adults with attention-deficit/hyperactivity disorder and delayed sleep: a case-control study. *J Sleep Res* 2013; 22: 607–16.

19 Wyatt JK, Stepanski EJ, Kirkby J. Circadian phase in delayed sleep phase syndrome: predictors and temporal stability across multiple assessments. *Sleep* 2006;29:1075–80.

20 Carpen JD, von Schantz M, Smits M, et al. A silent polymorphism in the PER1 gene associates with extreme diurnal preference in humans. *J Hum Genet* 2006; 51: 1122–5.

21 Palmer CR, Kripke DF, Savage HC Jr, et al. Efficacy of enhanced evening light for advanced sleep phase syndrome. *Behav Sleep Med* 2003; 1: 213–26.

22 Akerstedt T. Shift work and disturbed sleep/wakefulness. *Occup Med* 2003; 53: 89–94.

23 Flo E, Pallesen S, Magerøy N, et al. Shift work disorder in nurses--assessment, prevalence and related health problems. *PLoS ONE* 2012; 7: e33981.

24 Knutsson A. Health disorders of shift workers. *Occup Environ Med* 2003; 53: 103–8.

25 Folkard S, Tucker P. Shift work, safety and productivity. *Occup Med* 2003; 53: 95–101.

26 Wright KP Jr, Bogan RK, Wyatt JK. Shift work and the assessment and management of shift work disorder (SWD). *Sleep Med Rev* 2013; 17: 41–54.

27 Eastman CI, Burgess HJ. How to travel the world without jet lag. *Sleep Med Clin* 2009 4: 241–55.

28 Lockley SW, Dijk DJ, Kosti O, et al. Alertness, mood and performance rhythm disturbances associated with circadian sleep disorders in the blind. *J Sleep Res* 2008; 17: 207–16.

29 Hayakawa T, Uchiyama M, Kamei Y, et al. Clinical analyses of sighted patients with non-24-hour sleep-wake syndrome: A study of 57 consecutively diagnosed cases. *Sleep* 2005; 28: 945–52.

30 Wulff K, Dijk DJ, Middleton B, et al. Sleep and circadian rhythm disruption in schizophrenia. *Br J Psychiatry* 2012; 200(4): 308–16.

31 Myers E, Startup H, Freeman D. Cognitive behavioural treatment of insomnia in individuals with persistent persecutory delusions: A pilot trial. *J Behav Ther Exp Psychiatry* 2011; 42: 330–6.

32 McCurry SM, Ancoli-Israel S. Sleep dysfunction in Alzheimer's disease and other dementias. *Curr Treat Options Neurol* 2003; 5: 261–72.

33 Volicer L, Harper DG, Manning BC, et al. Sundowning and circadian rhythms in Alzheimer's disease. *Am J Psychiatry* 2001; 158: 704–11.

12

Parasomnias and Their Differentiation from Epilepsy

Chris Derry

Department of Clinical Neurosciences, Western General Hospital, Edinburgh, UK

Introduction

Accurately diagnosing attacks arising from sleep can be challenging, especially as there is a relatively wide differential diagnosis in this situation. Often the most difficult aspect is differentiating epileptic seizures, particularly those arising from the frontal lobes, from non-rapid eye movement (NREM) arousal parasomnias. In order to make an accurate diagnosis, a knowledge of the differential diagnosis is essential, along with an understanding of the role of the clinical history and investigations in the diagnostic process.

This chapter will address these areas and provide a practical approach to the diagnostic process.

Epileptic and Non-epileptic Conditions Presenting as 'attacks' from Sleep

Sleep-related Epilepsies

Most 'pure sleep epilepsies' (characterised by seizures arising exclusively or almost exclusively from sleep) are focal epilepsies which clinically manifest as complex partial or secondarily generalised seizures (see Chapter 19).

Tonic-clonic seizures are least likely to cause diagnostic confusion assuming a witnessed account is available. If not, unwitnessed features such as nocturnal tongue biting or urinary incontinence will often provide diagnostic clues.

More difficult are complex partial seizures (also known as 'focal seizures with dyscognitive features'). Such seizures can present in a range of ways, from brief arousals or periods of apparent confusion arising from sleep, to dramatic and bizarre seizures comprising complex or violent movements, limb posturing and vocalisation.

Sleep Disorders in Neurology: A Practical Approach, Second Edition.
Edited by Sebastiaan Overeem and Paul Reading.
© 2018 John Wiley & Sons Ltd. Published 2018 by John Wiley & Sons Ltd.

Frontal lobe epilepsy (FLE) most often causes the most diagnostic difficulty. While temporal lobe epilepsy is rarely a 'pure sleep epilepsy', and the presence of typical daytime seizures will usually help remove doubt over the nature of sleep-related events, this is not the case in FLE.

Seizures in FLE have a strong tendency to arise from sleep, and in some individuals occur exclusively, or almost exclusively, from sleep; this is often termed 'nocturnal frontal lobe epilepsy' (NFLE) [1]. More recently, however, the name 'sleep hypermotor epilepsy' (SHE) [2] has been adopted in place of NFLE, a change prompted by the fact that some individuals have typical seizure onset outside the frontal lobes [3].

The nature of seizures in NFLE/SHE can vary markedly from one individual to the next, and descriptions may seem extremely unusual or atypical for epilepsy. A description of the full range of possible features of frontal lobe seizure is covered elsewhere [4], but key properties include:

- Prominent bimanual or bipedal automatisms (such as cycling movements).
- Repetitive axial movements (such as rocking or twisting).
- Vocalisation (commonly screaming, but may also include coherent speech).
- Limb posturing.
- Retained (partial) awareness.
- Brief events (usually lasting less than 1 minute).
- Ambulation – standing or running (this is relatively uncommon).

In addition to their habitual seizures, individuals with NFLE also have frequent, brief arousals throughout NREM sleep (particularly stage N2). These are likely to be short 'fragments' of seizure activity, sufficient merely to cause arousal from sleep without progression to a 'full' seizure [5].

NFLE/SHE can therefore present in a variety of ways. At one end of the spectrum an individual can have dramatic events with screaming, running, and largely retained awareness; others may have more 'typical' frontal lobe seizures with stiffening (asymmetric tonic posturing) and kicking (bipedal automatisms); whilst others may have only frequent, brief, subtle arousals from sleep with associated daytime sleepiness. This wide variability often fuels diagnostic doubt when considering the possibility of NFLE/SHE in an individual with sleep-related attacks.

Non-epileptic Paroxysmal Events from Sleep

While excluding seizures is often a key consideration in this context, most individuals with attacks from sleep have a primary sleep disorder rather than epilepsy, and it is important to consider the range of conditions that can present in this manner. A full discussion of these is beyond the scope of this chapter, and is addressed elsewhere in this book, but conditions which may be confused with seizures are given below

NREM Arousal Parasomnias

NREM arousal parasomnias present with motor behaviours most frequently arising from slow wave sleep. As in NFLE/SHE there is a range of behaviours, from subtle to dramatic, and NREM arousal parasomnias are often subdivided according to the most prominent behaviours observed. 'Confusional arousals' are episodes of awakening with apparent confusion but little motor or emotional activity; 'sleepwalking' involves motor activity but little apparent emotion; and 'sleep terrors' are characterised by marked apparent fear or agitation. However, all these events are thought to reflect the same underlying process and there is considerable overlap between them.

NREM arousal parasomnias arise through a 'dissociation' of sleep states, and are best conceptualised as intrusions of wakeful behaviour into NREM sleep. The underlying mechanisms are not deeply understood, but genetic and maturational factors are clearly important. Other conditions causing a tendency to recurrent arousal (such as obstructive sleep apnoea, OSA) are sometimes identified as triggers. They usually begin in childhood, when they are very common, and tend to diminish in adolescence. While 15–20% of pre-adolescent children have had at least one episode of sleepwalking, only 1–4% of adults have ongoing NREM arousal parasomnias.

Due to the range of behaviours seen in both NFLE/SHE and NREM arousal parasomnias, these conditions are the most likely to cause diagnostic confusion in practice.

REM Sleep Behaviour Disorder

REM sleep behaviour disorder (RBD) results through a loss of physiological REM atonia, resulting in dream enactment ('oneiric') behaviours. It is strongly associated with neurodegenerative conditions, particularly parkinsonian conditions, and can predate the diagnosis by many years.

Onset of RBD is usually over the age of 50, and it has a strong male predominance. The events are often associated with clear dream recollection if the subject wakes during an event (which is not uncommon), and any observed behaviour is often concordant with the reported dream (e.g. running, punching, kicking). It is very unusual for an individual to stand or walk during these episodes. The patient typically remains lying down throughout although sometimes they may fall from the bed.

Overall the clinical presentation of RBD is usually sufficiently characteristic to prevent diagnostic confusion with NFLE/SHE.

Nocturnal Dissociative Seizures (Psychogenic Non-epileptic Seizures, 'Pseudoseizures')

Up to 60% of individuals with dissociative seizures report events from sleep. Video EEG studies show these arise from a 'pseudo-sleep' state, in which the EEG shows an awake pattern at onset even though the individual appears asleep behaviourally. Dissociative seizures restricted exclusively to pseudo sleep are uncommon, with most patients having events both in wakefulness and apparent sleep.

Nocturnal Panic

During panic attacks the patient typically wakes with a feeling of intense fear and associated tachycardia. Return to sleep is difficult and vivid recall of the events is usual. Nocturnal panic attacks occur in around half of people with an established panic disorder. Although a small subgroup of patients have symptoms predominantly from sleep, purely nocturnal panic attacks are uncommon.

Obstructive Sleep Apnoea

OSA is common, and when it presents in a typical fashion (excessive daytime sleepiness in an overweight patient, with a good witness account of snoring, choking and apnoeic periods), diagnostic confusion is unlikely. Sometimes, however, in less typical cases, recurrent arousals in OSA can be confused with the brief arousals of NFLE (and vice versa).

Rhythmic Movement Disorder

Rhythmic Movemement Disorder (RMD) condition is characterised by stereotyped repetitive movements of the head and neck most often occurring at sleep onset, stage 1 sleep and during short arousals in light sleep. The most common movements are repetitive head rolling, body rocking and head banging. It is very common in infants but usually resolves by around the age of 5. It is uncommon in adulthood, although can occur in association with autism or intellectual disability. It should not be confused with epilepsy, although the relative rarity of the condition in adulthood may occasionally lead to misdiagnosis. Furthermore, in adults, the events can sometimes be limited to REM sleep episodes. The bed partner is usually the main complainant.

Periodic Limb Movements During Sleep

Periodic limb movements during sleep (PLMS) should not usually be confused with epilepsy, but this can occasionally occur in atypical cases, especially if movements are particularly vigorous.

Sleep Starts (also Known as Hypnic Jerks)

These common, quasi-physiological jerks at the transition from wakefulness to sleep are frequently associated with a hallucination of movement (often a sensation of falling). It is unusual for this phenomenon to cause diagnostic confusion.

Conclusion

In general, if an adequate history can be obtained, it is relatively straightforward to distinguish these various events from epilepsy. When diagnostic doubt remains, standard polysomnography (PSG) is usually helpful in addressing OSA, RBD, PLMS, and RMD, for example.

In clinical practice, NREM arousal parasomnias and NFLE/SHE are the conditions most frequently confused (Table 12.1 [6]). Both present as paroxysmal episodes from sleep, with a range of behaviours that can include bizarre or dramatic features. Moreover, both can be associated with a positive family history. There is a strong hereditary component seen in parasomnias and a genetic form of NFLE/SHE exists, inherited in an autosomal dominant fashion and associated with a number of genetic mutations predominantly involving genes for the $\alpha 4\beta 2$ nicotinic acetylcholine receptor [7].

Diagnosing Sleep-related Attacks

History

Taking a careful history, with a witness account, is critical in the accurate diagnosis of any sleep-related events, and in many cases this will be sufficient to make a confident diagnosis without recourse to investigations.

When NFLE/SHE appears possible, and distinction from NREM arousal parasomnias is a key concern, several specific points should be addressed [8]; these are covered in Table 12.2.

Clinical Scales

There are several clinical scales which have been developed to assist clinicians in the diagnosis of NFLE/SHE and parasomnias.

Table 12.1 Summary of clinical and EEG/polysomnographic features of NFLE/SHE.

	Disorders of arousal (NREM arousal disorders e.g. sleepwalking, sleep terrors)	NFLE/ SHE
Age at onset	Usually <10 years	Variable; usually childhood or adolescence
Positive family history	60–90%	Up to 40%
Attacks per night (mean)	1 or 2	3 or more
Episode frequency/ month	<1–4	20–40
Clinical course (over years)	Tends to disappear by adolescence	Often stable with increasing age
Episode duration	Seconds to 30 minutes	Seconds to 3 minutes (often <2 minutes)
Semiology of movements	Variable complexity; not highly stereotyped (on video)	Stereotyped on video monitoring, often vigorous movements
Trigger factors	Sleep deprivation, febrile illness, alcohol, stress	Often none identified
Associated conditions	Obstructive sleep apnoea	Often none identified
Ictal EEG	Mixture of slow waves, alpha and fast activity; no epileptiform features	Often normal, or obscured by movement. Frankly epileptiform ictal rhythms in <50%
Time of episodes during sleep	First third of night, but usually after 90 minutes of sleep	Any time, but may occur within first 30–60 minutes
PSG sleep stages when events occur	NREM stage N3	Usually NREM stage N2

Source: Ref. [6].

For NFLE/SHE, the Frontal Lobe Epilepsy and Parasomnias (FLEP) scale has been developed and validated in two studies [8,9]. Both studies found the scale to have a high positive predictive and negative predictive value, although in one study a high number of indeterminate scores were generated (around 30%), and the authors highlighted that two subjects with epilepsy were scored as parasomnias. It can be a helpful screening tool, particularly in situations when obtaining objective confirmation of the diagnosis is difficult due to infrequent episodes or limited access to investigations, for example, although its limitations should be recognised.

An alternative scale, the Structured Interview for NFLE (SINFLE), has more recently been developed [10]. This has been reported to have a low sensitivity for detecting NFLE (59%) though a high specificity (95%), and as yet it has not been independently validated.

It is, however, important to recognise inherent limitations of these scales. They effectively represent a standardised method of history taking, covering the key elements of the conditions, and are best considered as screening tools for NFLE/SHE.

Table 12.2 Key points to clarify in the history.

What time of night do the events occur?

- NFLE/SHE seizures usually occur during stage 2 sleep, and hence can occur at any time of night. Seizures can, and often, occur after falling asleep (within 30 minutes), or just before waking in the morning, when stage 2 sleep is prevalent
- In contrast, NREM parasomnias arise from slow wave sleep, and as such usually occur at least 1–2 hours after falling asleep, but in the first half of the night, in periods when N3 sleep is most prevalent

How many events tend to occur in a single night?

- Individuals with NFLE often, though not always, report multiple attacks in one night. Typically between 3 events and 8 events may be reported in a single night, and sometimes even more; 'clustering' is also common
- In contrast, parasomnias infrequently occur more than once or twice per night, and clusters are less often reported
- It can be helpful to ask about both the 'typical' number of attacks in a night, as well as the most an individual has ever had in a single night.

Is there any recollection of the events?

- In NFLE/SHE awareness may be retained in some attacks, often associated with feelings of breathlessness or muscle spasm
- NREM parasomnias tend to be associated with no recollection, or occasionally a vague recollection of 'something' having happened, but with no detail.

What behaviours occur during the episodes?

- Features of arousal, vocalisation, wandering, fear and distress, may be seen in both conditions, and there are few specific individual features which discriminate between the conditions
- Stiffening and dystonic posturing are often seen in NFLE/SHE (reflecting involvement of the supplementary motor area) is very unusual in parasomnias
- A high degree of interaction with the environment (conversations with people, complex behaviours such as opening cupboards, turning on lights, etc.) is common in parasomnias and uncommon in NFLE/SHE (although is occasionally seen in the latter)

Are the events always the same?

- A high degree of stereotypy tends to favour NFLE/SHE, but getting a reliable history in this respect is not always easy

How long do the episodes last?

- NFLE seizures are usually very brief, lasting less than 1 minute, and often under 30 seconds
- NREM parasomnias can also be brief, but often last for several minutes; some may go on for 15 minutes or longer, with a waxing and waning quality

At what age did the events start?

- NFLE can begin at any age. The mean age of onset is 14 years, but onset in infancy or adulthood is common
- NREM parasomnias tend to appear in childhood, with a peak prevalence at between 5 years and 10 years

---

Sometimes, however, even the most careful history will not lead to a definitive diagnosis. In people who sleep alone there may be no collateral history available; in others, the presentation lacks key distinguishing features, or has elements that may favour either condition. In this situation, further investigations are required.

Investigations

There are a range of investigations which may be useful in clarifying the diagnosis of paroxysmal attacks. The availability of these to clinicians will vary, but more specialised tests such as long-term video electroencephalography (EEG) monitoring and PSG will generally require referral to a specialist unit. A summary flow chart of investigations is provided in Figure 12.1.

Routine and Sleep-deprived EEG

EEG, including recording periods of sleep, is generally recommended in the investigation of suspected NFLE/SHE [2]. However, it is important to recognise the diagnostic limitations of this investigation. Whilst the presence of epileptiform discharges strongly suggests a diagnosis of epilepsy, fewer than 50% of patients with NFLE have such EEG changes [1]. On the other hand, minor 'non-specific' EEG changes may be seen in both NFLE and parasomnias, such changes are entirely non-diagnostic, and the clinician must be careful not to 'over-interpret' these.

Neuroimaging

Whilst the finding of an epileptogenic lesion on neuroimaging favours a diagnosis of epilepsy in the appropriate clinical context, only a small minority of patients with NFLE/SHE have such a lesion [1]. Again, caution is required to avoid over-interpretation of non-specific or incidental findings.

Home Video

Video recording provides important diagnostic information in this context. Prior to or in the absence of easily available video-EEG/PSG studies, simple home video can be performed. While there are inherent limitations to recording episodes through home

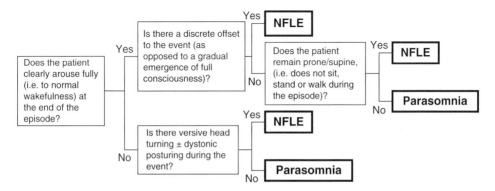

Figure 12.1 Flow chart to illustrate diagnostic process. Note that the diagnosis may be reached at any step along the process; however, further investigation is indicated if diagnostic uncertainty remains. NFLE, nocturnal frontal lobe epilepsy.

video, not least the problems in recording the onset of episodes, if adequate recording of events can be obtained this can be an effective way to establish the diagnosis. Key features on video are considered in the 'Video analysis of events' section below.

Standard PSG

If diagnostic doubt persists despite EEG, neuroimaging and home video, inpatient monitoring may be required.

Standard PSG generally involves monitoring for a single night, and with limited EEG channels. If events are recorded on video, this can be highly effective in the diagnosis, particularly as other key variables (such as sleep stage at onset) can be recorded, and the presence or absence of other potentially relevant conditions such as obstructive sleep apnoea hypopnoea syndrome established.

However, with only a single night of monitoring events may not be recorded. Also, the limited EEG montage makes the identification of ictal EEG rhythms more difficult.

Video-EEG Monitoring or Combined Video-EEG/PSG

Prolonged video-EEG monitoring, with or without full PSG, may be preferable to standard PSG in some situations, particularly of there is a high suspicion of NFLE/SHE and events are not occurring every night. This investigation will usually involve admission and monitoring for at least 96 hours, and often longer, increasing the chances of a seizure being recorded.

Even when seizures are captured using video-EEG monitoring, however, the ictal EEG may be non-diagnostic, with only around half of NFLE/SHE seizures being associated with a clear ictal rhythm [1]. In the remaining cases, a combination of prominent movement and muscle artifact produces non-diagnostic EEG changes with short seizure duration or deep seizure foci. Nevertheless, in such cases, careful analysis of the video recording can still provide confident diagnosis; this will be assessed in the next section.

Video Analysis of Events

As stressed previously, in many situations, a careful clinical history will be sufficient to make a confident diagnosis whereas investigation findings (such as interictal abnormalities or an ictal EEG rhythm during an event) may provide a definitive diagnosis of NFLE/SHE in other cases. However, there are difficult clinical scenarios in which the both history is equivocal and investigations unhelpful. Typically, parasomnias are associated with normal or non-specific findings on standard investigations, and the majority of individuals with NFLE/SHE also have normal EEG, neuroimaging and EEG [1]. Therefore, normal investigations are generally non-contributory and do not favour either diagnosis.

Even when events are recorded on video-EEG monitoring or video PSG, diagnostic doubt may remain, as only around half of NFLE/SHE seizures are associated with diagnostic ictal EEG.

In this situation, video analysis can be crucial, as the 'semiology' (observed clinical signs and behaviours) may be definitive. If typical features of frontal lobe epilepsy such

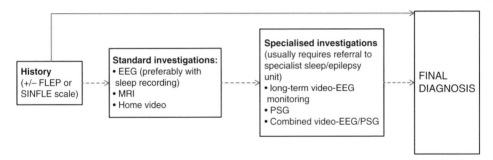

Figure 12.2 Diagnostic algorithm for distinguishing NFLE/SHE from parasomnias based on video recording only.

as asymmetric tonic posturing, and axial or bipedal automatisms are recorded, a confident diagnosis of NFLE/SHE may be possible even if no ictal rhythm is seen on EEG.

Conversely, a waxing and waning pattern of behaviours, a failure to arouse to full wakefulness after the event, and an indistinct offset to episodes favour a diagnosis of NREM parasomnia.

A detailed analysis of similarities and differences in the semiology of NFLE/SHE and parasomnias is beyond the scope of this chapter and can be found elsewhere [11]. However, an algorithm has been suggested to accurately distinguish NREM arousal parasomnias from NFLE/SHE seizures in one study that awaits replication (Figure 12.2).

Conclusion

Distinguishing sleep-related epileptic and non-epileptic paroxysmal episodes can be challenging. Differentiating between NFLE/SHE and NREM arousal parasomnias is often the most difficult aspect, but a careful history, potentially supplemented by the use of published ad hoc scales, may enable confident diagnosis in many cases.

Standard investigations, including EEG, magnetic resonance imaging, and PSG may sometimes give important diagnostic information, but these are often normal in both NFLE/SHE and parasomnias.

In difficult cases, recording of events on video-EEG/PSG is considered the gold standard diagnostic technique but this is not always available or achievable. Even when events are recorded, normal interictal and ictal scalp EEG does not exclude NFLE/SHE, meaning careful video analysis of events is essential.

Key Points

- The nature of seizures in NFLE/SHE can vary markedly from one individual to the next, and descriptions may seem extremely unusual or atypical for epilepsy.
- The distinction between nocturnal seizures and non-epileptic events (mainly parasomnias) can be difficult although a detailed and focused history is usually sufficient for a confident diagnosis.
- Video recording, ideally in the home environment, can be very helpful where there is diagnostic doubt.

References

1 Provini F, Plazzi G, Tinuper P, et al. Nocturnal frontal lobe epilepsy. A clinical and polygraphic overview of 100 consecutive cases. *Brain* 1999;122:1017–31.

2 Tinuper P, Bisulli F, Cross JH, et al. Definition and diagnostic criteria of sleep-related hypermotor epilepsy. *Neurology* 2016;86(19):1834–42.

3 Ryvlin P, Minotti L, Demarquay G, et al. Nocturnal hypermotor seizures, suggesting frontal lobe epilepsy, can originate in the insula. *Epilepsia* 2006;47(4):755–65.

4 Derry CP. The sleep manifestations of frontal lobe epilepsy. *Curr Neurol Neurosci Rep* 2011;11(2):218–26.

5 Nobili L, Sartori I, Terzaghi M, et al. Intracerebral recordings of minor motor events, paroxysmal arousals and major seizures in nocturnal frontal lobe epilepsy. *Neurol Sci* 2005;26(Suppl. 3):s215–9.

6 Derry CP, Duncan JS, Berkovic SF. Paroxysmal motor disorders of sleep: the clinical spectrum and differentiation from epilepsy. *Epilepsia* 2006;47(11):1775–91.

7 Marini C, Guerrini R. The role of the nicotinic acetylcholine receptors in sleep-related epilepsy. *Biochem Pharmacol* 2007;74(8):1308–14.

8 Derry CP, Davey M, Johns M, et al. Distinguishing sleep disorders from seizures: diagnosing bumps in the night. *Arch Neurol* 2006;63(5):705–9.

9 Manni R, Terzaghi M, Repetto A. The FLEP scale in diagnosing nocturnal frontal lobe epilepsy, NREM and REM parasomnias: data from a tertiary sleep and epilepsy unit. *Epilepsia* 2008;49(9):1581–5. doi: 10.1111/j.1528-1167.2008.01602.x.

10 Bisulli F, Vignatelli L, Naldi I, et al.Diagnostic accuracy of a structured interview for nocturnal frontal lobe epilepsy (SINFLE): a proposal for developing diagnostic criteria. *Sleep Med* 2012;13(1):81–7.

11 Derry CP, Harvey AS, Walker MC, et al. NREM arousal parasomnias and their distinction from nocturnal frontal lobe epilepsy: a video EEG analysis. *Sleep* 2009;32(12):1637–44.

13

Restless Legs Syndrome and Periodic Limb Movement Disorder

Thomas C. Wetter[1] and Christine Norra[2]

[1] *Department of Psychiatry and Psychotherapy, University of Regensburg, Regensburg, Germany*
[2] *LWL Hospital Paderborn and Department of Psychiatry, Psychotherapy and Preventive Medicine, Ruhr University Bochum, Bochum, Germany*

Introduction

Although widely varying in its severity, proactive questioning reveals that restless legs syndrome (RLS) is a very common phenomenon in a variety of populations. A term coined by Ekbom in 1945 [1], RLS (also named Willis–Ekbom disease) is characterised by an imperative desire to move the extremities, usually the legs, most often in association with unpleasant sensory phenomena. Relaxation or inactivity specifically worsens the symptoms whereas movement or vigorous rubbing relieves them, if only temporarily.

A key feature is that symptoms are worse or may occur uniquely in the late evening and night when sitting or lying in bed, often disrupting nocturnal sleep with subsequent significant daytime consequences like fatigue or sleepiness. Nocturnal sleep can additionally be disrupted by associated periodic limb movements (PLMs) which commonly coexist with RLS. PLMs are repetitive, usually stereotyped leg movements, most often bilateral, that resemble a slow version of the peripheral withdrawal reflex. In periodic limb movement disorder (PLMD), by definition, there needs to be a clinical consequence on sleep quality or daytime wakefulness caused by the leg movements, not attributable to any other sleep disorder. As such, it is often debated whether PLMD should be better assessed by movement disorder or sleep specialists. Indeed, the third edition of the International Classification of Sleep Disorders (ICSD-3) manual categorises both RLS and PLMD as 'sleep-related movement disorders' [2]. In any event, in the sleep clinic, it is not uncommon to diagnose PLMD in the absence of a clear history of abnormal leg movements or, indeed, with the condition never having been previously considered.

In the early 1980s, Coleman [3] was the first to propose standardised scoring criteria for PLMs that were modified by the World Association of Sleep Medicine (WASM) in 2006 and later by the American Academy of Sleep Medicine (AASM) in 2007 [4].

Sleep Disorders in Neurology: A Practical Approach, Second Edition.
Edited by Sebastiaan Overeem and Paul Reading.
© 2018 John Wiley & Sons Ltd. Published 2018 by John Wiley & Sons Ltd.

The latter criteria were recently included in the ICSD-3 definition of PLMD [2]. Still, whether PLMD in a relatively pure form represents a single disease entity or is part of the phenotypic spectrum of RLS remains a matter of controversy and debate.

Clinical Aspects

In 1995, the International RLS Study Group developed standardised criteria for the diagnosis of RLS which have been modified and updated [5] and partly included into the ICSD-3 criteria [2] (Table 13.1). The onset of RLS symptoms often follows a fluctuating course with periods of improvement or remission over a period of weeks, months, or even years. The precise expression of symptoms varies widely from patient to patient. Overall, however, the frequency and severity of symptoms tend to progress with age and permanent remissions are considered rare. To assess the severity of symptoms and to monitor treatment outcome, the International RLS Study Group rating scale for RLS may be applied, i.e. a 10-item questionnaire instrument with a Likert scale ranging symptoms of RLS from none to very severe (0–4 points). Scoring criteria are: mild (score 1–10); moderate (score 11–20); severe (score 21–30); and very severe (score 31–40) [6]. More specifiers for the clinical course of RLS have been established: in chronic-persistent RLS symptoms when not treated would occur on average at least twice weekly for the past year whereas in intermittent RLS less than twice a week for the past year with at least five lifetime events [5].

Table 13.1 Diagnostic criteria for restless legs syndrome according to ICSD-3.

Criteria A–C must be met

A) An urge to move the legs, usually accompanied by or thought to be caused by uncomfortable and unpleasant sensations in the legs.[1,2] These symptoms must:

   1) Begin or worsen during periods of rest or inactivity such as lying down or sitting.

   2) Be partially or totally relieved by movement, such as walking or stretching, at least as long as the activity continues;[3] and

   3) Occur exclusively or predominantly in the evening or night rather than during the day.[4]

B) The above features are not solely accounted for as symptoms of another medical or a behavioural condition (e.g. leg cramps, positional discomfort, myalgia, venous stasis, leg oedema, arthritis, habitual foot tapping).

C) The symptoms of RLS cause concern, distress, sleep disturbance, or impairment in mental, physical, social, occupational, educational, behavioural, or other important areas of functioning.[5]

Notes

1) Sometimes the urge to move the legs is present without the uncomfortable sensations, and sometimes the arms or other parts of the body are involved in addition to the legs.

2) For children, the description of these symptoms should be in the child's own words.

3) When symptoms are very severe, relief by activity may not be noticeable but must have been previously present.

4) As a result of severity, treatment intervention, or treatment-induced augmentation, the worsening in the evening or night may not be noticeable but must have been previously present.

5) For certain research applications, such as genetic or epidemiological studies, it may be appropriate to omit criterion C. If so, this should be clearly stated in the research report.

Source: Ref. [2]. Reproduced with permission of Elsevier.

When using standardised diagnostic criteria population-based surveys have consistently shown that between 5% and 10% of the general population in various parts of Europe and North America have the cardinal and defining symptoms of RLS [7]. Females are twice as likely to be affected, and about 20–30% of females will experience RLS to varying degrees during pregnancy. However, the lack of recognition of RLS by primary care physicians as an identifiable and treatable phenomenon undoubtedly leads to underdiagnosis or even misdiagnosis. Many patients, particularly, but not always, at the mild end of the spectrum also fail to seek medical advice.

In elderly populations, co-morbid medical conditions including hypertension, cardiovascular disease, stroke, fibromyalgia or irritable bowel syndrome as well as polypharmacy may confuse accurate diagnosis. Mental health co-morbidities such as mood disorders, especially depression and anxiety disorders, may also contribute to the complex picture with substantial impact on quality of life. Conversely, although prevalence studies suggest low rates in children, RLS certainly exists and may account for symptoms wrongly attributed to 'growing pains' or attention deficit hyperactivity disorder (ADHD).

PLMs are a common polysomnographic finding even in the absence of complaints of sleep disruption, particularly in the elderly. A PLM index >5 (which is arbitrarily regarded as abnormal) can be found in up to 45% of subjects older than 60 years [8]. PLMs are also found, possibly incidentally, in a large variety of sleep disorders including insomnia, sleep apnoea, hypersomnia, narcolepsy, Parkinsonism, and rapid eye movement (REM) sleep behaviour disorder. However, the association is particularly tight with RLS (a PLM index >5 is present in 80–90% of RLS patients). Although PLMs are common, PLMD, namely, PLMs with symptomatic sleep disruption, is thought to be relatively rare. A large-scale study using a telephone interview and the ICSD criteria from 1990 established prevalence rates of 3.9% in a random multinational population sample [9]. In PLMD, although PLMs may be associated with an EEG arousal or a brief awakening (Figure 13.1), subjects are often unaware of excessive limb movements or even sleep disruption and it is the observation of the bed partner that suggests their presence.

Pathophysiological Aspects

RLS is usually divided into idiopathic (primary) and symptomatic (secondary) forms although the clinical presentation is identical. Approximately 50% of the patients with the idiopathic form report a positive family history with at least one affected first-degree relative. Typically, patients with a positive family history have a much younger age of onset and there is sometimes a suggestion of 'anticipation' with an earlier onset in subsequent generations. Large pedigrees with familial RLS also suggest a strong genetic contribution to RLS. Meanwhile, several chromosomal loci and some common genetic variants within regions including MEIS1 or BTBD9 have been identified as genetic predisposition (for a review see Ref. [10]). In a recent meta-analysis, 13 novel-risk loci associated with RLS were identified confirming MEIS1 as the strongest risk factor [11].

In contrast to idiopathic RLS, there are many potential causes or contributors to secondary RLS, usually occurring later in life, occasionally in association with clinical abnormalities on examination. The commonest associations are pregnancy, especially

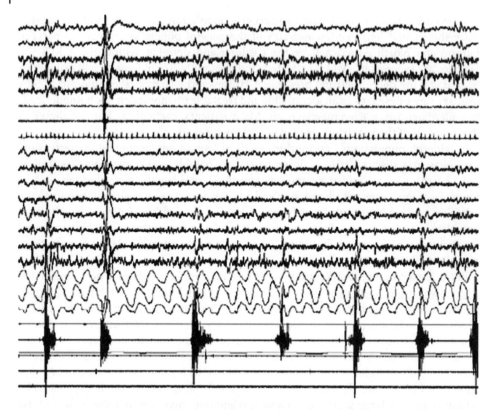

Figure 13.1 This 90-second epoch of a nocturnal polysomnography of a patient with periodic limb movement disorder contains seven periodic leg movements during sleep. The overall PLMs index was 48/h. The PLMs (in this epoch only present in the right leg) occur every 10–15 seconds during sleep stage 2. Each leg movement is associated with an EEG arousal.

in the later trimesters with complete relief of symptoms after delivery; anaemia due to iron or folic acid deficiency; and end-stage renal disease. At least 20–30% of uremic patients meet the clinical criteria for the diagnosis of RLS. In addition, peripheral neuropathies (even if subclinical), radiculopathies, rheumatoid arthritis, and Isaac syndrome have all been identified as provoking RLS. Nerve conduction studies may reveal a peripheral or spinal cord origin. It remains debatable whether Parkinson's disease is an independent RLS risk factor although RLS is undoubtedly recognised in this patient group.

Based on worsening of RLS symptoms by dopaminergic antagonists, SPECT and PET studies of the nigrostriatal pre- and postsynaptic receptor binding potentials have shown conflicting results, possibly reflecting a subtle receptor dysfunction of the central dopaminergic system (for a review see Ref. [12]). Consequently, it is important to consider that certain drugs including dopamine D2 receptor blocking agents, some antidepressants such as selective serotonin reuptake inhibitors (SSRIs), serotonin and norepinephrine reuptakte inhibitors (SNRIs), mirtazapine or atypical antipsychotics may evoke or worsen RLS and/or PLMD. Also, antihistamines may exacerbate RLS symptoms possibly due to increase of hypocretin-1 (orexin A) that is mediated by histamine and interacts with the dopaminergic system [13].

Central nervous iron deficiency with subsequent dysfunctional dopaminergic system is now considered a major etiologic factor of RLS. Of possible relevance, iron acts as a cofactor of tyrosine hydroxylase converting levodopa to dopamine. Thus, abnormalities of the iron metabolism have been suggested to be involved in reduced brain iron and ferritin concentrations (cerebrospinal fluid), as well as dopamine D2 receptor dysfunction in patients with RLS [14,15]. Moreover, there is a potential pathophysiological link between RLS and ADHD with similar features, notably, dopaminergic hypoactivity, iron deficiency and shared genetic polymorphisms [16].

Altogether, genetic risk factors at one end and major environmental or co-morbid disease at the other end seem to represent the spectrum of interaction with evolution of RLS [17].

Diagnostic Procedures

RLS is a clinical diagnosis based solely on history of symptoms. However, investigations are often appropriate to exclude secondary causes and to differentiate RLS from similar disorders that may mimic elements of RLS. Table 13.2 outlines a suggested scheme for investigations. If a peripheral neuropathy is suspected from history or clinical findings such as areflexia and nerve conduction studies a search for treatable underlying causes may be worthwhile. Full polysomnography is rarely needed and of little use in diagnosing RLS. However, it can be useful in quantifying the severity and extent of associated PLMs in the context of RLS or PLMD and their disruptive effects on sleep architecture.

The diagnosis of PLMD ideally requires objective measurement of PLMs by nocturnal polysomnography, or actigraphy if there is sufficient expertise for confident interpretation of the data. The diagnostic criteria for PLMD according to the ICSD-3 [2] and scoring of PLMs as defined by the AASM [4] are summarised in Tables 13.3 and 13.4. According to the International (IRLSSG) and European (EURLSSG) Restless Legs Syndrome Study Group criteria, PLMs include at least four consecutive candidate leg movements (CLMs) with an intermovement interval of ≥10 seconds and ≤90 seconds without any CLM preceded by an interval of <10 seconds interrupting the PLM series. The criteria also state the duration of any PLM (monolateral or bilateral) should be between 0.5 seconds and 10 seconds [18]. The differential diagnosis of PLMD includes other involuntary movements occurring during sleep such as normal phenomena at the sleep–wake transition (e.g. hypnic jerks), as well as sleep-related epilepsy, propriospinal myoclonus, REM sleep behaviour disorder, rhythmic movement disorders of sleep, or nocturnal paroxysmal dystonia. In addition, sleep-related breathing disorders and

Table 13.2 Clinical testing for restless legs syndrome.

Tests considered mandatory: haemoglobin, urea, creatinine and electrolytes, serum ferritin and total iron binding capacity

Tests occasional helpful when there are clinical pointers: thyroid function tests, glucose, B12 and folate levels, nerve conduction studies

Tests rarely helpful unless clear indication or diagnostic confusion: cerebrospinal fluid analysis for inflammatory markers, video-polysomnography, actigraphy

---

Table 13.3 Diagnostic criteria for periodic limb movement disorder.

Criteria A–D must be met

A) Polysomnography demonstrates PLMS, as defined in the most recent version of the American Academy of Sleep Medicine (AASM) Manual for the Scoring of Sleep and Associated Events.

B) The frequency is >5/hour in children or >15/hour in adults.[1]

C) The PLMS cause clinically significant sleep disturbance or impairment in mental, physical, social, occupational, educational, behavioural, or other important areas of functioning.[2,3]

D) The PLMS and the symptoms are not better explained by another current sleep disorder, medical or neurological disorder, or mental disorder (e.g. PLMS occurring with apnoeas or hypopnoeas should not be scored).[4,5]

Notes

1) The PLMS index must be interpreted in the context of a patient's sleep-related complaint. In adults, normative values greater than five per hour have been found in studies that did not exclude respiratory event-related arousals (using sensitive respiratory monitoring) and other causes for PLMS. Data suggest a partial overlap of PLMS index values between symptomatic and asymptomatic individuals, emphasising the importance of clinical context over an absolute cut-off value.

2) If PLMS are present without clinical sleep disturbance or daytime impairment, the PLMS can be noted as a polysomnographic finding, but criteria are not met for a diagnosis of PLMD.

3) The presence of insomnia or hypersomnia with PLMS is not sufficient to establish the diagnosis of PLMD. Studies have shown that in most cases the cause of the accompanying insomnia or hypersomnia is something other than the PLMS. To establish the diagnosis of PLMD, it is essential to establish a reasonable cause-and-effect relationship between the insomnia or hypersomnia and the PLMS. This requires that other causes of insomnia such as anxiety or other causes of hypersomnia such as obstructive sleep apnoea or narcolepsy are ruled out. PLMS are common, but PLMD is thought to be rare in adults.

4) PLMD cannot be diagnosed in the context of RLS, narcolepsy, untreated obstructive sleep apnoea, or REM sleep behaviour disorder; PLMS occur commonly in these conditions but the sleep complaint is more readily ascribed to the accompanying disorder. The diagnosis of RLS takes precedence over that of PLMD when potentially sleep-disrupting PLMS occur in the context of RLS. In such cases, the diagnosis of RLS is made and the PLMS are noted.

5) When it is reasonably certain that the PLMS has been induced by medication, and full criteria for PLMD are met, it is preferred that the more specific diagnosis of PLMD be used, rather than 'Sleep related movement disorder due to a medication or substance'.

PLMD, periodic limb movement disorder; PLMS, periodic limb movement during sleep; RLS, restless legs syndrome.
Source: Ref. [2]. Reproduced with permission of Elsevier.

associated general restlessness following apnoea-related arousals may mimic PLMD. For such differentiation, full polysomnography including video monitoring of movements may be needed.

A number of conditions other than RLS must be considered in the differential diagnosis of altered sensations in the legs with positive sensory phenomena. These include disorders of the peripheral nervous system such as small fibre sensory neuropathies and syndromes reflecting irritation or compression of peripheral nerves. Nocturnal leg cramps, 'painful legs and moving toes', and vascular insufficiency can occasionally be mistaken for RLS. Altered lower limb sensations and motor restlessness are also reported in patients with general anxiety disorders and ADHD. Akathisia in association with antipsychotic medication may superficially resemble RLS but patients do not

Table 13.4 Definition of PLMS according to the American Academy of Sleep Medicine [4].

A) A LM event is characterised by the following aspects:
  1) Minimum duration: 0.5 seconds.
  2) Maximum duration: 10 seconds.
  3) Minimum amplitude: 8 μV increase in EMG voltage above resting EMG.
  4) Onset: time-point when minimum amplitude is reached.
  5) End: marked when EMG amplitude is below 2 μV above resting EMG for at least 0.5 seconds.
B) A PLM series is defined as follows:
  1) Minimum of four consecutive LM events.
  2) Minimum period between LMs: 5 seconds.
  3) Maximum period between LMs: 90 seconds.
  4) LM in different legs separated by <5 seconds between LM onset is regarded as a single LM.

LM, leg movement.

report any circadian rhythm in the urge to move their legs. Furthermore, any witnessed movements tend to be continuous and are relatively unconcerning to the subject.

Given the improvement of RLS symptoms in some patients with a single dose of a dopaminergic agent such as levodopa, some authorities advocate that such a drug challenge can be used to help diagnosis. It is claimed to have a high sensitivity and specificity in subjects with RLS and is considered as a supportive feature although is not a widespread practice [19].

Management

General Aspects

The decision to start treatment should always depend on an individual's severity and frequency of symptoms and the degree to which they interfere both with daily activities and nocturnal sleep. Clearly if an underlying potentially treatable cause is revealed, specific therapies such as iron replacement are appropriate. Most authorities recommend an empirical trial of iron replacement if ferritin levels are below 50 or 75 μg/l even in the absence of anaemia. Folic acid replacement has also been shown to be of benefit in pregnancy or, obviously, in folic acid deficiency.

Non-pharmacological treatment may consist of specific physical strategies such as moving the legs in certain patterns or applying various sensory stimuli. However, exercise (for uremic RLS) as well as pneumatic compression devices are currently considered to be likely efficacious for the treatment of RLS and this approach rarely helps significantly if symptoms are more severe. Similarly, recommended modifications of sleep hygiene and lifestyle such as limiting alcohol and avoiding nicotine or caffeine rarely improve the situation for any length of time. Medication with RLS inducing or worsening properties (e.g. antidepressants, dopamine-blocking agents, sedating antihistamines) should be identified and if possible reduced or withdrawn without causing the patient harm. However, if antidepressants are necessary, the symptoms can usually be treated in the same way as primary RLS [20].

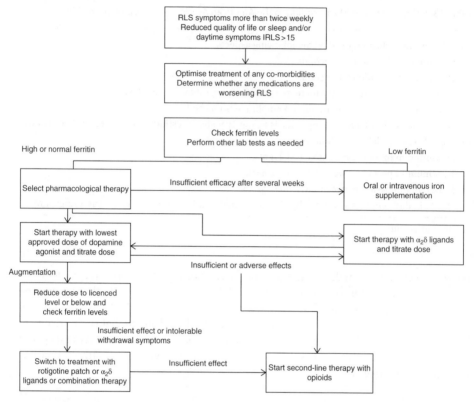

Figure 13.2 Flowchart outlining a general strategy for the initation of pharmacological therapy for RLS, and management of augmentation based on clinical experience. *Source:* Adapted from Ref. [23]. Reproduced with permission of Springer Nature.

Pharmacological agents are often needed for adequate symptom control in RLS and, more controversially, PLMD. Effective treatments have been demonstrated in a number of large-scale multicentre trials over the last few years (for reviews see Refs [21,22]). Dopaminergic drugs, including levodopa and dopamine agonists, are currently regarded as the first-line treatment option in moderate to severe RLS. In chronic persistent RLS, $\alpha_2\delta$ ligands may also be considered. For the treatment of refractory RLS, a combination therapy (dopamine agonist and $\alpha_2\delta$ ligand) or high-potency opioids may be considered [20]. Refractory RLS is characterised by unresponsiveness to monotherapy with tolerable doses of first-line agents due to reduction in efficacy, augmentation, or adverse effects (Figure 13.2 [23]).

Therapy of PLMD, if indicated, is assumed to be similar to the treatment of RLS, although there are insufficient placebo-controlled treatment trials specifically targeting PLMD (for a review see Ref. [24]).

Dopaminergic Agents

Levodopa

Evidence-based guidelines have identified levodopa as effective in the treatment of RLS [21,22,24]. Levodopa plus a decarboxylase inhibitor (carbidopa or benserazide) generally results in robust initial relief with the first dose. Controlled studies have shown the efficacy of levodopa both in idiopathic and uremic RLS. In subsequent comparative studies, levodopa was found to be effective in reducing RLS, but was inferior to prami-pexole and ropinirole in that respect. To avoid augmentation, a serious problem with dopaminergic treatment, the daily dosage should be lower than 300 mg/day. Adverse events may also include dry mouth, nausea, vomiting, headache or drug-induced insomnia, and sleep disruption, especially in the elderly. Early morning rebound of symptoms may occur, necessitating a second dosing during the night or the prescrip-tion of a sustained-release formula. Thus, levodopa can be recommended for patients with intermittent but not daily RLS.

Dopamine Agonists

Dopamine agonists are regarded as first-line treatment for moderate to severe primary RLS, especially if daily treatment is required. This is due to their well-documented effectiveness and overall good tolerability (for reviews see Refs [21,22,24]). The available dopamine agonists differ considerably with respect to pharmacokinetics (e.g. half-life), dopamine receptor profiles, potential serious side effects, availability of long-term experience, and licensing status. If dopamine agonists are considered, there is a need to increase the dosage slowly to avoid side effects, making these drugs less suitable to use on an intermittent basis.

Concerns regarding the development of 'sleep attacks', following observations in Parkinson patients started on low-dose dopamine agonists, do not seem to be a major concern in RLS. However, although probably more common in levodopa treatment, long-term studies suggest that augmentation may also occur with most of the dopamine agonists. In addition, some patients may experience impulse control disorders, such as pathological gambling [20].

Non-ergot Derivatives

Pramipexole has been shown to be effective in reducing sensory restless legs symptoms and PLMs in controlled and open-label trials for time spans between one night and several months [25]. Titration of pramipexole is usually started at 0.125 mg and increased every few days. Most patients require 0.75 mg or less, and patients taking higher doses should be carefully monitored for adverse effects, especially augmentation (Table 13.5).

Several placebo-controlled and open-label studies have shown that ropinirole is effec-tive in significantly improving both the subjective of RLS and objective measurements of its consequences for periods of up to 52 weeks [26]. Ropinirole is generally well toler-ated with early response to treatment initiation at first dose. Ropinirole is usually started at 0.25 mg although most cases require around 2 mg with maximum doses in individual patients of up to 4 mg.

Table 13.5 Non-ergot dopamine agonists for the treatment of restless legs syndrome.

	Receptor subtype	Half-life (h)	Starting dose (mg)	Daily dose range (mg)	Common side effects
Pramipexole	D2/D3	8–12	0.088	0.125–0.75	Nausea; headache; fatigue; vomiting
Ropinirole	D2/D3	~6	0.25	1–4	Similar to pramipexole

Rotigotine is designed to be administered as a transdermal patch for 24 hours continuous dopaminergic stimulation. A multicentre controlled study has shown that rotigotine applied once a day for 6 months (dose range 1–3 mg over 24 hours) significantly relieved the night- and daytime symptoms of idiopathic RLS [27]. Application site reactions were the most common adverse events in comparison with oral agonists in which nausea can be a significant and limiting side effect.

Ergot Derivatives

Although both pergolide and cabergoline have proven efficacy in reducing sensory RLS symptoms and PLMs both at sleep onset and during the night in placebo-controlled trials, they are rarely used in current practice. This is mostly due to concerns over potentially serious long-term side effects such as cardiac valvulopathies, constrictive pericarditis, and pleuropulmonary fibrosis. These problems have been well documented in Parkinson's disease treated with pergolide and cabergoline. Given the relative safety of non-ergot compounds, it is rarely appropriate to use pergolide or cabergoline in non-progressive, relatively benign conditions such as RLS or PLMD.

Augmentation

Unfortunately, all dopaminergic agents have the potential for causing 'augmentation' of RLS symptoms in which restlessness and associated sensory phenomena occur earlier in the day, often in a more severe form and involving additional body parts such as the arms. A detailed description of the key features of augmentation according to a WASM consensus report [28] is given in Table 13.6. Augmentation may develop as early as during the first month and in up to 82% of patients taking levodopa [29]. The occurrence typically correlates with higher daily doses (e.g. levodopa >300 mg). In terms of dopamine receptor agonists (pramipexole, ropinirole, rotigotine) augmentation may

Table 13.6 Key features of augmentation.

A or B and C for at least 1 week and a minimum of 5 days per week

A) Shifting of RLS symptoms to a period of time 2 h earlier than was the typical period of daily onset of symptoms before pharmacological intervention

B) Two or more of the following features:
- An increased overall intensity of the urge to move or sensation that is temporally related to an increase in daily medication dosage
- A decreased overall intensity of the urge to move or sensation that is temporally related to a decrease in the daily medication dosage
- The latency to RLS symptoms at rest is shorter than the latency with initial therapeutic response or before treatment
- The urge to move or sensations are extended to previously unaffected limbs or body parts
- The duration of treatment effect is shorter than the duration with initial therapeutic response
- Periodic limb movements while awake either occur for the first time or are worse than with initial therapeutic response or before treatment

C) No other medical, psychiatric, behaviour, or pharmacological factors explain the exacerbation of RLS

Source: Ref. [28]. Reproduced with permission of Elsevier.

also occur, but probably less frequently compared with levodopa treatment and possibly less common with rotigotine than with other dopamine agonists, which have a shorter duration of action.

As a consequence of augmentation, it may be necessary to discontinue levodopa and switch to dopamine agonists. If augmentation develops with dopamine agonists it may be helpful to reduce and/or to split the dosage to an earlier time or to switch to a rotigotine patch, a longer acting agonist. However, the physician should be aware that even low dose dopaminergics can cause augmentation. If augmentation still occurs it is necessary to switch to $\alpha_2\delta$ ligands or a combination therapy. In the case of insufficient effects, a second-line therapy with opioids may be necessary (Figure 13.2) [23].

Opioids

Opioids are generally considered as a second-line treatment of RLS. They are recommended in persistent or refractory RLS if symptoms fail to respond to dopaminergic medication or in cases where tolerance or augmentation are major issues [20]. Low- and high potency opioids such as oxycodone, tilidine, tramadol and methadone are successfully used in clinical practice although a number of patients take codeine bought from retail pharmacies as a non-prescribed drug (Table 13.7). High potency opioids may be very effective in the management of refractory RLS; in particular, a long-acting form of oxycodone may be most appropriate as shown in a recent randomised controlled trial [30]. Prolonged-release oxycodone–naloxone is approved for RLS therapy in Europe. Side effects of opioids include nausea and constipation, dizziness, sedation, nocturnal confusion, and worsening or even the development of sleep-related breathing disorders. Screening overnight oxymetry or polysomnography should be considered in the case of suspected sleep apnoea. Escalation of dose or dependency may not seem to be a major risk of long-term administration in the absence of a history of substance abuse [20]. Generally, these drugs are well tolerated at the recommended doses. It is likely that opioids perhaps in combination with dopaminergic agents, will improve symptom relief further in patients at the severe end of the RLS spectrum.

Table 13.7 Opioids for the treatment of restless legs syndrome. With the exception of oxycodone/naloxone opioids are not approved for RLS therapy in Europe.

Agent	Initial dose (mg)	Usual daily dose range (mg)
Oxycodone/naloxone	5	5–40 twice daily
Tilidine/naloxone Controlled release	50/4	50/4–200/16
Tramadol	50	50–200
Methadone	5	5–40
Propoxyphene	65	100–500
Dihydrocodeine	30	60–120

α$_2$δ Ligands: Pregabalin, Gabapentin and Other Anticonvulsants

Pregabalin (an analogue of γ-aminobutyric acid) or the structurally related compound gabapentin (α$_2$δ calcium channel ligands) may sometimes be considered as a drug of first line, particularly in patients with prominent unpleasant or frankly painful sensory symptoms. Both drugs are approved for the treatment of neuropathic pain and seizures, and pregabalin is also licensed for treatment of anxiety disorders. Also, pregabalin especially improves sleep disturbances in RLS patients. Randomised controlled randomised studies have shown favourable effects of gabapentin enacarbil (a prodrug of gabapentin, approved in the USA and Japan) and pregabalin [31,32]. Many patients require 900 to 1800 mg gabapentin daily, but doses up to 2700 mg can be used. Effective pregabalin doses are usually in the range of 150–450 mg/day. Class specific side effects include dizziness, somnolence and headache. These drugs may also directly enhance slow wave sleep which is characteristically deficient in RLS and PLMD. Combination with drugs mentioned previously such as dopamine agonists can be a useful strategy, however, controlled studies are lacking.

In idiopathic RLS, subjective relief of RLS symptoms has also been demonstrated with other anticonvulsants such as valproic acid, but the number of PLMs did not change. Carbamazepine may ameliorate subjective symptoms, but, again, recorded PLMs remain unchanged.

Benzodiazepines and Other Hypnotics

Clonazepam is regarded as an alternative treatment strategy in RLS and PLMD and is used to improve sleep continuity in a relatively non-specific manner. Combination treatment options that include clonazepam (0.5–2 mg) may suit individual patients. However, these longer acting agents may result in more adverse effects (e.g. cognitive impairment or risk of falls at night). In severe sleep onset insomnia or sleep fragmentation, the shorter acting hypnotics such as zolpidem (5–10 mg), or zaleplon (5–10 mg) may be helpful, usually on an intermittent basis [20].

Iron

Because iron deficiency is common in RLS, oral iron supplementation is an established treatment. Low ferritin concentration has been associated with an increased severity of RLS and treatment has been shown to improve symptoms. In addition, very low ferritin levels increase the risk of treatment complications, specifically augmentation. Serum ferritin levels – an indirect measure of brain iron status – should be at least 50 µg/l, and transferrin saturation not less than 20%. Therefore, RLS patients with low ferritin levels should be treated with iron supplementation before starting dopaminergic therapy (Figure 13.2). A common therapeutic regimen two to three times a day is 325 mg of ferrous sulfate combined with 100–200 mg of vitamin C to enhance absorption. Follow-up ferritin level determinations are needed initially every 3–6 months [20]. Oral iron therapy can cause constipation, nausea and abdominal discomfort. These side effects can be minimised by lowering the dose or by taking the iron with food. There is still insufficient evidence to draw conclusions on the efficacy of oral iron preparations for RLS patients. Likely efficacious are i.v. formulations of iron (e.g. iron sucrose 400–1000 mg four or five times or ferrocarboxymaltose 500–1000 mg once) though not yet approved for RLS therapy. This treatment may be considered for those patients whose iron deficiency is unambiguous and who are refractory to pharmacotherapy. Augmentation has not been reported. However, not all patients with iron deficiency benefit from iron supplementation. The current recommended treatment is to administer iron supplements to patients with iron deficiency and RLS, irrespective of whether they have associated anaemia [23]. Potential serious anaphylaxis and other adverse events have to be considered.

Magnesium supplementation may show beneficial effects in mildly affected RLS patients with a postulated magnesium deficiency.

Key Points

- RLS (Willis–Ekbom disease) is a common and underdiagnosed condition with a wide spectrum of severity.
- In the diagnostic work-up, it is important to search for potentially treatable causes for secondary RLS, such as iron deficiency.
- PLMs are very often present in patients with RLS but their clinical relevance is often unclear.
- When moderate or severe, RLS is a treatable condition and dopamine agonists are regarded as first-line treatment.
- For patients with severe RLS, opioid drugs are an option as second-line treatment.
- Because iron deficiency is common in RLS, ferritin levels should be checked. In patients with low ferritin levels, iron supplementation should be the first-line therapy.
- Augmentation is an important 'side effect' of dopaminergic agents, and sometimes difficult to treat.
- If sensory symptoms predominate, evidence suggests that pregabalin or gabapentin is effective often in combination with dopaminergic treatment.

References

1 Ekbom KA. Restless legs: a clinical study. *Acta Med Scand* 1945;158 (Suppl.):1–122.

2 American Academy of Sleep Medicine. International Classification of Sleep Disorders, 3rd edn. Darien, IL: American Academy of Sleep Medicine, 2014.

3 Coleman RM, Pollak CP, Weitzman ED. Periodic movements in sleep (nocturnal myoclonus): relation to sleep disorders. *Ann Neurol* 1980;8:416–421.

4 American Academy of Sleep Medicine. The AASM Manual for the Scoring of Sleep and Associated Events: Rules, Terminology and Technical Specifications, 1st edn. Westchester, IL: American Academy of Sleep Medicine, 2007.

5 Allen RP, Picchietti DL, Garcia-Borreguero D, et al. Restless legs syndrome/Willis–Ekbom disease diagnostic criteria: updated International Restless Legs Syndrome Study Group (IRLSSG) consensus criteria – history, rationale, description, and significance. *Sleep Med* 2014;15:860–873.

6 The International Restless Legs Syndrome Study Group. Validation of the International Restless Syndrome Study Group rating scale for restless legs syndrome. *Sleep Med* 2003;4:121–132.

7 García-Borreguero D, Egatz, R, Winkelmann J, et al. Epidemiology of restless legs syndrome: the current status. *Sleep Med Rev* 2006;10:153–167.

8 Ancoli-Israel S, Kripke DF, Klauber MR, et al. Periodic limb movements in sleep in community-dwelling elderly. *Sleep* 1991; 14:496–500.

9 Ohayon MM, Roth T. Prevalence of restless legs syndrome and periodic limb movement disorder in the general population. *J Psychosom Res* 2002;53:547–554.

10 Freeman AA, Rye DB. The molecular basis of restless legs syndrome. *Curr Opin Neurobiol* 2013;23:895–900.

11 Schormair B, Zhao C, Bell S, et al. Identification of novel risk loci for restless legs syndrome in genome-wide association studies in individuals of European ancestry: a meta-analysis. *Lancet Neurol* 2017;16:898–907.

12 Wetter TC, Klösch G. Functional neuroimaging of dopamine, iron, and opiates in restless legs syndrome. In: Neuroimaging of Sleep and Sleep Disorders, Nofzinger E, Maquet P and Thorpy MJ, eds. Cambridge: Cambridge University Press, 2013, pp. 363–374.

13 Allen RP, Mignot E, Ripley B, et al. Increased CSF hypocretin-1 (orexin-A) in restless legs syndrome. *Neurology* 2002;59:639–641.

14 Connor JR, Wang XS, Allen RP, et al. Altered dopaminergic profile in the putamen and substantia nigra in restless legs syndrome. *Brain* 2009;132:2403–2412.

15 Earley CJ, Connor JR, Beard JL, et al. Abnormalities in CSF concentrations of ferritin and transferrin in restless legs syndrome. *Neurology* 2000;54:1698–1700.

16 Walters AS, Silvestri R, Zucconi M, et al. Review of the possible relationship and hypothetical links between attention deficit hyperactivity disorder (ADHD) and the simple sleep related movement disorders, parasomnias, hypersomnias, and circadian rhythm disorders. *J Clin Sleep Med* 2008;4:591–600.

17 Trenkwalder C, Allen R, Högl B, et al. Restless legs syndrome associated with major diseases: A systematic review and new concept. *Neurology* 2016;86:1336–1343.

18 Ferri R, Fulda S, Allen RP, International and European Restless Legs Syndrome Study Groups (IRLSSG and EURLSSG). World Association of Sleep Medicine (WASM) 2016 standards for recording and scoring leg movements in polysomnograms developed by a joint task force from the International and the European Restless Legs Syndrome Study Groups (IRLSSG and EURLSSG). *Sleep Med* 2016; 26:86–95.

19 Stiasny-Kolster K, Kohnen R, Möller JC, et al. Validation of the 'L-Dopa test' for diagnosis of restless legs syndrome. *Mov Disord* 2006;21:1333–1339.

20 Silber MH, Becker M, Earley C, et al. Willis–Ekbom Disease Foundation revised consensus statement on the management of restless legs syndrome. *Mayo Clin Proc* 2013;88:977–986.

21 Hornyak M, Scholz H, Kohnen R, et al. What treatment works best for restless legs syndrome? Meta-analyses of dopaminergic and non-dopaminergic medications. *Sleep Med Rev* 2014;18:153–164.

22 Garcia-Borreguero D, Silber MH, Winkelman JW, al. Guidelines for the first-line treatment of restless legs syndrome/Willis-Ekbom disease, prevention and treatment of dopaminergic augmentation: a combined task force of the IRLSSG, EURLSSG, and the RLS-foundation. *Sleep Med* 2016;21:1–11.

23 Trenkwalder C, Winkelmann J, Inoue Y, et al. Restless legs syndrome – current therapies and management of augmentation. *Nat Rev Neurol* 2015;11:434–445.

24 Aurora RN, Kristo DA, Bista SR, et al. The treatment of restless legs syndrome and periodic limb movement disorder in adults – an update for 2012: Practice parameters with an evidence-based systematic review and meta-analyses. *Sleep* 2012;35:1039-1062.

25 Merlino A, Serafini F, Robiony M, et al. Clinical experience with pramipexole in the treatment of restless legs syndrome. *Expert Opin Drug Metabol* 2008;4:225–235.

26 Bogan RK. Ropinirole treatment for restless legs syndrome. *Expert Opin Pharmacother* 2008;9:611–623.

27 Trenkwalder C, Beneš H, Poewe W, et al. Efficacy of rotigotine for treatment of moderate-to-severe restless legs syndrome: a randomised, double-blind, placebo-controlled trial. *Lancet Neurol* 2008;7:595–604.

28 García-Borreguero D, Allen RP, Kohnen R, et al. Diagnostic standards for dopaminergic augmentation of restless legs syndrome: Report from a World Association of Sleep Medicine – International Restless Legs Syndrome Study Group consensus conference at the Max Planck Institute. *Sleep Med* 2007;8:520–530.

29 Allen RP, Earley CJ. Augmentation of the restless legs syndrome with carbidopa/levodopa. *Sleep* 1996;19:205–203.

30 Trenkwalder C, Beneš H, Grote L, et al. Prolonged release oxycodon-naloxone for treatment of severe restless legs syndrome after failure of previous treatment: a double-blind, randomised, placebo-controlled trial with an open-label extension. *Lancet Neurol* 2013;12:1141–1150.

31 Winkelman JW, Bogan RK, Schmidt MH, et al. Randomized polysomnography study of gabapentin enacarbil in subjects with restless legs syndrome. *Mov Disord* 2011; 26:2065–2072.

32 Allen RB, Chen C, Garcia-Borreguero D, et al. Comparison of pregabalin with pramipexole for restless legs syndrome. *N Engl J Med* 2014;370:621–631.

Part Three

Sleep in Neurological Disorders

14

Sleep Disorders in Parkinson's Disease and Other Parkinsonian Syndromes

Isabelle Arnulf[1], Valérie Cochen De Cock[2], Paul Reading[3] and Marie Vidailhet[4]

[1] Sleep Disorders Unit, Pitié-Salpêtrière Hospital (APHP), Sorbonne University, Paris, France
[2] Department of Neurology and Sleep Disorders, Clinique Beau Soleil, Montpellier, France
[3] Department of Neurology, James Cook University Hospital, Middlesbrough, UK
[4] Movement Disorders Unit, Pitié-Salpêtrière Hospital (APHP), CRICM UMR 975, and Paris 6 University, Paris, France

Introduction

Over the last two decades, the notion that idiopathic Parkinson's disease (PD) is predominantly a motor disorder simply reflecting nigrostriatal dopamine deficiency has been increasingly revised. As the disease advances, the non-motor aspects of PD are now considered at least as disabling as the more obvious motor deficits and are generally more difficult to manage. Alongside the well-established cognitive, neuropsychiatric, and autonomic problems seen in PD, significant sleep-related symptoms are now routinely assessed and sometimes treated. Although severe sleep disturbance is seen as a relatively new element to the spectrum of possible symptoms in PD, it is interesting to acknowledge that James Parkinson himself was aware that patients were often 'constantly sleepy' and 'exhausted'.

The whole gamut of sleep disorders may be seen in PD, occasionally in the same patient. Insomnia, particularly an inability to maintain the state of sleep, is extremely common. There are numerous potential causes for poor quality nocturnal sleep in PD including significant difficulties in moving around the bed during nocturnal awakenings secondary to hypokinesia. Excessive daytime sleepiness (EDS) can clearly result from poor overnight sleep, but is probably mainly caused by the underlying neurodegenerative process. Even when severe, EDS is often unreported by patients who often seem unaware of the extent of their somnolence. Finally, nocturnal disturbances such as parasomnias, particularly rapid eye movement sleep behaviour disorder (RBD), and prolonged confusional episodes are also a significant issue for many patients and carers alike.

Because of the potential complexity of sleep–wake problems in PD, it is difficult to define a typical symptom profile or, indeed, to construct simple protocols and guidelines for management. A further confound is that conventional PD drug treatment may fuel or even cause sleep-related symptoms. In reaching diagnostic conclusions, assuming

Sleep Disorders in Neurology: A Practical Approach, Second Edition.
Edited by Sebastiaan Overeem and Paul Reading.
© 2018 John Wiley & Sons Ltd. Published 2018 by John Wiley & Sons Ltd.

a detailed history is available, it is debatable what further useful information is gained from detailed sleep investigations other than clarifying the severity of the problem. Despite these caveats, it is argued that treatment options will exist for the vast majority of PD patients with sleep-related symptoms. However, treatments need to be tailored to individual patients and an empirical approach is often necessary, in the absence of formal evidence-based trial data.

In other parkinsonian syndromes (PSs), sleep disorders are also frequent and often severe. In multiple system atrophy (MSA), the most prevalent PS, the full spectrum of sleep disturbances can be seen with insomnia, EDS, RBD and also sleep-disordered breathing, frequently exacerbated by nocturnal stridor. Nocturnal stridor is associated with life-threatening episodes of respiratory failure causing sudden death during sleep and should, therefore, be treated promptly. In dementia with Lewy Bodies (DLB), RBD is so frequent that it has become one of the diagnostic criteria. In progressive supranuclear palsy (PSP), a tauopathy in contrast to the previous synucleinopathies, sleep disturbances may show a somewhat different spectrum. While insomnia and sleepiness are common, RBD is much less frequently encountered. Finally, there is a rare but interesting toxic tauopathy, 'Guadeloupian parkinsonism', caused by ingestion of soursop, a tropical fruit in which patients have a PSP-like syndrome with a particular spectrum of sleep disorders.

Clinical Epidemiology

Every study addressing the issue has confirmed that sleep disorders are both highly frequent and disturbing to patients with PSs, as well as their carers. In a community-based survey, 60% of PD patients complained of severely disturbed sleep, significantly more than in patients with diabetes mellitus (45%), or in aged controls (33%) [1]. There was no difference between groups regarding difficulty falling asleep but PD patients were twice as likely to report frequent (39%) or early morning (24%) awakenings than the other groups. Furthermore, when present, these problems were described as more distressing. The proportion of PD patients affected by 'broken sleep' rises to 76% in hospital samples [2].

Repeated sleep-related violence and nocturnal injuries are reported by 15% of PD patients [3]. RBD, usually reflecting violent or unpleasant dream enactment, is increasingly recognised and affects between 30% and 60% of patients [4,5]. In RBD, there is a striking and unexplained male predominance [6,7] in those who exhibit RBD without clinical parkinsonism, referred to as idiopathic RBD. The latter are at major (92%) risk of developing either PD or a similar neurodegenerative disorder in the fullness of time [8–10].

Case-controlled epidemiological studies performed in various countries addressing EDS have consistently found higher levels of somnolence in PD populations compared with age- and sex-matched controls [11–13]. The prevalence of significant EDS is probably around 30% although the figure varies between 16% and 74% in the published studies. It is even possible that a symptom of EDS may be a harbinger of PD as sleepy adults in a large Asian longitudinal study were 3.3 times more likely to develop PD in later life [14]. Of note, patients with idiopathic RBD have higher levels of daytime sleepiness than age-matched controls, sometimes reaching the level observed in patients with advanced

PD [15]. Very severe sleepiness such that patients fall asleep without recognising the prior imperative to sleep may affect a proportion of patients (1–4%) [16,17]. Such so-called 'sleep attacks' have led to major concerns regarding safe driving, particularly in generally less physically disabled younger patient groups.

Compared with PD, sleep disorders are even more frequent in MSA. As many as 70% of patients with MSA have significant sleep complaints, including sleep fragmentation (53%), early waking (33%), and insomnia (20%) [18]. EDS is present in about 50% of such patients [19]. Although the prevalence of restless legs syndrome (RLS) is only a little higher than the general population, periodic limb movements (PLMs) are recorded in almost all patients with severe MSA patients [18]. Nocturnal hallucinations seem to be much less common in MSA compared with PD but RBD affects 90–100% of patients [20,21], and may precede the onset of MSA by years [22]. Interestingly, RBD has been reported to disappear as the disease inevitably progresses [23]. Sleep apnoea is estimated to affect up to 37% of MSA patients [18–20] and nocturnal stridor from 13 to 69% of them [19,24,25].

Large epidemiological studies exploring sleep in PSP are not available although a case series with polysomnography (PSG) measurements showed severe insomnia in all sub-jects. Total sleep time dropped to between 2 hours and 6 hours with an average time awake per night of more than 4 hours [26]. Clinically, RBD is present in less than 15% of patients with PSP. Rapid eye movement (REM) sleep without atonia is detected by PSG a little more often, affecting about 30% of patients. The prevalence and severity of EDS is comparable with that found in PD [27]. Finally, in Guadeloupean parkinsonism, most patients complain about insomnia and, surprisingly, given its nature as a tauopathy, the majority have RBD confirmed on PSG [27].

Signs and Symptoms

Insomnia

A relative inability to fall and stay asleep appears a natural and inevitable consequence of normal aging. However, in parkinsonian patients, there are frequently additional factors which significantly worsen sleep. In general, there is a correlation between the degree of insomnia and the severity of motor symptoms although it is unclear how much dopamine deficiency per se contributes to the problem. In addition, advanced patients tend to be taking increased amounts of PD medication which may confound the picture and contribute to insomnia. A systematic and directed interview is probably the most effective method of assessing insomnia as sleep monitoring rarely reveals specific causes.

Particularly in patients with moderate to severe PD, special attention should be directed to disruptive nocturnal sensory and motor symptoms. Discomfort during the night is particularly common in PD patients and can have many causes. Symptoms of restless legs may affect 12–21% patients [28,29] although occasionally the combination of leg pain and additional akathisia in PD may mimic true RLS. Painful dystonia is also well described, particularly classical 'early morning dystonia'. Occurring during the latter part of the night, usually after a normal awakening, this typically presents as long-lasting, postural contractions of the toes in flexion or extension, sometimes with internal rotation of the ankle. The dystonic postures and associated discomfort make mobilisation difficult and may cause anxiety, inhibiting any attempts to return to sleep. Dystonia affecting other body parts such as the neck and back muscles may also occur only at night, presumably when cerebral dopamine levels are lower.

Nocturnal bradykinesia may also significantly disrupt sleep in some PD patients and should be addressed. An inability to turn in bed, adjust the pillows or leave the bed to urinate, for example, may produce prolonged arousals. The act of voiding urine may take many minutes and need to be repeated through the night, especially if incomplete or if there is associated confusion. Whether bladder instability contributes to nocturia in PD patients or whether the desire to pass urine occurs only after sleep is fragmented for other reasons remains uncertain. In any event, PD patients have, on average, twice as many nocturnal awakenings as controls [12] with most reporting between two and five prolonged arousals, lasting 30–40% of the nocturnal period [30,31].

More complex PSs are generally poorly levodopa responsive such that nocturnal symptoms linked to their 'off' state might be expected to be even worse. Further, in MSA, severe urinary dysfunction with associated frequent nocturia and often incontinence can be a major contributor to poor sleep.

The issue of mood disorder in PD is complex but is likely to impact on sleep quality as an independent factor in some cases. In particular, anxiety may increase nocturnal arousals and depression may disrupt sleep or its timing. In general, poor sleep quality in PD appears to correlate with depression and anxiety scores [32]. Anxiety is also likely to be enhanced by nocturnal bradykinesia.

The role of dopaminergic therapy in causing insomnia should also be considered. Agonists taken at bedtime may effectively act as stimulants and delay sleep onset [33]. The consequences of using supra-optimal doses of dopamine agonists and levodopa day and night should also be addressed in certain patients. Although often in denial, such patients often stay awake and are hyperactive at night, using computers, gambling, or engaging in other compulsive activities. This condition is identified as the dopamine dysregulation syndrome and affects up to 11% of patients with PD [34].

Many PD patients have great difficulty in waking at a conventional hour with early rising a particular problem. A circadian disorder typical for PD, perhaps mimicking advanced sleep phase syndrome, has been reported using actigraphy [35].

Excessive Daytime Sleepiness

EDS in PD can be reported by patients or only noticed by the carer as a significant symptom. In fact, it seems likely that PD patients are particularly poor at recognising their levels of sleepiness and will frequently even deny sleep episodes captured during objective investigations such as the Multiple Sleep Latency Test (MSLT) [36]. Napping after lunch is very common in PD patients and is often perceived as beneficial. In severe cases, the levels of sleepiness can resemble those seen in narcolepsy with sudden naps during activities such as eating a meal, walking, attending work, and, of particular concern, while driving a car. Sleep attacks can sometimes be confused with fainting caused by orthostatic or postprandial hypotension, symptoms associated with the dysautonomia seen in PD or, more commonly, MSA.

The Epworth sleepiness score (ESS) has been assessed specifically in PD [37] and scores above 10, as in other populations, usually suggest a significant problem. However, the ESS is poorly predictive of sleep attacks [16], perhaps due to the potential discordance between subjective and objective sleepiness witnessed in many PD patients [38]. Some authors have added specific questions to the ESS designed for PD, addressing the ability to fall asleep when driving, eating, working or performing regular housework activities [16], that might better predict the risk of driving-related accidents.

Finally, sleepiness in PD could be the result of a circadian dysfunction. The 24-hour melatonin rhythm, a marker of endogenous circadian rhythmicity has been shown to be blunted in patients with PD compared with controls. Those patients reporting sleepiness appear to have particularly impaired rhythms [39].

Sleep-disordered Breathing

Given the wide availability of effective treatments options, it is important to enquire about severe snoring and symptoms compatible with obstructive sleep apnoea (OSA) in PD that could be involved either in symptoms of insomnia or daytime sleepiness. Although PD patients tend to be thinner than control groups, the prevalence of OSA is about the same as in the general population. Other mechanisms might be involved in obstruction in these patients such as neuromuscular oropharyngeal dysfunction or an increased tendency to be supine in sleep secondary to hypokinesia, fuelling gravity-driven collapse of the tongue and pharyngeal soft tissue with subsequent airway occlusion [40].

In MSA, besides uncomplicated OSA, central alveolar hypoventilation is relatively common and could be secondary to the degeneration of pontomedullary respiratory centres. Patients with MSA may also develop severe nocturnal stridor, caused by a combination of vocal cord paralysis and excessive adductor activation during inspiration. Nocturnal stridor can occur in all clinical stages of the disease and is occasionally a presenting symptom [41]. It is characterised as a harsh, high-pitched, inspiratory crowing sound. It can be very loud, often disturbing the sleep of the bed partner. Although very distinct from normal heavy snoring, the two can occur together and even 'mix', making the diagnosis less easy. In a patient with PS, the presence of a nocturnal stridor is a reliable marker for MSA.

Nocturnal motor disturbances

Excessive motor activity during sleep in PD may range from repetitive jerks of the lower limbs reflecting PLMs to less stereotyped and more vigorous activity involving any body part in RBD. Movements in RBD tend to be brief or explosive, often incorporating the upper limbs in defensive manoeuvres. Punching, catching invisible objects, and slapping are typical activities, usually with the eyes closed. Purposeful use of nearby objects is exceptional and any violence or injury caused by the disturbance occurs incidentally. The lower limbs tend to be less involved although kicking and bicycling are frequently witnessed. Standing up and walking are very rare during RBD-related movements [7], although some RBD cases also exhibit associated sleepwalking behaviours arising from non-REM sleep [5]. Vocalisation is common and may precede motor activity in the limbs. Groaning, swearing and crying are typical although laughing and conversational speech are increasingly recognised. Intriguingly, motor activity and speech during RBD is often more fluid than appears possible during waking hours in generally bradykinetic patients with advanced PD [5] and MSA [42]. Subjects can usually be woken relatively easily from an RBD event and congruent dream activity is generally recalled, particularly in typically aggressive episodes. Although injury to the spouse may result, the violent dream often centres on protecting a loved one from animal or human aggressors.

In the presence of significant cognitive impairment, PD patients, especially in those with associated dementia, display prolonged confusional episodes arising from sleep, sometimes with associated hallucinatory and delusional intrusions. These events may resemble a form of 'disorder of arousal', akin to a non-REM sleep parasomnia although probably have a different underlying neurobiology. The term 'status dissociatus' is sometimes used, implying a loss of boundaries between wake and sleep.

Diagnostic Procedures

A directed interview with knowledge of the spectrum of potential sleep–wake problems seen in PD and other PSs, as well as the relative role of motor, cognitive and therapeutic factors is the key to successful diagnosis and treatment (Table 14.1). Three specific scales, the PD Sleep Scale, the SCOPA-sleep and PD Sleep Scale-2 (PDSS-2) can be helpful for research purposes addressing sleep issues in PD [43–45] but are no substitute for a detailed clinical history. The timing of drug doses can be relevant especially in assessing insomnia, especially if nocturnal symptoms might reflect dopaminergic

Table 14.1 Some relevant probes to assess sleep problems in Parkinson's disease and parkinsonian syndrome.

- How long does it take for you to fall asleep after switching off the lights in the evening? (>30 min implies significant sleep onset insomnia)
- Do you wake early and find it difficult to return to sleep?
- Do you have frequent awakenings at night?
- Are you confused or 'not yourself' during these awakenings?
- Does it take a long time for you to pass urine at night?
- How often do you need to urinate at night?
- Can you resume sleep easily after being awake during the night?
- How long do you sleep at night?
- Do you experience painful foot dystonia ('curled up toes') in the early morning?
- Do you have pain in some parts of your body during the night?
- Do you experience restlessness in the legs?
- Are you a snorer? Has your partner witnessed long gaps in your breathing?
- Are you talking, shouting, or swearing while asleep?
- Do you have nightmares (e.g. being attacked, defending your family against aggressors)?
- Has your partner observed you moving, kicking, or punching while asleep?
- Do you have hallucinations at night (seeing somebody or an animal in the bedroom)?
- Do you fall asleep when inactive during the day?
- Are you driving a car? Do you struggle to stay awake whilst driving?
- Do you experience partial hallucinations during the daytime (the feeling that there is somebody behind you, or that an animal or a person passes by you)?

underactivity. If RLS or PLMD are thought likely contributors, as in other patient groups, it is always worthwhile checking ferritin levels for iron deficiency as a reversible precipitant.

If EDS has been recognised, reducing any sedative drugs including opiate painkillers, long-acting benzodiazepines and sedative antidepressants should be first considered. Recent changes in dopaminergic therapy, particularly agonists, may also coincide with striking somnolence. Some younger patients appear to exhibit idiosyncratic reactions to agonists such that they suddenly develop EDS at narcoleptic levels [30]. Changing or discontinuing agonist therapies may help in this situation.

The precise roles of nocturnal sleep monitoring in PD and subsequent daytime investigations such as a MSLT are uncertain. Even if previously unexpected severe OSA or PLMs are revealed, their relevance to the overall sleep–wake disturbance is often unclear. However, the full extent of the sleep–wake dysregulation across a 24-hour period may be clearly demonstrated by investigations and the concept of 'secondary' narcolepsy has arisen in severely affected PD patients. Although the sleep–wake profile and investigation results may mimic those of idiopathic narcolepsy, in the absence of cataplexy, the underlying mechanisms are probably different. Video and audio observation at night may provide key information and allow differentiation of motor (bradykinesia, tremor, restless legs, PLM, RBD), behavioural (dopamine dysregulation syndrome) and respiratory (particularly stridor) problems in PD and PS.

If prominent jerks or violent behaviours, suggestive of PLMs or RBD, respectively, are reported, a first step is to check the drug history. The majority of antidepressants, including serotonin reuptake inhibitors, venlafaxine and mirtazapine, can exacerbate general motor restlessness, PLMs and RBD. Even if RBD appears extremely likely from the history, many authorities advocate detailed nocturnal sleep and video monitoring to address the possibility of prolonged apnoeic events in REM sleep triggering motor restlessness or abnormal arousals.

It should be mentioned that there may be particular problems with interpreting PSG data, particularly in advanced PD patients and especially if automated systems are used. Dissociated sleep states, including RBD, are frequently seen and phenomena such as continuous alpha background rhythm, non-specific sleep artifacts, and continuous eye movements during sleep combine to make accurate or reliable sleep staging very difficult (Table 14.2).

Management

Insomnia

Perhaps appropriately, there are no protocols or formal guidelines for treating insomnia in relation to PD and a flexible experience-based approach is much more useful than one hoping to rely on population-based trial data (Table 14.3). Simple measures to improve overnight comfort may often be overlooked. Examples include the use of sheets and bedclothes that slip easily and pyjamas without buttons. Similarly, having medication, water and other items such as a phone within easy reach of the bed may make a useful difference. Some parkinsonian patients develop rigid patterns of behaviour with respect to sleep–wake habits and drug taking. For example, some will set alarm clocks

Table 14.2 Abnormal findings on polysomnography and Multiple Sleep Latency Test in Parkinson's disease and parkinsonian syndrome.

	Abnormalities	Indicates
EEG		
	Slow (<8 Hz) alpha rhythm during relaxed wakefulness	Possible cortical degeneration Frequently associated with RBD
	Continuous alpha rhythm during all sleep stages	Unknown. Complicates the scoring process (not to be confused with complete insomnia)
Eye movements		
	Can be present during stage N2	Sleep dissociation. Complicates the scoring process. No associated clinical problem
	Square-wave jerks during wakefulness and REM sleep	Raises possibility of progressive supranuclear palsy as diagnosis.
Chin muscle tone		
	Enhanced tonic activity during REM sleep	REM sleep without atonia, preceding or associated with RBD
	Increased twitching during REM sleep	Possible vocalisation
Leg EMG		
	Frequent, periodic 0.5- to 10-s bursts	Periodic leg movement syndrome, possibly associated with restless legs syndrome
	4–6 Hz bursts	Parkinsonian tremor persists in sleep (can be seen on the chin too)
	2 Hz left/right alternating bursts	Alternative leg movement activity
	Long-lasting, prominent activity	Dystonia of leg muscles.
	Complex vigorous movements during REM	RBD
Respiratory sensors		
	Apnoeas	Sleep apnoea syndrome
	Stridor (inspiratory, harsh sound)	Multiple system atrophy more likely, reconsider diagnosis Treat stridor
MSLT		
	Mean latency lower than 8 min	Objective sleepiness demonstrated
	Plus two or more sleep onset REM periods (usually without atonia)	Criteria for secondary narcolepsy met

EEG, electroencephalography; EMG, electromyography; MSLT, Multiple Sleep Latency Test; RBD, rapid eye movement sleep behaviour disorder; REM, rapid eye movement.

Table 14.3 Management suggestions for sleep problems in Parkinson's disease patients.

Symptom	Possible problem	Proposed management
Frequent (>2) micturitions at night		
Normal volumes	Sleep apnoea syndrome	Check for sleep apnoea and treat appropriately
Small volumes, poor stream	Prostatism	Refer to urologist
Small volumes, good stream	Parkinsonism-associated polyuria	Consider intranasal desmopressin in the evening
		Have a bottle for collecting urine in the bedside table or an overnight sheath for males
Difficulty initiating sleep		
Early in the evening	Lights off too early (patient going to bed fatigued but not necessarily sleepy)	Switch off lights later
	Anxiety or behavioural insomnia	Sleep hygiene
		Treat anxiety
		Evening melatonin
		Zolpidem, zopiclone
Associated restlessness	Restless legs syndrome	Check for low ferritin (<75 mcg/L)
		Remove antidepressant drugs if possible
		If the diagnosis is uncertain, consider polysomnography with monitoring of leg movements
		Try gabapentin
		Try an opiate such as Tramadol 100 mg if not confused
Late in the night	Altered circadian cycle	Sleep hygiene,
		Decrease levodopa/ dopamine agonists in the evening
		Melatonin at the end of the afternoon
Late in night, hyperactive or hypomanic	Dopamine dysregulation syndrome	Remove dopamine agonists, levodopa monotherapy
		Neuropsychological assessment and follow up
Difficulty resuming or maintaining sleep		
With cramps, muscle pain, slowness	Nocturnal akinesia	Try immediate release levodopa with a glass of water during awakening
		Try long-acting dopamine agonists before bed
With restlessness	Restless legs syndrome	Check for low ferritin
		Remove antidepressant drugs
		Try gabapentin
		Try tramadol 100 mg if not confused

(Continued)

Table 14.3 (Continued)

Symptom	Possible problem	Proposed management
With anxiety	Anxiety disorder	Try evening sedative antidepressant
With low mood	Depressive disorder	Actively treat depression
Nightmares, agitation		
Confused at night when awake	Hallucinatory intrusions	Remove/reduce the evening dose of dopamine agonist and any other psychoactive agents (particularly tricyclics)
		Check for sleep apnoea;
		Try antipsychotic such as quetiapine/clozapine
Kicks, shouts, slaps	RBD	Secure the bed environment
		Reduce antidepressants
		Assess likelihood of sleep apnoea and consider performing video-polysomnography before treating
		Try clonazepam 0.5–2 mg in the evening
		Try melatonin 2–6 mg in the evening
Daytime sleepiness		
Falls asleep unexpectedly	Sleep attacks	Assess whether drug-related, particularly dopamine agonists, and remove/change
		Counsel for driving
Excessive and troublesome EDS		Explore levels of sleepiness and ask partner
		Consider polysomnography and MSLT
		Ask about associated hallucinations
		Treat sleep apnoea if moderate/severe
		Decrease/stop dopamine agonist during daytime and other potentially sedative drugs
		Consider L dopa instead of dopamine agonist
		Try daytime modafinil or methylphenidate
		Consider sodium oxybate before bed in severe cases

EDS, excessive daytime sleepiness; MSLT, Multiple Sleep Latency Test; RBD, rapid eye movement sleep behaviour disorder.

to take their first PD drug prescribed at a precise early morning time and then have difficulty in resuming sleep. Others might retire to bed at a fixed hour but be unable to fall asleep, generating further anxiety. In such cases, advice to be more flexible with sleep and drug timings may be beneficial.

Improving the continuity of sleep by manipulating dopaminergic therapy can often be successful, especially in the presence of likely dystonias or hypokinetic symptoms disturbing nocturnal sleep. Long-acting agonists such as the rotigotine patch before bed may improve both motor dysfunctions and sleep disturbances [46]. Simple use of levodopa (200 mg) taken mid-evening was assessed in an early study and found to reduce excessive nocturnal movement and improve subjective sleep quality [47]. However, randomised comparisons with sustained release levodopa preparations are lacking. Immediate release levodopa may also be used with success for prolonged nocturnal arousals. Alternatively, if there are symptoms suggesting nocturnal over-arousal or intrusive dreams, for example, reducing dopaminergic treatments late in the day may help the situation.

Even if it is not a primary sleep 'toxin', nocturia is a frequent symptom of concern that may lead to practical difficulties with micturition, especially if confusion is present. One simple strategy is to use a bottle or bedpan or even a condom catheter, in males, averting the need to leave the bed. The use of desmopressin spray to suppress urinary output is probably safe and may be worthy of consideration in some PD patients.

Hypnotic drugs and neuroleptics are sometimes used in attempts to improve sleep continuity in PD although published evidence to guide drug choice is very limited. Single, small, unblinded trials of zolpidem, clozapine for nocturnal akathisia, and quietapine have shown a benefit on sleep in PD patients. Even in the absence of RBD, clonazepam (0.5–2 mg) can be used empirically, especially if the risk of sleep apnoea is low. In clinical practice, low doses of sedative antidepressants such as amitriptyline (5–10 mg) are frequently used with variable and often unpredictable success rates. Many antidepressants, particularly tricyclics, however, can worsen sleep quality even if sleep time is prolonged.

Patients with varying degrees of cognitive impairment, nocturnal hallucinations and confusional arousals present particular problems for drug therapy. If adjustment or reductions of existing therapy have not helped, additional use of antipsychotic agents such as quetiapine (12.5–100 mg) or clozapine (12.5–50 mg) is favoured by some, even though the latter requires regular monitoring for the rare adverse event of agranulocytosis. Increasing anecdotal evidence suggests that cholinesterase inhibitors such as rivastigmine, perhaps delivered via a transdermal patch (9.5 mg), are very useful in this difficult group and may help to restore sleep continuity. However, care should be taken with this approach as some patients develop nightmares or even hallucinations, presumably as a result of increased REM sleep density induced by cholinergic drugs.

The role of subthalamic (STN) stimulation in improving insomnia symptoms has received recent attention. Certainly, if hypokinesia or dystonias are prominent symptoms at night, it appears to improve sleep efficiency substantially [48]. The resulting reductions in dopaminergic therapy that usually follow STN stimulation may also improve sleep quality in some.

Restless Legs Syndrome

In the absence of iron deficiency, the treatment of nocturnal RLS in PD may be complex and there is little published guidance.

Anticonvulsants such as gabapentin and pregabalin may improve the sensory discomfort and, if there are no significant neuropsychiatric problems, opiates may be used successfully [18]. Although increasing nocturnal dopamine stimulation would seem logical in this situation, some hold the theory that nocturnal RLS in PD reflects the phenomenon of 'augmentation' secondary to excessive dopamine daytime stimulation. This might be supported by the development, in some, of RLS several years after the motor symptoms of parkinsonism. If this hypothesis were true, paradoxical reduction of daytime dopaminergic drugs would be a more appropriate approach.

Sleep-disordered Breathing

In PD, conventional treatment of OSA with continuous positive airway pressure (CPAP) has been shown as effective in reducing the apnoea–hypopnea index, oxygen desaturations and also objective sleepiness, increasing the patients mean sleep latency on MSLT [49]. However, disappointingly in this study, subjective sleepiness and quality of life measures were not demonstrated. Moreover, CPAP therapy in patients with PD often poses practical problems with device manipulation and carers are often needed for assistance [50].

In patients with MSA, if stridor is present, treatment should not be delayed given the reported risk of respiratory failure and sudden death during sleep [18]. CPAP is an effective non-invasive treatment to eliminate stridor [50–52]. While untreated stridor is associated with short survival [51], this is not seen in stridor patients treated with CPAP. Experience with botulinum toxin injected inside the laryngeal adductor muscles is limited [53]. This therapy is invasive and may increase the risk of bronchial aspiration, aggravate dysphonia and dysphagia. When CPAP is not tolerated or effective and severe stridor persists, even in wakefulness, tracheostomy should be considered taking into account the patient's quality of life and life expectancy.

In central alveolar hypoventilation during sleep, adaptive servo-ventilation (ASV) may be necessary [54].

Rapid Eye Movement Sleep Behaviour Disorder

In clinically significant RBD, patients should secure their bed environment and protect their partner, perhaps by placing a pillow between them, using twin beds, or having the mattress directly on the floor. Removing nearby objects such as tables and lamps is also sensible. If existing drug treatments such as antidepressants are thought contributory, they should be stopped if possible. Furthermore, if investigations confirm significant sleep-related breathing disorders, the use of a nasal positive airway pressure device can sometimes reduce the abnormal nocturnal behaviours and the need for active drug treatment.

Pharmacotherapy is appropriate in most subjects but there is a lack of randomised, double blind, placebo-controlled studies. By consensus, clonazepam is widely regarded as the first-line treatment (0.5–2 mg), especially if sleep apnoea has been excluded or treated, with good efficacy and reasonable tolerance [55]. There is debate whether other hypnotic agents are as effective as clonazepam in RBD or whether clonazepam has a pharmacological profile that provides particular benefit.

Increasing evidence suggests that melatonin is also effective and well tolerated in RBD, probably in a dose range of 2–9 mg. Of interest, the drug appears to partially restore normal muscle atonia during REM sleep in PD patients [56,57], in contrast to clonazepam which simply attenuates the phenomenon, perhaps reducing violent jerks to minor twitches. Despite anecdotal reports of success, dopaminergic agents, in general, do not alter RBD in symptomatic patients [6,58].

Excessive Daytime Sleepiness

If EDS is a symptom of concern to patients or their care givers, initial efforts should be directed to reducing potential sedative drugs including dopamine agonists, sedative antidepressants, opioids and clonazepam, if possible. The utility of planned short daytime naps has not been assessed systematically but appears to benefit some. The use of wake-promoting therapy is often appropriate if simple measures have failed to help. Perhaps due to the complexities and variable causes of EDS in PD, the published evidence regarding the success of drugs such as modafinil is mixed [59]. However, modafinil is generally safe, even in the elderly, and an empirical trial of therapy is often warranted. An overall positive response rate in approximately 30% of patients might be expected. More traditional psychostimulants such as methylphenidate have been used less frequently although might be especially useful if atypical depression, anhedonia or apathy are prominent additional symptoms.

A new approach to EDS in PD mirrors that used in narcolepsy. In particular, there is early uncontrolled trial evidence that nocturnal sodium oxybate may help to consolidate sleep in PD and subsequently improve daytime wakefulness, as in narcoleptics. Significant reductions in Epworth scores from 16 to 9 were reported [60].

Conclusions

It is clear that virtually every aspect of the sleep–wake cycle can be disrupted in PD and PS, especially in advanced cases. Interactions between drug therapies and the underlying disease process can interfere with sleep and daytime wakefulness such that manipulations in pharmacotherapy may improve one aspect but worsen another. In view of the potential complexity and multifactorial nature of the sleep problems in PD, perhaps contrary to expectations, treatments can frequently benefit subjects and improve quality of life, especially for carers. It should be emphasised that any management pathway, particularly involving drugs, should be flexible and individualised. With increasing awareness of sleep–wake issues in PD and PS, it is difficult to know when a movement disorder specialist should involve the expertise of a specific sleep clinic. However, a multidisciplinary approach is probably the best solution if resources allow.

> **Key Points**
>
> - Virtually any sleep-related problem across a 24-hour period can occur in PD and PSs, particularly in advanced cases with additional neuropsychiatric symptomology.
> - Some patients develop paradoxical severe daytime sleepiness with dopamine replacement therapy, particularly after starting low dose agonists.
> - A major cause of overnight sleep disruption is motor disability.
> - RBD with violent dream enactment is particularly common in PD patients and often precedes daytime motor symptoms.
> - Treatment of sleep-related problems in PD should be individualised to the specific symptoms elicited from a detailed 24-hour history.
> - Manipulating (nocturnal) dopaminergic therapy can be useful, as can providing hypnotic agents to improve overnight sleep and/or wake-promoting drugs during the day.
> - Nocturnal stridor may suggest the diagnosis of multiple system atrophy and should be actively treated by continuous positive airway pressure as a matter of urgency.

References

1 Tandberg E, et al. A community-based study of sleep disorders in patients with Parkinson's disease. *Mov Disord* 1998;13(6):895–9.

2 Lees AJ, et al. The night-time problems of Parkinson's disease. *Clin Neuropharmacol* 1988;11:512–9.

3 Comella C, et al. Sleep-related violence, injury, and REM sleep behavior disorder in Parkinson's disease. *Neurology* 1998;51:526–9.

4 Gagnon JF, et al. REM sleep behavior disorder and REM sleep without atonia in Parkinson's disease. *Neurology* 2002;59(4):585–9.

5 De Cock VC, et al. Restoration of normal motor control in Parkinson's disease during REM sleep. *Brain* 2007;130(Pt 2):450–6.

6 Iranzo A, et al. Characteristics of idiopathic REM sleep behavior disorder and that associated with MSA and PD. *Neurology* 2005;65(2):247–52.

7 Scaglione C, et al. REM sleep behaviour disorder in Parkinson's disease: a questionnaire-based study. *Neurol Sci* 2005;25(6):316–21.

8 Schenck CH, Mahowald MW. REM sleep behavior disorder: clinical, developmental, and neuroscience perspectives 16 years after its formal identification in SLEEP. *Sleep* 2002;25(2):120–38.

9 Iranzo A, et al. Rapid-eye-movement sleep behaviour disorder as an early marker for a neurodegenerative disorder: a descriptive study. *Lancet Neurol* 2006;5(7):572–7.

10 Postuma RB, et al. Quantifying the risk of neurodegenerative disease in idiopathic REM sleep behavior disorder. *Neurology* 2009 14;72(15):1296–300.

11 Ondo WG, et al. Daytime sleepiness and other sleep disorders in Parkinson's disease. *Neurology* 2001;57(8):1392–6.

12 Tan E, et al. Evaluation of somnolence in Parkinson's disease: comparison with age- and sex-matched controls. *Neurology* 2002;58:465–8.

13 Ghorayeb I, et al. A nationwide survey of excessive daytime sleepiness in Parkinson's disease in France. *Mov Disord* 2007;22(11):1567–72.

14 Abbott RD, et al. Excessive daytime sleepiness and subsequent development of Parkinson disease. *Neurology* 2005;65(9):1442–6.

15 Arnulf I, et al. Sleepiness in idiopathic REM sleep behavior disorder and Parkinson disease. *Sleep* 2015;38(10):1529–35.

16 Hobson D, et al. Excessive daytime sleepiness and sudden-onset sleep in Parkinson Disease. A survey by the Canadian Movement Disorder Group. *JAMA* 2002;287:455–63.

17 Korner Y, et al. Predictors of sudden onset of sleep in Parkinson's disease. *Mov Disord* 2004;19(11):1298–305.

18 Ghorayeb I, Bioulac B, Tison F. Sleep disorders in multiple system atrophy. *J Neural Transm* 2005; 112(12):1669–1675.

19 Ghorayeb I, et al. Sleep disorders and their determinants in multiple system atrophy. *J Neurol Neurosurg Psychiatry* 2002;72(6):798–800.

20 Vetrugno R, et al. Sleep disorders in multiple system atrophy: a correlative video-polysomnographic study. *Sleep Med* 2004;5(1):21–30.

21 Plazzi G, et al. REM sleep behavior disorders in multiple system atrophy. *Neurology* 1997;48(4):1094–7.

22 Tison F, Wenning G, Quinn N, Smith S. REM sleep behaviour disorder as the presenting symptom of multiple system atrophy. *J Neurol Neurosurg Psychiatry* 1995;58:379–80.

23 Tachibana N, Oka Y. Longitudinal change in REM sleep components in a patient with multiple system atrophy associated with REM sleep behavior disorder: paradoxical improvement of nocturnal behaviors in a progressive neurodegenerative disease. *Sleep Med* 2004;5:155–8.

24 Wenning GK, et al. Multiple system atrophy: a review of 203 pathologically proven cases. *Mov Disord* 1997;12:133–47.

25 Yamaguchi M, Arai K, Asahina M, Hattori T. Laryngeal stridor in multiple system atrophy. *Eur Neurol* 2003;49(3):154–9.

26 Aldrich MS, et al. Sleep abnormalities in progressive supranuclear palsy. *Ann Neurol* 1989;25:577–81.

27 De Cock VC, et al. REM sleep behavior disorder in patients with Guadeloupean parkinsonism, a tauopathy. *Sleep* 2007;30(8):1026–32.

28 Ondo W, et al. Exploring the relationship between Parkinson disease and restless legs syndrome. *Arch Neurol* 2002;59:421–4.

29 Nomura T, et al. Prevalence and clinical characteristics of restless legs syndrome in Japanese patients with Parkinson's disease. *Mov Disord* 2006;21(3):380–4.

30 Factor SA, et al. Sleep disorders and sleep effect in Parkinson's disease. *Mov Disord* 1990;5:280–5.

31 Van Hilten B, et al. Sleep disruption in Parkinson's disease. Assessment by continuous activity monitoring. *Arch Neurol* 1994;51:922–8.

32 Borek LL, et al. Mood and sleep in Parkinson's disease. *J Clin Psychiatry* 2006;67(6):958–63.

33 Comella CL, et al. Nocturnal activity with nighttime pergolide in Parkinson disease: a controlled study using actigraphy. *Neurology* 2005;64(8):1450–1.

34 Lawrence A, et al. Compulsive use of dopamine replacement therapy in Parkinson's disease: reward systems gone awry? *Lancet Neurol* 2003;2:595–604.

35 Whitehead D, et al. Circadian rest-activity rhythm in Parkinson's disease patients with hallucinations. *Mov Disord* 2008;23:1137–45.

36 Merino-Andreu M, et al. Unawareness of naps in Parkinson's disease and in disorders with excessive daytime sleepiness. *Neurology* 2003;60(9):1553–4.

37 Hagell P, Broman JE. Measurement properties and hierarchical item structure of the Epworth Sleepiness Scale in Parkinson's disease. *J Sleep Res* 2007;16(1):102–9.

38 Cochen De Cock V, et al. Daytime sleepiness in Parkinson's disease: a reappraisal. *PLoS ONE* 2014;9(9):e107278.

39 Videnovic A, et al. Circadian melatonin rhythm and excessive daytime sleepiness in Parkinson disease. *JAMA Neurol* 2014;71(4):463–9.

40 Cochen De Cock V, et al. Supine sleep and obstructive sleep apnea syndrome in Parkinson's disease. *Sleep Med* 2015;16(12):1497–501.

41 Kew J, Gross M, Chapman P. Shy-Drager syndrome presenting as isolated paralysis of vocal cord abductors. *Br Med J* 1990; 300(6737):1441.

42 De Cock VC, et al. The improvement of movement and speech during rapid eye movement sleep behaviour disorder in multiple system atrophy. *Brain* 2011;134:856–62.

43 Chaudhuri KR, et al. The Parkinson's disease sleep scale: a new instrument for assessing sleep and nocturnal disability in Parkinson's disease. *J Neurol Neurosurg Psychiatry* 2002;73(6):629–35.

44 Marinus J, et al. Assessment of sleep and sleepiness in Parkinson disease. *Sleep* 2003;26(8):1049–54.

45 Trenkwalder C, et al. Parkinson's disease sleep scale – validation of the revised version PDSS-2. *Mov Disord* 2011;26(4):644–52.

46 Trenkwalder C, et al.; Recover Study Group. Rotigotine effects on early morning motor function and sleep in Parkinson's disease: a double-blind, randomized, placebo-controlled study (RECOVER). *Mov Disord* 2011;26(1):90–9.

47 Leeman AL, et al. Parkinson's disease in the elderly: response to and optimal spacing of night time dosing with levodopa. *Br J Clin Pharmacol* 1987;24(5):637–43.

48 Arnulf I, et al. Improvement of sleep architecture in PD with subthalamic nucleus stimulation. *Neurology* 2000;55:1732–5.

49 Neikrug AB, et al. Continuous positive airway pressure improves sleep and daytime sleepiness in patients with Parkinson disease and sleep apnea. *Sleep* 2014 1;37(1):177–85.

50 Iranzo A, Santamaria J, Tolosa E. Continuous positive air pressure eliminates nocturnal stridor in multiple system atrophy. Barcelona Multiple System Atrophy Study Group. *Lancet* 2000;356(9238):1329–30.

51 Iranzo A, et al. Long-term effect of CPAP in the treatment of nocturnal stridor in multiple system atrophy. *Neurology* 2004;63(5):930–2.

52 Ghorayeb I, Yekhlef F, Bioulac B, Tison F. Continuous positive airway pressure for sleep-related breathing disorders in multiple system atrophy: long-term acceptance. *Sleep Med* 2005;6(4):359–62.

53 Silber MH, Levine S. Stridor and death in multiple system atrophy. *Mov Disord* 2000;15(4):699–704.

54 Randerath WJ, et al. Adaptive servo-ventilation in patients with coexisting obstructive sleep apnoea/hypopnoea and Cheyne-Stokes respiration. *Sleep Med* 2008;9(8):823–30.

55 Gagnon JF, et al. Update on the pharmacology of REM sleep behavior disorder. *Neurology* 2006;67(5):742–7.

56 Kunz D, Bes F. Melatonin as a therapy in REM sleep behavior disorder patients: an open-labeled pilot study on the possible influence of melatonin on REM-sleep regulation. *Mov Disord* 1999;14(3):507–11.

57 Dowling GA, et al. Melatonin for sleep disturbances in Parkinson's disease. *Sleep Med* 2005;6(5):459–66.

58 Olson EJ, et al. Rapid eye movement sleep behaviour disorder: demographic, clinical and laboratory findings in 93 cases. *Brain* 2000;123(Pt 2):331–9.

59 Ondo WG, et al. Modafinil for daytime somnolence in Parkinson's disease: double blind, placebo controlled parallel trial. *J Neurol Neurosurg Psychiatry* 2005;76(12):1636–9.

60 Ondo WG, et al. Sodium oxybate for excessive daytime sleepiness in Parkinson's disease: an open-label polysomnographic study. *Arch Neurol* 2008;65:1337–40.

15

Sleep in Dementia and Other Neurodegenerative Diseases

Alex Iranzo[1-3]

[1] Neurology Service, Hospital Clínic de Barcelona, Barcelona, Spain
[2] Institut d'Investigació Biomèdiques August Pi i Sunyer (IDIBAPS), Barcelona, Spain
[3] Centro de Investigación Biomédica en Red sobre Enfermedades Neurodegenerativas (CIBERNED), Barcelona, Spain

Introduction

Sleep is affected in a range of neurodegenerative disorders, sometimes to great extent. In this chapter, sleep disorders occurring in the two most common dementias, namely Alzheimer's disease (AD) and dementia with Lewy bodies (DLB) are discussed, as well as Huntington's disease (HD) and the hereditary ataxias.

Alzheimer's Disease

Sleep Symptomatology

Sleep disturbances are highly common in AD and may occur at any stage of the disease. Sleep-related problems arise from multiple factors including: the degenerative process itself, damaging areas which modulate sleep (such as the suprachiasmatic nucleus in the hypothalamus); associated psychiatric disturbances (e.g. depression, agitation); medical issues (e.g. infections, pain) and side effects of medication. Impaired sleep almost certainly affects the quality of life of patients, relatives and caregivers alike, potentially leading to patient institutionalisation. Sleep disorders include sleep onset insomnia, sleep fragmentation, early morning awakenings, daytime sleepiness characterised by frequent napping, nocturnal hallucinations and confusional nocturnal wandering [1,2]. Perhaps the most common sleep problem in AD is an exaggerated tendency to phase delay the sleep–wake rhythm. The pattern is similar but much more severe than that seen in normal ageing. In extreme cases, AD patients present with the 'sundowning' syndrome which is characterised by agitation, confusion and aggressiveness in the dark hours of the evening and at night. In the middle of the night patients may experience confusional awakenings with nocturnal wandering and agitation.

Sleep Disorders in Neurology: A Practical Approach, Second Edition.
Edited by Sebastiaan Overeem and Paul Reading.
© 2018 John Wiley & Sons Ltd. Published 2018 by John Wiley & Sons Ltd.

Interestingly, rapid eye movement sleep behaviour disorder (RBD) seems to be rare in AD. One study involving 15 AD patients showed that RBD is uncommon [2], perhaps because brainstem damage is not prominent. Restless legs syndrome (RLS) also seems to be very prominent, although its frequency may be underestimated since an RLS diagnosis requires patients to describe the symptoms themselves. The frequency of obstructive sleep apnoea is high, affecting between 40% and 70% and may aggravate cognitive dysfunction in AD.

Pathophysiology

Population-based studies suggest that poor sleep quality is associated with an increased risk of dementia. An association has also been found with obstructive sleep apnoea. In addition, the APOE-4 allele is a risk factor for both AD and sleep apnoea. Exciting recent studies suggest that sleep disruption may directly affect AD pathophysiology. Animal studies suggest that sleep loss may hamper beta-amyloid clearance in the brain, and more recently, sleep deprivation was shown to increase beta-amyloid in healthy humans [1].

Diagnosis and Treatment

Actigraphy can be used to characterise circadian rhythm disturbances in AD, as well as sleep fragmentation with nocturnal unrest. Polysomnography typically shows reduced total sleep time and sleep efficiency, increased sleep onset latency and wake time after sleep onset, reduced deep sleep and rapid eye movement (REM) sleep amounts, and increased light sleep amount. In advanced cases, sleep scoring is difficult due to the absence of a clear alpha rhythm during wakefulness and loss of sleep spindles and K complexes.

Medication side effects should always be considered as a cause of sleep disruption. Acetylcholinesterase inhibitors, such as donepezil and rivastigmine, are used primarily as symptomatic agents at mild and moderate stages of the disease. They may all induce sleep onset insomnia. Conversely, the frequent use of typical and atypical antipsychotics, usually for agitation or behavioural problems, may induce hypersomnia.

Treatment of sleep disorders in AD is challenging and should be individualised. Melatonin and phototherapy can be considered in subjects with circadian dysrhythmia. Nocturnal agitation, hallucinations, confusional awakenings and nocturnal wandering may improve with atypical antipsychotic agents at bedtime (quetiapine, clozapine, olanzapine, risperidone). Sleep-disordered breathing can be treated with continuous positive airway pressure, but this typically requires intensive coaching of the patient in how to use the equipment. Insomnia, when required, can be usefully treated with trazodone or other sedative antidepressants at bedtime. Modafinil may improve daytime sleepiness in selected cases.

Dementia with Lewy Bodies

DLB is clinically characterised by dementia, parkinsonism, recurrent visual hallucinations and fluctuations in cognition and alertness. The combination of brainstem and cortical Lewy bodies is necessary for the pathological diagnosis of DLB [3].

Studies Evaluating Sleep in DLB

Overall, insomnia, circadian rhythm disorders with early awakening, nocturnal hallucinations and confusional nocturnal wandering are frequent in DLB, as is daytime sleepiness. In contrast, sleep apnoea and RLS seem to be no more common than in the general population of similar age. RBD is very common and may antedate the onset of dementia by several years. As RBD is rare in other forms of dementia, such as AD or frontotemporal dementia, the detection of RBD in a patient with dementia points toward a diagnosis of DLB.

In a large multicentre study, Bliwise et al. [4] compared nocturnal sleep disturbances between 339 patients with DLB and 4192 patients with AD.Nocturnal sleep disturbances were reported more frequently in DLB (63%) than in AD (27%) and were not linked to disease stage or the presence of depressive symptoms, apathy, hallucinations, delusions or agitation. Pao et al. [5] reviewed the polysomnographic findings of 78 DLB patients with sleep-related complaints. Seventy-five (96%) patients had histories of dream-enactment behaviours with confirmation of RBD using polysomnography (PSG) in 62 patients. The remaining 13 subjects did not attain any REM sleep, and hence RBD could not be formally confirmed. Terzaghi et al. [6] evaluated the clinical and video-PSG findings of 29 consecutive DLB patients with a mean age of 75 years and a mean disease duration of 3 years. Eleven (38%) patients reported insomnia, 23 (79%) hallucinations at night, 19 (65%) episodes suggestive of confusional arousals, and 18 (62%) episodes suggestive of RBD. RLS was reported only by one patient. Excessive daytime sleepiness was present in 17 (59%). Disruptive motor behaviours during sleep were found in 70% and consisted of RBD in 11 subjects, confusional episodes from non-REM (NREM) sleep in 7, and arousal-related episodes from REM or NREM sleep mimicking RBD in 2. Of note, these REM and NREM sleep enactment behaviours have also been described to occur in PD associated with dementia [7].

Rapid Eye Movement Sleep Behaviour Disorder in DLB

As stated, available data indicate that RBD is very common in DLB, may be the first symptom of the disease, and can in fact be considered a 'red flag' for the diagnosis. The current diagnostic criteria for DLB now include RBD as a suggestive feature [3,8]. This statement was initially based on a single retrospective study involving 37 consecutive patients with dementia plus RBD [9]. Of these, 23 fulfilled the 1996 consensus criteria for probable DLB and all fulfilled the criteria for possible DLB [3]. In a cohort of 234 autopsy-confirmed dementia patients followed longitudinally, a history of probably or definite RBD was present in 76% of 98 with autopsy-confirmed DLB. In contrast, only 6 of the 136 patients without autopsy-confirmed DLB exhibited RBD. Thus, inclusion of RBD improves the diagnostic accuracy of DLB [8].

Dugger et al. [10] compared the clinical characteristics of 71 DLB patients with RBD and 19 without RBD. Those with RBD were predominantly male, had shorter duration of dementia, earlier onset of parkinsonism and visual hallucinations, and less AD-related pathology on autopsy. The subgroup of patients in whom RBD developed before cognitive impairment were characterised by an earlier onset of visual hallucinations and parkinsonism, more severe baseline parkinsonism and shorter duration of dementia. Studies have now also shown that patients initially diagnosed with idiopathic RBD frequently are diagnosed with DLB and other synucleinopathies (mainly PD and less frequently multiple system atrophy [MSA]) with time. We reported that in a cohort of 44 idiopathic RBD subjects, 36 (82%) were eventually diagnosed with a defined neurodegenerative syndrome; 14 with DLB, 16 with PD, 1 with MSA and 5 with mild cognitive impairment [11]. The median interval between the diagnosis of mild cognitive impairment and the diagnosis of DLB was 2 years.

Treatment

Treatment of sleep-related symptoms in DLB is challenging and controlled evidence is lacking. A similar approach to that in advanced PD is appropriate and the reader is therefore referred to Chapter 14 for further details.

Huntington's Disease

HD is an autosomal dominant neurodegenerative disorder characterised by progressive dementia, chorea and psychiatric disturbances as a result of expanded CAG repeats in the Huntington gene. Pathological studies demonstrate severe atrophy of the caudate and putamen, and to a lesser extent, of the cortex [12].

Sleep Disruption in HD

Sleep disorders are common among patients with HD, particularly in advanced stages. Patients and caregivers usually report poor sleep quality with sleep fragmentation and frequent awakenings at night. Possibly as a result, excessive daytime sleepiness is common. In addition, apparent circadian rhythm disorders are described, typically of the advanced phase type, resulting in early morning awakenings [13–17]. A more disrupted and fragmented sleep is seen in premanifest gene carriers when compared with controls [18]. Interestingly, a transgenic model of HD in mice has disrupted circadian rhythms that worsen as the disease progresses, suggesting a progressive impairment of the suprachiasmatic nucleus in the hypothalamus [19].

In a community survey study with 292 patients, sleep problems were reported by 87% and were rated as important by 62% [13]. Overall, PSG studies show reduced sleep efficiency, increased wake time after sleep onset, increased percentage of light sleep, increased REM sleep latency and reduced percentage of slow wave sleep and REM sleep [14,20–23]. In HD, sleep complaints and PSG abnormalities increase with disease severity and duration. PSG studies have shown a low incidence of sleep apnoea [23–25] and RBD [14,20] in patients with HD. Multiple sleep latency tests were performed in only one study, showing reduced sleep latency in 4 of 25 patients (16%) and no REM sleep periods [14].

In pathological studies, a mean reduction of hypocretin cells of 27–30% was observed in the hypothalamus while the melanin-concentrating hormone cell number was not affected [26]. In general, HD patients do not have a narcoleptic phenotype however, because cataplexy is absent, Multiple Sleep Latency Test testing does not typically show sleep onset of REM sleep periods and hypocretin-1 levels in the cerebrospinal fluid were found to be normal [27–30).

Rapid Eye Movement Sleep Behaviour Disorder and RLS

The presence of RBD in HD was only investigated by clinical history and PSG in a few studies. In one study involving 25 patients only three (12%) had video-PSG-confirmed RBD [14]. In another study with 30 patients RBD or REM sleep without atonia was not detected, despite two subjects with an increased score on a RBD questionnaire [20]. It should be noted that abnormal behaviours during sleep in HD may be caused by RBD mimics such as violent opisthotonos-like movements during arousals from REM and NREM sleep [31] and severe periodic limb movements in sleep (PLMS) [32].

In a series of 25 patients, only one had RLS. A periodic limb movement (PLM) index greater than 15 was found in 6 (24%) [14] although PLMs did not result in fragmented sleep. In contrast, one study with six patients found a high mean PLM index of 123 that fragmented sleep architecture [23]. In an additional study with 30 patients, RLS was detected in 2 patients while PLM during sleep and wakefulness was observed in all 30 patients [20].

Hereditary Ataxias

Hereditary ataxias are genetic neurodegenerative disorders with a variable mode of inheritance, including autosomal dominant (e.g. spinocerebellar ataxias [SCAs]), autosomal recessive (e.g. ataxia telangectasia, Friedreich ataxia) and X-linked (e.g. fragile X tremor ataxia syndrome). Although these diseases predominantly affect the spinocerebellar tracts, cerebellum and brainstem, other structures in the brain are frequently involved. Clinically, they are characterised by progressive ataxia and a potential plethora of neurological symptoms and signs such as polyneuropathy and parkinsonism [33,34]. The occurrence and clinical relevance of sleep disorders have received relatively little attention, although several reports have addressed the presence of RBD and RLS.

Rapid Eye Movement Sleep Behaviour Disorder in Hereditary Ataxias

Although generally recognised as an accompaniment to parkinsonian syndromes, RBD also appears highly prevalent in other neurodegenerative conditions, including hereditary ataxias.

Spinocerebellar ataxia type 3 (SCA3 or Machado–Joseph disease) is an autosomal dominant disorder linked to CAG-trinucleotide repeat expansions in the ataxin-3 gene. Neurodegeneration involves the cerebellum, spinocerebellar tracts and brainstem [33]. In one study, 20 of 53 (38%) reported symptoms were suggestive of RBD [35]. One study described a presumed presence of RBD in 12 of 22 (56%) SCA3 patients. However, diagnosis was based on a questionnaire, patients were not interviewed by the authors and PSG was not performed and this may have resulted in confusion of RBD with other parasomnias [36]. We described the presence of video-PSG-confirmed RBD in five of nine (55%) consecutive Spanish SCA3 patients, four men and one woman, with a mean age of 48 years and a mean ataxia duration of 14 years. In two patients RBD preceded the ataxia onset by 10 and 8 years. Clinical RBD severity was mild or moderate [37]. In subsequent series using PSG, RBD or REM sleep without atonia was found in 45–73% of cases ([38–40].

In SCA2, a cerebellar syndrome characterised by CAG repeat expansion in the SCA2 gene with saccade slowing and gaze palsy, two studies have evaluated the presence of

RBD by clinical history and PSG. One study evaluated eight patients from five German families with sleep interviews and video-PSG. All but one reported good quality sleep. None of the patients and bed partners reported symptoms that might suggest RBD such as violent nightmares, frequent vocalisations or aggression during sleep. Video-PSG, however, showed subclinical RBD (increased submental electromyographic activity not associated with abnormal behaviours) in three patients, normal REM sleep in two and an apparent absence of REM sleep in three [41]. In another study, four of five SCA2 patients of three different Austrian families had increased electromyographic activity during REM sleep in the video-PSG. These four patients exhibited a mild form of RBD consisting of prominent myoclonic jerks in the absence of complex behaviours [42]. RBD was not observed in 36 presymptomatic SCA2 patients from Cuba [43], while RBD was shown in only 2 of 32 (6%) symptomatic patients from the same origin [44].

Restless Legs Syndrome

Studies found RLS in patients with SCA1, SCA2, SCA3 and SCA6 who were not treated with dopaminergic or antidopaminergic drugs (Table 15.1). The highest frequency of RLS has been found in SCA3, ranging from 30 to 55% of the cases, a proportion consistently higher than that seen in control populations. PSG in SCA1, SCA2, SCA3 and SCA6 has generally revealed a high number of PLMS in patients with or without RLS [35,37,40,42,44–50]. Most SCA patients, however, were unaware of their leg movements and PLMS were usually not associated with arousals.

Results from one study [45] in 89 patients found RLS in 2 of 11 (18%) SCA2 patients, 23 of 51 (45%) SCA3 patients, and 1 of 21 (5%) SCA6 patients, whereas none of the 6 SCA1 patients studied had symptoms. RLS was usually severe, although standard dopaminergic therapy was effective in 14 of 16 patients. In another study, RLS in 58 patients with SCA1, SCA2 and SCA3 was more frequent than in 40 age-matched controls (28% versus 10%) (51). RLS was present in 3 of the 13 SCA1 (23%), 6 of the 22 SCA2 (27%), and 7 of the 23 SCA3 (30%). Ataxia always preceded RLS onset. RLS was not associated with CAG repeat length, ataxia onset, and abnormalities in nerve conduction electromyography and somatosensory evoked potentials. Our group found RLS in 5 of 9 SCA3 patients (55.5%) and in none of the 9 matched controls. In another study, 4 of 10 SCA patients without parkinsonism suffered from RLS (1 of 4 SCA1, 1 of 4 SCA2, and 2 of 2 SCA3) [50]. RLS was not associated with peripheral neuropathy. The mean PLMS index was increased in all three types, particularly in SCA3 where the mean PLMS index was 134 [50]. In one study evaluating the sleep quality of eight SCA2 patients, all but one reported good sleep, none reported RLS and PSG detected a PLMS index greater than five in only one subject (PLMS index of 10) [41]. In 44 patients with SCA3, RLS was found in 21 (51%) [40]. In 47 SCA3 subjects RLS was found in 44% and the mean PLMS index was 22 [49]. In asymptomatic SCA2 carriers RLS and PLMS are very rare [43] whereas in manifested patients RLS occurs in 25% and PLMS in 37% [44].

The reason why RLS occurs in subjects with autosomal dominant SCAs is unknown. Peripheral neuropathy and length of the CAG repeat expansion have not been associated with RLS in SCA1, SCA2 and SCA3 [45,51]. Conversely, in patients with idiopathic and familial RLS no expanded CAG repeats were identified in the SCA1, SCA2, SCA3, SCA6, SCA7 and SCA17 loci [50,52].

Central dopaminergic dysfunction may be suspected given the reported response to levodopa in some subjects with SCAs [45,51]. In SCA3, there is neurodegeneration in

Table 15.1 Studies evaluating the frequency of restless legs syndrome in hereditary ataxias.

Year	Country	Ref.	SCA1 (n)	RLS in SCA1 (%)	SCA2 (n)	RLS in SCA2 (%)	SCA3 (n)	RLS in SCA3 (%)	SCA6 (n)	RLS in SCA6 (%)	RLS in Friedreich ataxia (n, %)	RLS in controls (%)
1998	Germany	[45]	6	0	11	18	51	45	21	5	NA	NA
2001	Germany	[46]	13	23	22	27	23	30	NA	NA	NA	10
2003	Spain	[37]	NA	NA	NA	NA	9	55.5	NA	NA	NA	0
2006	Austria	[47]	NA	NA	NA	NA	NA	NA	5	40	NA	NA
2006	Austria	[42]	NA	NA	5	0	NA	NA	NA	NA	NA	NA
2006	Germany	[40]	4	25	4	25	2	100	NA	NA	NA	NA
2009	Brazil	[35]	NA	NA	NA	NA	53	20.7	NA	NA	NA	4.7
2011	Austria	[46]	NA	NA	NA	NA	NA	NA	NA	NA	16, 50	NA
2011	Germany	[48]	NA	NA	NA	NA	NA	NA	NA	NA	28, 32	0
2014	Brazil	[40]	NA	NA	NA	NA	44	51	NA	NA	NA	NA
2016	Brazil	[49]	NA	NA	NA	NA	47	44	NA	NA	NA	NA

NA, not available; RLS, restless legs syndrome.

both the substantia nigra and basal ganglia, and functional neuroimaging studies show decreased transporter binding in the nigrostriatal dopamine pathway in patients with and without extrapyramidal signs [53] and decreased [^{18}F]fluorodopa uptake in the putamen [54]. Furthermore, nigrostriatal dopaminergic impairment is suspected in SCA2, SCA3 and SCA6 since some patients develop parkinsonism that responds to levodopa and functional studies in these patients demonstrated reduction of presynaptic striatal dopamine transporters [55–59]. Interestingly, a functional neuroimaging study in SCA1, SCA2 and SCA3 patients with RLS showed normal postsynaptic striatal D2 receptor availability in the striatum suggesting that the postsynaptic striatal system is not involved in the origin of RLS [50]. A lower content of iron may also influence the occurrence of RLS since the substantia nigra echogenicity size (measured by transcranial sonography evaluating the iron content) is lower in SCA3 patients with RLS than without RLS [60].

Sleep-disordered Breathing in Hereditary Ataxias

Generally, PSG studies in patients with autosomal dominant SCAs and ataxia telangectasia have shown that obstructive sleep apnoea is not a common finding but it may occur in SCA1 [61] and other ataxias.

We evaluated sleep-disordered breathing in nine SCA3 patients by PSG and laryngoscopy during wakefulness. Stridor secondary to vocal cord abductor paralysis occurred in one patient who required emergency tracheotomy in the emergency room because of subacute respiratory failure. In another two patients, laryngoscopy disclosed partial vocal cord abduction restriction that was unilateral. These two patients did not have stridor, dyspnoea or dysphonia and PSG excluded obstructive sleep apnoea [37]. Vocal cord abductor paralysis has also been described in SCA1 [62]. Neuropathological changes in SCA3 patients with dysphonia include neuronal loss in the nucleus ambiguus [63]. Thus, vocal cord abductor dysfunction in SCA3 may result from neuronopathy of the nucleus ambiguus impairing the recurrent laryngeal nerve fibres that mainly innervate the posterior cricoarytenoid muscle. This is supported by the findings of a study showing neurogenic atrophy of the intrinsic laryngeal muscles in SCA3 patients with vocal cord abduction palsy [64].

Key Points

- In AD, the sleep–wake cycle can be severely disturbed although there is no pathognomonic pattern. Medication side effects and sleep-disordered breathing may be important in individual patients.
- Patients suffering from DLB frequently have significant daytime somnolence and very disturbed nocturnal sleep with nocturnal confusion and REM sleep parasomnias as particular problems. Management approaches are the same as for severe parkinsonism.
- HD may produce severe sleep–wake disturbance especially if advanced. Disorganisation of circadian rhythm control appears most characteristic with advancement of the sleep phase and general sleep fragmentation as typical features.
- The well described association of RBD with parkinsonian syndromes may also extend to the hereditary ataxias, especially SCA3 (Machado–Joseph disease).
- Sleep-related breathing disorders are not routinely seen in the hereditary ataxias although neurogenic vocal cord paralysis with associated stridor has been reported in SCA3 and SCA1.

References

1 Videnovic A, Lazar AS, Barker RA, Overeem S. 'The clocks that time us' – circadian rhythms in neurodegenerative disorders. *Nature Reviews Neurology* 2014;10(12):683–93.

2 Gagnon JF, Petit D, Fantini ML, et al. REM sleep behavior disorder and REM sleep without atonia in probable Alzheimer disease. *Sleep* 2006;29(10):1321–5.

3 McKeith IG, Dickson DW, Lowe J, et al. Diagnosis and management of dementia with Lewy bodies: third report of the DLB Consortium. *Neurology* 2005;65(12):1863–72.

4 Bliwise DL, Mercaldo ND, Avidan AY, et al. Sleep disturbance in dementia with Lewy bodies and Alzheimer's disease: a multicenter analysis. *Dementia and Geriatric Cognitive Disorders* 2011;31(3):239–46.

5 Pao WC, Boeve BF, Ferman TJ, et al. Polysomnographic findings in dementia with Lewy bodies. *The Neurologist* 2013;19(1):1–6.

6 Terzaghi M, Arnaldi D, Rizzetti MC, et al. Analysis of video-polysomnographic sleep findings in dementia with Lewy bodies. *Movement Disorders* 2013;28(10):1416–23.

7 Ratti PL, Terzaghi M, Minafra B, et al. REM and NREM sleep enactment behaviors in Parkinson's disease, Parkinson's disease dementia, and dementia with Lewy bodies. *Sleep Medicine* 2012;13(7):926–32.

8 Ferman TJ, Boeve BF, Smith GE, et al. Inclusion of RBD improves the diagnostic classification of dementia with Lewy bodies. *Neurology* 2011;77(9):875–82.

9 Boeve BF, Silber MH, Ferman TJ, et al. REM sleep behavior disorder and degenerative dementia: an association likely reflecting Lewy body disease. *Neurology* 1998;51(2):363–70.

10 Dugger BN, Boeve BF, Murray ME, et al. Rapid eye movement sleep behavior disorder and subtypes in autopsy-confirmed dementia with Lewy bodies. *Movement Disorders* 2012;27(1):72–8.

11 Iranzo A, Tolosa E, Gelpi E, et al. Neurodegenerative disease status and post-mortem pathology in idiopathic rapid-eye-movement sleep behaviour disorder: an observational cohort study. *The Lancet Neurology* 2013;12(5):443–53.

12 Novak MJ, Tabrizi SJ. Huntington's disease. *British Medical Journal* 2010;340:c3109.

13 Taylor N, Bramble D. Sleep disturbance and Huntingdon's disease. *The British Journal of Psychiatry* 1997;171:393.

14 Arnulf I, Nielsen J, Lohmann E, et al. Rapid eye movement sleep disturbances in Huntington disease. *Archives of Neurology* 2008;65(4):482–8.

15 Videnovic A, Leurgans S, Fan W, et al. Daytime somnolence and nocturnal sleep disturbances in Huntington disease. *Parkinsonism & Related Disorders* 2009;15(6):471–4.

16 Baker CR, Dominguez DJ, Stout JC, et al. Subjective sleep problems in Huntington's disease: A pilot investigation of the relationship to brain structure, neurocognitive, and neuropsychiatric function. *Journal of the Neurological Sciences* 2016;364:148–53.

17 Morton AJ. Circadian and sleep disorder in Huntington's disease. *Experimental Neurology* 2013;243:34–44.

18 Lazar AS, Panin F, Goodman AO, et al. Sleep deficits but no metabolic deficits in premanifest Huntington's disease. *Annals of Neurology* 2015;78(4):630–48.

19 Morton AJ, Wood NI, Hastings MH, et al. Disintegration of the sleep-wake cycle and circadian timing in Huntington's disease. *The Journal of Neuroscience* 2005;25(1):157–63.

20 Piano C, Losurdo A, Della Marca G, et al. Polysomnographic findings and clinical correlates in Huntington disease: A cross-sectional cohort study. *Sleep* 2015;38(9):1489–95.

21 Hansotia P, Wall R, Berendes J. Sleep disturbances and severity of Huntington's disease. *Neurology* 1985;35(11):1672–4.

22 Wiegand M, Moller AA, Lauer CJ, et al. Nocturnal sleep in Huntington's disease. *Journal of Neurology* 1991;238(4):203–8.

23 Silvestri R, Raffaele M, De Domenico P, et al. Sleep features in Tourette's syndrome, neuroacanthocytosis and Huntington's chorea. *Neurophysiologie Clinique/Clinical Neurophysiology* 1995;25(2):66–77.

24 Bollen EL, Den Heijer JC, Ponsioen C, et al. Respiration during sleep in Huntington's chorea. *Journal of the Neurological Sciences* 1988;84(1):63–8.

25 Banno K, Hobson DE, Kryger MH. Long-term treatment of sleep breathing disorder in a patient with Huntington's disease. *Parkinsonism & Related Disorders* 2005;11(4):261–4.

26 Aziz A, Fronczek R, Maat-Schieman M, et al. Hypocretin and melanin-concentrating hormone in patients with Huntington disease. *Brain Pathology* 2008;18(4):474–83.

27 Petersen A, Gil J, Maat-Schieman ML, et al. Orexin loss in Huntington's disease. *Human Molecular Genetics* 2005;14(1):39–47.

28 Meier A, Mollenhauer B, Cohrs S, et al. Normal hypocretin-1 (orexin-A) levels in the cerebrospinal fluid of patients with Huntington's disease. *Brain Research* 2005;1063(2):201–3.

29 Baumann CR, Hersberger M, Bassetti CL. Hypocretin-1 (orexin A) levels are normal in Huntington's disease. *Journal of Neurology* 2006;253(9):1232–3.

30 Gaus SE, Lin L, Mignot E. CSF hypocretin levels are normal in Huntington's disease patients. *Sleep* 2005;28(12):1607–8.

31 Neutel D, Tchikviladze M, Charles P, et al. Nocturnal agitation in Huntington disease is caused by arousal-related abnormal movements rather than by rapid eye movement sleep behavior disorder. *Sleep Medicine* 2015;16(6):754–9.

32 Piano C, Bentivoglio AR, Cortelli P, Della Marca G. Motor-related sleep disorders in Huntington disease. A comment on: Neute et al.: 'Nocturnal agitation in Huntington disease is caused by arousal-related abnormal movements rather than by rapid eye movement sleep behavior disorder' by Neutel et al. *Sleep Medicine* 2016;20:172–3.

33 Wolf NI, Koenig M. Progressive cerebellar atrophy: hereditary ataxias and disorders with spinocerebellar degeneration. *Handbook of Clinical Neurology* 2013;113:1869–78.

34 van de Warrenburg BP, Sinke RJ, Kremer B. Recent advances in hereditary spinocerebellar ataxias. *Journal of Neuropathology & Experimental Neurology* 2005;64(3):171–80.

35 D'Abreu A, Franca M, Jr, Conz L, et al. Sleep symptoms and their clinical correlates in Machado-Joseph disease. *Acta Neurologica Scandinavica* 2009;119(4):277–80.

36 Friedman JH, Fernandez HH, Sudarsky LR. REM behavior disorder and excessive daytime somnolence in Machado-Joseph disease (SCA-3). *Movement Disorders* 2003;18(12):1520–2.

37 Iranzo A, Munoz E, Santamaria J, et al. REM sleep behavior disorder and vocal cord paralysis in Machado-Joseph disease. *Movement Disorders* 2003;18(10):1179–83.

38 Chi NF, Shiao GM, Ku HL, Soong BW. Sleep disruption in spinocerebellar ataxia type 3: a genetic and polysomnographic study. *Journal of the Chinese Medical Association* 2013;76(1):25–30.

39 Pedroso JL, Braga-Neto P, Felicio AC, et al. Sleep disorders in Machado-Joseph disease: a dopamine transporter imaging study. *Journal of the Neurological Sciences* 2013;324(1–2):90–3.

40 dos Santos DF, Pedroso JL, Braga-Neto P, et al. Excessive fragmentary myoclonus in Machado-Joseph disease. *Sleep Medicine* 2014;15(3):355–8.

41 Tuin I, Voss U, Kang JS, et al. Stages of sleep pathology in spinocerebellar ataxia type 2 (SCA2). *Neurology* 2006;67(11):1966–72.

42 Boesch SM, Frauscher B, Brandauer E, et al. Disturbance of rapid eye movement sleep in spinocerebellar ataxia type 2. *Movement Disorders* 2006;21(10):1751–4.

43 Rodriguez-Labrada R, Velazquez-Perez L, Ochoa NC, et al. Subtle rapid eye movement sleep abnormalities in presymptomatic spinocerebellar ataxia type 2 gene carriers. *Movement Disorders* 2011;26(2):347–50.

44 Velazquez-Perez L, Voss U, Rodriguez-Labrada R, et al. Sleep disorders in spinocerebellar ataxia type 2 patients. *Neurodegenerative Diseases* 2011;8(6):447–54.

45 Schols L, Haan J, Riess O, et al. Sleep disturbance in spinocerebellar ataxias: is the SCA3 mutation a cause of restless legs syndrome? *Neurology* 1998;51(6):1603–7.

46 Frauscher B, Hering S, Hogl B, et al. Restless legs syndrome in Friedreich ataxia: a polysomnographic study. *Movement Disorders* 2011;26(2):302–6.

47 Boesch SM, Frauscher B, Brandauer E, et al. Restless legs syndrome and motor activity during sleep in spinocerebellar ataxia type 6. *Sleep Medicine* 2006;7(6):529–32.

48 Synofzik M, Godau J, Lindig T, et al. Restless legs and substantia nigra hypoechogenicity are common features in Friedreich's ataxia. *Cerebellum* 2011;10(1):9–13.

49 Silva GM, Pedroso JL, Dos Santos DF, et al. NREM-related parasomnias in Machado-Joseph disease: clinical and polysomnographic evaluation. *Journal of Sleep Research* 2016;25(1):11–15.

50 Reimold M, Globas C, Gleichmann M, et al. Spinocerebellar ataxia type 1, 2, and 3 and restless legs syndrome: striatal dopamine D2 receptor status investigated by [11C] raclopride positron emission tomography. *Movement Disorders* 2006;21(10):1667–73.

51 Abele M, Burk K, Laccone F, et al. Restless legs syndrome in spinocerebellar ataxia types 1, 2, and 3. *Journal of Neurology* 2001;248(4):311–4.

52 Konieczny M, Bauer P, Tomiuk J, et al. CAG repeats in Restless Legs syndrome. *American Journal of Medical Genetics. Part B, Neuropsychiatric Genetics* 2006;141b(2):173–6.

53 Yen TC, Lu CS, Tzen KY, et al. Decreased dopamine transporter binding in Machado-Joseph disease. *Journal of Nuclear Medicine* 2000;41(6):994–8.

54 Taniwaki T, Sakai T, Kobayashi T, et al. Positron emission tomography (PET) in Machado-Joseph disease. *Journal of the Neurological Sciences* 1997;145(1):63–7.

55 Tuite PJ, Rogaeva EA, St George-Hyslop PH, Lang AE. Dopa-responsive parkinsonism phenotype of Machado-Joseph disease: confirmation of 14q CAG expansion. *Annals of Neurology* 1995;38(4):684–7.

56 Khan NL, Giunti P, Sweeney MG, et al. Parkinsonism and nigrostriatal dysfunction are associated with spinocerebellar ataxia type 6 (SCA6). *Movement Disorders* 2005;20(9):1115–9.

57 Lu CS, Wu Chou YH, Yen TC, et al. Dopa-responsive parkinsonism phenotype of spinocerebellar ataxia type 2. *Movement Disorders* 2002;17(5):1046–51.

58 Wilkins A, Brown JM, Barker RA. SCA2 presenting as levodopa-responsive parkinsonism in a young patient from the United Kingdom: a case report. *Movement Disorders* 2004;19(5):593–5.

59 Wullner U, Reimold M, Abele M, et al. Dopamine transporter positron emission tomography in spinocerebellar ataxias type 1, 2, 3, and 6. *Archives of Neurology* 2005;62(8):1280–5.

60 Pedroso JL, Bor-Seng-Shu E, Felicio AC, et al. Severity of restless legs syndrome is inversely correlated with echogenicity of the substantia nigra in different neurodegenerative movement disorders. a preliminary observation. *Journal of the Neurological Sciences* 2012;319(1–2):59–62.

61 Dang D, Cunnington D. Excessive daytime somnolence in spinocerebellar ataxia type 1. *Journal of the Neurological Sciences* 2010;290(1–2):146–7.

62 Shiojiri T, Tsunemi T, Matsunaga T, et al. Vocal cord abductor paralysis in spinocerebellar ataxia type 1. *Journal of Neurology, Neurosurgery, and Psychiatry* 1999;67(5):695.

63 Yuasa T, Ohama E, Harayama H, et al. Joseph's disease: clinical and pathological studies in a Japanese family. *Annals of Neurology* 1986;19(2):152–7.

64 Isozaki E, Naito R, Kanda T, et al. Different mechanism of vocal cord paralysis between spinocerebellar ataxia (SCA 1 and SCA 3) and multiple system atrophy. *Journal of the Neurological Sciences* 2002;197(1–2):37–43.

16

Myotonic Dystrophy

Bart Willem Smits[1] and José Enrique Martínez-Rodríguez[2]

[1] Department of Neurology, Maasstadziekenhuis, Rotterdam, The Netherlands
[2] Neurology Service, Hospital del Mar, IMAS, IMIM, Barcelona, Spain

Introduction

Myotonic dystrophy (MD) is one of the commonest inherited neuromuscular disorders in adults. The defining and characteristic symptoms include muscle dystrophy and myotonia. Dystrophy results in weakness and focal atrophy of the affected skeletal muscles, while myotonia is characterised by delayed relaxation after contraction.

Although usually characterised as a neuromuscular disorder, MD should be really regarded as a multi-organ disease, with involvement of the eye, heart, endocrine system as well as the brain.

Although MD was recognised more than 100 years ago, it was not until 1994 that it was appreciated that it comprises two genetically very distinct disorders [1]. MD type 1 (MD1), also known as Steinert's disease is caused by an unstable CTG repeat expansion in the 3' untranslated region of the DMPK gene on chromosome 19q13. In contrast, MD type 2 (MD2), originally referred to as proximal myotonic myopathy (PROMM), is related to a CTG expansion in the zinc finger protein 9 gene on chromosome 3q.

Despite the striking overlap in phenotypes, both disorders have several specific clinical features (Table 16.1) [2]. The most striking difference is prominent involvement of the central nervous system in MD1, as demonstrated by several neuro-imaging and neuropathological studies [3,4]. Moreover, sleep disorders have long been recognised as an important and early feature in MD1, often preceding other more recognisable systemic manifestations [5,6]. In recent years a growing number of reports on sleep disorders in MD2 have appeared. It appears however that there are considerable differences between the type and impact of sleep disturbances between the two MD types. Both disorders will therefore be discussed separately in this chapter.

Sleep Disorders in Neurology: A Practical Approach, Second Edition.
Edited by Sebastiaan Overeem and Paul Reading.
© 2018 John Wiley & Sons Ltd. Published 2018 by John Wiley & Sons Ltd.

Table 16.1 Clinical manifestations in the myotonic dystrophies.

	Adult-onset myotonic dystrophy type 1	Myotonic dystrophy type 2
Genetics		
Inheritance	Autosomal dominant	Autosomal dominant
Anticipation	Pronounced	Exceptionally rare
Congenital form	Yes	No
Chromosome	19q13.3	3q21.3
Locus	DMPK	CNBP
Expansion mutation	(CTG)n	(CCTG)n
Location of the expansion	3' untranslated region	Intron 1
Core features		
Clinical myotonia	Typical in adult onset	Present in less than 50%
Myotonia on electromyography	Generally present	Absent and variable in many patients
Muscle weakness	Disability often by age 30–50	Disability at age 60–85
Cataracts	Generally present	Present in a few patients at diagnosis
Localisation of muscle weakness		
Face or jaw	Generally present	Usually absent
Ptosis	Often present	Rare, mild, or moderate
Bulbar (dysphagia)	Generally present later in life	Not present
Respiratory muscles	Generally present later in life	Exceptionally rare cases
Distal limb muscle	Generally prominent	Flexor digitorum profundus in some
Proximal limb muscle	Can be absent for many years	Main disability in most patients, late onset
Sternocleidomastoid muscle	Generally prominent	Prominent in few patients
Muscular symptoms		
Myalgic pain	Absent or moderate	Most disabling symptom in many patients
Muscle strength variations	Occasional	Can be considerable
Visible muscle atrophy	Face, temporal, extremities	Usually absent
Calf hypertrophy	Absent	Present in at least 50%
Laboratory findings		
Serum creatine kinase	Normal-to-moderate increase	Normal-to-moderate increase

Table 16.1 (Continued)

	Adult-onset myotonic dystrophy type 1	Myotonic dystrophy type 2
Muscle biopsy findings		
Fibre atrophy	Smallness of type 1 fibres	Highly atrophic type 2 fibres
Nuclear clump fibres	In late stage only	Scattered early before weakness
Sarcoplasmic masses	Very frequent in distal muscles	Very rare
Ring fibres	Frequent	May occur
Internal nuclei	Massive in distal muscle	Variable and mainly in type 2 fibres
Cardiac symptoms		
Conduction defects	Common	Highly variable, absent to severe
Other neurological symptoms		
Tremors	Absent	Prominent in many patients
Behavioural changes	Common	Not apparent
Other features		
Manifest diabetes	Occasional	Infrequent
Frontal balding in men	Generally present	Exceptional
Incapacity (work and activities of daily living)	Typically after age 30–35 years	Rarely younger than 60 years, unless severe pain
Life expectancy	Reduced	Normal

Myotonic Dystrophy Type 1

Clinical Epidemiology

Four subtypes can be recognised in MD1, with an overall prevalence of approximately 1:8000: the congenital, childhood-onset, adult-onset and the late-onset oligosymptomatic types. Disease onset and severity are directly correlated with the number of CTG repeats although clinical features can vary considerably between subtypes. The congenital and childhood-onset types are mainly characterised by central nervous system involvement, while symptoms of the late-onset type can be limited to late-onset cataracts and mild skeletal muscle atrophy [4]. The adult-onset type is considered the 'typical' MD1 phenotype. As this is also the most common type, the remainder of this chapter focuses on adult-onset MD1.

Signs and Symptoms

Weakness and wasting predominantly affects the distal limbs and oculopharyngeal musculature. Atrophy and weakness of the temporalis muscles, frontal baldness, ptosis and a 'long face' produce the characteristic facial appearance. Myotonia is a core feature, most easily observed in the hands, and clinically manifest by an inability to release objects quickly.

Central nervous system involvement has been known since the earliest clinical descriptions of the disease [7]. Typically, this includes mild cognitive impairments as well as a variety of behavioural and personality traits such as apathy and decreased motivation, persistence or cooperation [8]. As a result, patients often do not spontaneously report their complaints or, alternatively, trivialise them. Furthermore, adherence to treatment and follow-up visits is often low [9]. Any doctor treating MD1 patients should be aware of this, as these personality traits pose a risk of underestimating and therefore undertreating the patient's condition.

Cardiac (conduction) abnormalities are common and a major cause of mortality [10]. Endocrine disturbances (testicular atrophy, insulin resistance) and gastrointestinal dysfunction are also often encountered. Many MD1 patients are increasingly disabled by the fifth or sixth decade after an insidious and long disease course. Life expectancy is reduced in MD1, largely due to increased rate of respiratory and cardiovascular pathology.

Sleep Disorders in MD1

Excessive Daytime Sleepiness

Excessive daytime sleepiness (EDS) has been noted as one of the main symptoms in MD1, with a prevalence between 33% and 77% [5,11]. EDS can occur at any point along the course of the disease, often preceding other systemic manifestations [6]. However, it is rare for this aspect of a patient's symptoms to be picked up early, as many physicians typically pay little attention to sleepiness when taking a medical history. Conversely, if attending a sleep clinic, MD1 may be missed in the early stage, when physicians do not have this diagnosis in mind when assessing a patient with daytime sleepiness. In MD1, it is likely that EDS is often interpreted as lack of motivation, laziness, apathy or loss of interest given that these traits are also common at any stage of the disease [11,12]. Paradoxically, apathy may also be a reason why patients often do not spontaneously complain of sleepiness per se. Indeed, it is common for relatives to notice excessive sleepiness and unplanned naps in subjects who, themselves, may appear unaware of any significant problem [12].

The severity of EDS in MD1 can be comparable with that seen in primary hypersomnias such as narcolepsy. Indeed, on the background of fairly continuous excessive sleepiness during the day, sudden episodes of irresistible sleep or 'sleep attacks' are not infrequent.

Clinically, it may be difficult to distinguish EDS from the common complaint of fatigue in MD1, and both symptoms may co-occur. Moreover, the reliability of the Epworth sleepiness scale (ESS), the most commonly used for rating EDS, is low in MD1. As an alternative, the Daytime Sleepiness scale (DSS) has been designed specifically for evaluating EDS in MD1 [13].

The severity of sleepiness is only weakly correlated with the degree of muscular impairment [5]. Similarly, other variables such as age, anthropometric data, gender, number of CTG repeats, or disease duration are not clearly correlated with the severity of EDS. Therefore, EDS has been proposed to reflect an intrinsic central dysfunction of the brain areas controlling the sleep–wake cycle that may be involved in the neurodegenerative process of MD1.

Sleep-related Breathing Disorders

Recent studies reported a prevalence of sleep apnoea in MD1 of 55–86%, with up to 30% having severe apnoea (Apnoea–Hypopnoea Index, AHI > 30) [14–17]. Obstructive apnoeas are the predominant type, although central or mixed apnoeas are also encountered. Obstructive apnoeas in MD1 patients are thought to result from weakness and hypotonia of upper-airway muscles. Features often encountered in 'primary' obstructive sleep apnoea (OSA) such as increased neck circumference or a crowded oropharynx are less important factors in MD1. Moreover, sleep apnoea in MD1 is characterised by a striking absence of typical clinical markers, such as snoring, nocturia, morning headache or non-restorative sleep. Also, there is no correlation with levels of muscle weakness, daytime respiratory function, cardiac involvement, the number of CTG repeats, nor with subjective daytime fatigue or sleepiness. In fact, EDS often persists after appropriate treatment of the sleep-disordered breathing, which further supports the concept that EDS is primarily caused by dysfunction of sleep regulatory circuits in the central nervous system.

Restless Legs and Periodic Leg Movements

An increased index of periodic limb movements during sleep (PLMI > 5/ hour) is found in 25–61% of MD1 patients [15,16,18]. Periodic limb movements during sleep in MD1 are associated with microarousals. Periodic limb movements during wakefulness and restless legs are reported by about one quarter of MD1 patients [15]. Periodic limb movements are however not associated with EDS or with subjective sleep quality and are mostly unrelated to respiratory events.

Other Sleep Disorders

Studies using the Multiple Sleep Latency Test (MSLT) have shown at least one sleep onset rapid eye movement (REM) period in about half of MD1 patients and at least two in about one third [15]. Questionnaire-based studies indicate an increased frequency of REM sleep behaviour disorder or narcolepsy-like symptoms (hypnagogic hallucinations, sleep paralysis and even cataplexy). However, these results were not confirmed in studies which assessed subjective sleep complaints by means of an interview by an experienced physician [15,17].

Diagnostic Procedures

Sleep-related symptoms should be part of every clinical interview with a MD1 patient. This includes assessment of EDS, indicators of sleep-related breathing disorders and any other nocturnal sleep disorder. Physicians should keep in mind that MD1 patients do not always recognise EDS as a medical problem or trivialise their complaints. It is therefore advised to confirm the patient's answers with a relative.

Given the fact that subjective complaints are poor predictors of an underlying sleep disorder and that an AHI > 30 invariably warrants treatment regardless of symptoms, it is preferable to perform polysomnography in all MD1 patients reporting sleep-related symptoms [9].

Figure 16.1 outlines the general procedure to follow in the evaluation of sleep disorders in a patient with MD1. The first step is to assess the possibility of potentially

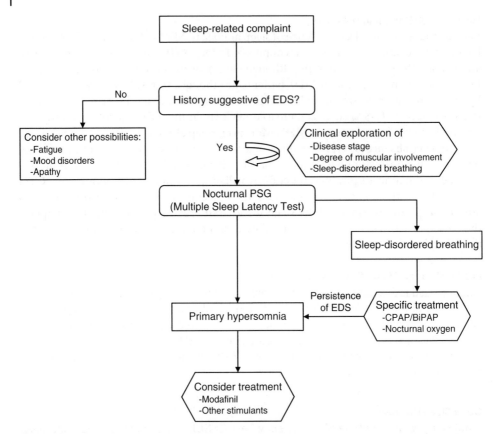

Figure 16.1 Flow chart for the diagnosis and management of excessive daytime sleepiness (EDS) in MD1. BiPAP, bi-level positive airway pressure; CPAP, continuous positive airway pressure; PSG, polysomnography.

treatable causes such as sleep-disordered breathing. As a general rule, an MD1 patient cannot be diagnosed with central hypersomnia if a complete sleep study has not been performed first.

MSLT findings are poor predictors of subjective sleep complaints and are therefore unlikely to influence the choice of treatment [15]. Hypocretin-1 measurements are not generally useful in the clinical workup of EDS in MD1, as only a subset of patients with EDS show clearly decreased levels.

When considering a sedated endoscopy or a surgical intervention for sleep-disordered breathing, special consideration should be given to the increased anesthesiological risks in MD1 patients.

Management

Significant sleep-related breathing disorders invariably justify treatment. Treatment can give symptom control but also is likely to prolong survival and improve quality of life [9]. First-line treatment is positive airway pressure, with conventional continuous positive airway pressure (CPAP) as a starting point. However, the use of CPAP may be limited by the degree of muscle weakness and bi-level positive airway pressure (BiPAP) therapy is regularly indicated. Oxygen therapy should always be considered in patients with significant nocturnal breathing disorders, although it should be used with caution, and preferably with input from a respiratory physician. Further details can be found in Chapter 17.

If breathing disorders are not present, or when adequate treatment does not appear to eliminate EDS, pharmacologic treatment with stimulants should be considered in patients with disability due to EDS. Both amphetamine-like stimulants and modafinil have been used to good effect in the treatment of EDS in MD1 [19,20]. Methylphenidate 10–40 mg is effective, but may be limited by side effects. Furthermore, tolerance has been observed in some patients. Small open-label trials of modafinil (200–400 mg/day) showed that the drug is well tolerated and without significant side effects. Moreover, tolerance has not been reported with modafinil in MD1. Before starting any stimulant treatment in a patient with MD1, in view of potential cardiac complications, a cardiologist should ideally be consulted and an appropriate workup performed.

Myotonic Dystrophy Type 2

Clinical Epidemiology

The prevalence of MD2 is less established, but recent literature suggests it is at least as common as MD1 [21]. Since symptoms can be non-specific, especially early in the disease, it is possible that many patients are not yet diagnosed. The prevalence of MD2 is therefore likely to increase with the passage of time.

Signs and Symptoms

The phenotype of MD2 is highly variable, ranging from mild proximal weakness and a slightly elevated serum creatine kinase in elderly patients to marked disability and cardiac death in early adult life. An overview of the clinical features is given in Table 16.1. Myalgia is a prominent symptom and often precedes weakness. Pain in MD2 is often generalised, resembling fibromyalgia, and does not respond well to pain medication [22].

Muscle weakness is typically proximal. Weakness of facial, bulbar and respiratory muscles is rare. The calves can become hypertrophic. Myotonia can be mild or even absent, both clinically and electrophysiologically. (Lethal) cardiac involvement is reported, but is less frequent than in MD1. Cognitive and social skills are typically normal or mildly affected at most.

Sleep disturbances have only recently been recognised in MD2. In general, studies are characterised by small sample sizes and much of the data have not yet been verified.

Sleep Disorders in MD2

Excessive Daytime Sleepiness
There is conflicting evidence about EDS in MD2. ESS scores are comparable with controls [14,23,24]. In contrast, MD2 patients have higher DSS scores, indicating increased daytime sleepiness [23,25]. Despite this uncertainty about the exact frequency or severity of EDS in MD2, it is likely to be less than that seen in MD1.

Sleep-related Breathing Disorders
An increased AHI is found in about half of MD2 patients [14,25,26]. As in MD1, most apnoeas are obstructive. AHI and the oxygen desaturation index are inversely correlated with vital capacity and maximal inspiratory pressure [14].

Restless Legs and Periodic Leg Movements
At least half of MD2 patients meet the criteria for restless legs syndrome (RLS) [23,27]. RLS in MD2 is associated with EDS and is an independent predictor of decreased subjective sleep quality. One quarter to one third of MD2 patients have a PLMI > 15, most of whom also report RLS. These periodic limb movements are however mostly associated with apnoeas, and it remains unknown whether periodic limb movements in MD2 are an isolated manifestation or mainly related with breathing events [23].

Other Sleep Disorders
Subjective sleep quality (Pittsburg Sleep Quality Index score) is decreased in the majority of MD2 patients [14,24,25]. Poor sleep quality is confirmed by polysomnographic recordings demonstrating decreased sleep efficiency, relative time in slow wave and REM sleep. In addition to the high prevalence of classical sleep disorders, pain also seems to be an important determinant of impaired sleep quality.

There are a few reports of REM sleep without atonia and/or REM sleep behaviour disorder in MD2 patients, all in patients with moderate to severe OSA [25].

Diagnostic Procedures

Any doctor treating MD2 patients should be aware of the increased prevalence of sleep disturbances.

When assessing subjective sleep quality, special attention should be paid to the influence of pain. It is advised to perform specific enquiries about present and past analgesia use with evaluation of current analgesic therapy.

Dedicated assessment of RLS is also appropriate. Although ferritin levels are routinely measured in RLS, it may be particularly important in MD2, since low ferritin levels are found in half of MD2 patients with RLS [23,27].

A polysomnogram is indicated if the patient complains about poor sleep quality, non-restorative sleep, EDS, leg movements during sleep or symptoms of sleep apnoea.

It is worth mentioning that there are no specific anesthesiological complications associated with MD2

Management

There are no clinical trials that have specifically studied the effect of treatment of sleep disorders in MD2. With the current evidence, sleep disorders in MD2 should be treated as in otherwise healthy subjects.

Subjective sleep quality might be improved by pain medication, although pain in MD2 is notoriously refractory to analgesics.

One small study reported a good response to CPAP in three out of four patients with OSA [26]. In patients with RLS, ferritin levels should be normalised, if low. If ferritin levels are normal, consider a trial of dopamine agonists.

Key Points

- EDS of central origin can be a defining feature of MD1, and appears very early in the course of the disease.
- MD1 patients often trivialise their complaints. Check the answers with a relative or keep asking until you are convinced that you have the correct information.
- MD1 patients with debilitating EDS of presumed central origin can be treated with stimulants (after a thorough cardiac workup), which is often very rewarding.
- Sleep-related breathing disorders and periodic limb movements during sleep are common in both MD1 and MD2.
- Nocturnal sleep quality is severely affected by pain in MD2. Make sure your patient has optimal analgesics.

References

1 Thornton CA, Griggs RC, Moxley RT. Myotonic dystrophy with no trinucleotide repeat expansion. *Ann Neurol* 1994; 35: 269–272.

2 Udd B, Krahe R. The myotonic dystrophies: molecular, clinical, and therapeutic challenges. *Lancet Neurol* 2012; 11: 891–905.

3 Glantz RH, Wright RB, Huckman MS, et al. Central nervous system magnetic resonance imaging findings in myotonic dystrophy. *Arch Neurol* 1988; 45: 36–37.

4 Harper PS. Myotonic Dystrophy, 3rd edn. W.B. Saunders: Philadelphia, 2001.

5 Laberge L, Bégin P, Montplaisir J, et al. Sleep complaints in patients with myotonic dystrophy. *J Sleep Res* 2004; 13: 95–100.

6 Ashizawa T. Myotonic dystrophy as a brain disorder. *Arch Neurol* 1998; 55: 291–293.

7 Aidie WJ, Greenfield JG. Dystrophia myotonica (myotonia atrophica). *Brain* 1923; 46: 73–127.

8 Winblad S, Lindberg C, Hansen S. Temperament and character in patients with classical myotonic dystrophy type 1 (DM-1). *Neuromuscul Disord* 2005; 15: 287–292.

9 Nugent AM, Smith IE, Shneerson JM. Domiciliary-assisted ventilation in patients with myotonic dystrophy. *Chest* 2002; 121: 459–464.

10 Groh WJ, Groh MR, Saha C, et al. Electrocardiographic abnormalities and sudden death in myotonic dystrophy type 1. *N Engl J Med* 2008; 358: 2688–2697.

11 Rubinsztein JS, Rubinsztein DC, Goodburn S, et al. Apathy and hypersomnia are common features of myotonic dystrophy. *J Neurol Neurosurg Psychiatry* 1998; 64: 510–515.

12 Phemister JC, Small JM. Hypersomnia in dystrophia myotonica. *J Neurol Neurosurg Psychiatry* 1961; 24: 173–175.

13 Laberge L, Gagnon C, Jean S, et al. Myotonic dystrophy: a study of reliability fatigue and daytime sleepiness rating scales. *J Neurol Neurosurg Psychiatry* 2005; 76: 1403–1405.

14 Bianchi ML, Losurdo A, Di Blasi C, et al. Prevalence and clinical correlates of sleep disordered breathing in myotonic dystrophy types 1 and 2. *Sleep Breath* 2013; 18: 579–589.

15 Yu H, Laberge L, Jaussent I, et al. Daytime sleepiness and REM sleep characteristics in myotonic dystrophy: a case-control study. *Sleep* 2011; 34: 165–70.

16 Pincherle A, Patruno V, Raimondi P, et al. Sleep breathing disorders in 40 Italian patients with Myotonic dystrophy type 1. *Neuromuscul Disord* 2012; 22: 219–24.

17 Laberge L, Bégin P, Dauvilliers Y, et al. A polysomnographic study of daytime sleepiness in myotonic dystrophy type 1. *J Neurol Neurosurg Psychiatry* 2009; 80: 642–646.

18 Romigi A, Izzi F, Pisani V, et al. Sleep disorders in adult-onset myotonic dystrophy type 1: a controlled polysomnographic study. *Eur J Neurol* 2011; 18: 1139–1145.

19 van der Meche FGA, Bogaard JM, van der Sluys JC, et al. Daytime sleep in myotonic dystrophy is not caused by sleep apnea. *J Neurol Neurosurg Psychiatry* 1994; 57; 626–628.

20 Damian MS, Gerlach BS, Schmidt F, et al. Modafinil for excessive daytime sleepiness in myotonic dystrophy. *Neurology* 2001; 56: 794–796.

21 Udd B, Meola G, Krahe R, et al. 140th ENMC International Workshop: myotonic dystrophy DM2/PROMM and other myotonic dystrophies with guidelines on management. *Neuromuscul Disord* 2006; 16: 403–413.

22 George A, Schneider-Gold C, Zier S, et al. Musculoskeletal pain in patients with myotonic dystrophy type 2. *Arch Neurol.* 2004; 61:1938–1942.

23 Lam EM, Shepard PW, St Louis EK, et al. Restless legs syndrome and daytime sleepiness are prominent in myotonic dystrophy type 2. *Neurology* 2013; 81: 157–164.

24 Tieleman AA, Knoop H, van de Logt AE, et al. Poor sleep quality and fatigue but no excessive daytime sleepiness in myotonic dystrophy type 2. *J Neurol Neurosurg Psychiatry* 2010; 81: 963–967.

25 Romigi A, Albanese M, Placidi F, et al. Sleep disorders in myotonic dystrophy type 2: a controlled polysomnographic study and self-reported questionnaires. *Eur J Neurol* 2014; 21: 929–934.

26 Bhat S, Sander HW, Grewal RP, et al. Sleep disordered breathing and other sleep dysfunction in myotonic dystrophy type 2. *Sleep Med* 2012; 13: 1207–1208.

27 Shepard P, Lam EM, St Louis EK, et al. Sleep disturbances in myotonic dystrophy type 2. *Eur Neurol* 2012; 68: 377–380.

17

Sleep Disorders in Neuromuscular Disease

Sushanth Bhat[1] and Johan Verbraecken[2]

[1] *JFK Neuroscience Institute, Hackensack Meridian Health-JFK Medical Center, Edison, USA*
[2] *Department of Pulmonary Medicine and Multidisciplinary Sleep Disorders Centre, Antwerp University Hospital and University of Antwerp, Antwerp, Belgium*

Introduction

Sleep disorders, while common in patients with neuromuscular diseases, are often overlooked. This may be because sleep complaints are not volunteered by the patient or elicited by the clinician, or because the symptoms, such as insomnia, excessive limb movements in sleep or daytime sleepiness are wrongly attributed to the underlying neuromuscular disease process itself. However, most sleep dysfunction co-morbid with neuromuscular diseases is easily diagnosed and effectively treated, potentially improving quality of life and favourably influencing morbidity and mortality. This chapter reviews sleep disorders that occur with common neuromuscular diseases and summarises the latest diagnostic recommendations and treatment strategies. Sleep dysfunction that occurs with myotonic dystrophy is discussed in Chapter 16.

Sleep-disordered breathing (SDB), whether obstructive or central sleep apnoea or nocturnal hypoventilation, is by far the most common cause of sleep dysfunction in patients with neuromuscular diseases. However, restless legs syndrome (RLS), periodic limb movements of sleep (PLMS), rapid eye movement sleep behaviour disorder (RBD) and even narcolepsy-type syndromes may also occur with specific diseases. These will be described in greater detail in the sections that follow.

Sleep and Breathing

The difference in respiratory control mechanisms during wakefulness and sleep explains the exquisite vulnerability of patients with neuromuscular diseases to SDB. The purpose of respiration is to maintain arterial blood gases (ABGs), specifically the partial pressures of oxygen and carbon dioxide (PaO_2 and $PaCO_2$, respectively), in a narrow range. Accordingly, chemoreceptors must be sufficiently sensitive to changes in PaO_2 and $PaCO_2$, posterior airway (pharyngeal dilator and tongue muscle) tone must be adequate

Sleep Disorders in Neurology: A Practical Approach, Second Edition.
Edited by Sebastiaan Overeem and Paul Reading.
© 2018 John Wiley & Sons Ltd. Published 2018 by John Wiley & Sons Ltd.

to allow air passage, respiratory control centres in the medulla must initiate inspiration to create a negative thoracic pressure sufficient to draw air into the lungs, and inspiratory muscles (primarily the diaphragm, but also accessory muscles such as the external intercostals and the sternocleidomastoideus) must generate sufficient force to ensure that an adequate volume of air enters the lungs. Expiration occurs passively from the natural elastic recoil of the lungs after the inspiratory muscles have ceased contraction, although expiratory muscles, mainly the internal intercostals and the rectus abdominis, may be active during periods of high demand.

During wakefulness, *volitional control* (originating in the cerebral cortex and mediated by descending pathways into the brainstem) ensures initiation of inspiration and high muscle tone in the posterior airway, and accessory muscle recruitment aids the diaphragm in ensuring adequate tidal volume, preventing respiratory compromise. In sleep, this volitional control is lost, with breathing regulated purely by the *metabolic* (or 'autonomic') pathway (which while also active during wakeful state, plays a subservient role). This pathway is maintained via a feedback loop, with inputs from the peripheral and central chemoreceptors relaying to the respiratory centres in the medulla, the 'pacemaker' for inspiration. In sleep, chemoreceptor responsiveness to changes in PaO_2 and $PaCO_2$ is blunted, more markedly in rapid eye movement (REM) sleep than in non-rapid eye movement (NREM) sleep, and progressive muscle atonia increases upper airway resistance and decreases tidal volumes, again most markedly in REM sleep, where all pharyngeal dilators and respiratory muscles with the exception of the diaphragm are paralysed. REM sleep, a particularly dynamic phase, is additionally characterised by wide autonomic swings resulting in irregular breathing and fluctuating tidal volumes. The net result is a physiological fall in PaO_2 (of about 3–10 mm Hg, reflected by a decrease in arterial oxygen saturation, SaO_2, of about 2–3%) and a rise in $PaCO_2$ (of about 2–8 mm Hg) in sleep in healthy individuals which is of little clinical consequence with intact respiratory muscle function. However, patients with neuromuscular diseases, in whom muscle tone is already compromised, may suffer severe derangements of ABGs in sleep due to *nocturnal alveolar hypoventilation*, with the attendant long-term cardiovascular risk and impact on daytime functioning. This results in *sleep hypoxaemia* (characterised by low baseline arterial oxygenation in sleep), usually initially present exclusively or most severely in REM sleep, but occurring in NREM sleep and finally in wakefulness as the underlying neuromuscular condition worsens.

In neuromuscular diseases there may also be superimposed *obstructive sleep apnoea* (OSA), with recurrent episodes of loss of upper airway tone causing partial or complete airway closure in sleep, impeding airflow and resulting in sleep fragmentation and repeated oxygen desaturations. Weight gain due to inactivity and muscular weakness, state-dependent decrease in neural drive to the upper airway dilators, and vibratory mechanical damage to these muscles and their sensory nerves may all worsen OSA. On overnight polysomnography (PSG), respiratory events in adults must be at least 10 seconds long to be scored. *Hypopnoeas* are characterised by diminished airflow with continued respiratory effort and require a 30% reduction in airflow with a 3% oxygen desaturation or an arousal [1]. With apnoeas, there is complete cessation in airflow; during an *obstructive apnoea*, respiratory effort persists, whereas during a *central apnoea*, it ceases. Central apnoeas imply an absence of the neurological drive to breathe, as may be seen in narcotic use, in congestive heart failure (CHF) as part of Cheyne–Stokes respirations, or with neurological conditions such as strokes, multiple sclerosis, or Arnold–Chiari malformations. *Mixed apnoeas* begin as central apnoeas and end as obstructive apnoeas. The Apnoea–Hypopnoea Index (AHI) measures the average number of respiratory events per hour of sleep on a polysomnogram (OSA is described as mild with an AHI between 5/hour and 15/hour, moderate between 15/hour and 30/hr, and severe greater than 30/hour). OSA leads *event-related hypoxaemia*, characterised by the occurrence of repeated episodes of falls in SaO2 (often measured by a surrogate, pulse oximetry, the SpO2) resulting from airflow limitation as a result of increased upper airway resistance, as is typical in OSA, or as a result of cessation of breathing, as seen with central sleep apnoea. Oxygen resaturation with event termination brings the SaO2 back to baseline. Muscle atonia lies at the heart of both nocturnal hypoventilation and OSA; expectedly, many patients with neuromuscular diseases exhibit sleep hypoxaemia with superimposed respiratory-event related hypoxaemia.

Initial Clinical Approach

Detection of sleep dysfunction in patients with neuromuscular diseases requires a high index of suspicion and familiarity with common manifestation of symptoms. A detailed sleep history, preferably with the input of the bed partner, encompassing specific enquiries about snoring and witnessed apnoeas, sleep initiation or maintenance insomnia, nocturnal orthopnoea, frequent awakenings with choking/gasping in sleep, morning headaches, cognitive impairment and sleepiness during the day is imperative. The Epworth Sleepiness Scale (ESS) [2] and the Sleep-disordered Breathing in Neuromuscular Disease Questionnaire (SiNQ)-5 [3] are useful additional tools. However, some patients may appear asymptomatic despite having seemingly significant SDB. Abnormal behaviour, excessive movements in sleep, and dream-enacting behaviour must be carefully elicited. Table 17.1 summarises the symptoms that should alert the clinician to possible underlying sleep dysfunction.

The physical examination may reveal several clues. Risk factors for OSA include narrow oropharyngeal passages due to tonsillar hypertrophy, retrognathia/micrognathia,

Table 17.1 Some signs and symptoms of sleep-disordered breathing in neuromuscular diseases.

Nocturnal
- Snoring
- Witnessed apnoeas and choking/gasping in sleep
- Frequent unexplained arousals from sleep
- Restless sleep
- Abnormal movements in sleep

Daytime
- Excessive daytime sleepiness and/or fatigue
- Morning headaches
- Cognitive complaints, mood symptoms
- In children, failure to thrive and declining school performance
- Signs of cardiovascular sequelae of chronic nocturnal hypoxia (e.g. pedal oedema and raised jugular venous pressure)

macroglossia or high arching palates, large neck circumferences (greater than 17 in. in men and 16 in. in women), and increased body mass indices (25–29 kg/m^2 being considered overweight, 30 kg/m^2 and above being considered obese). Overt signs of respiratory distress (rapid, shallow breathing, use of accessory muscles of respiration, tachypnoea with trouble completing full sentences, paradoxical breathing and supine orthopnoea) suggest weakness of inspiratory muscles, raising the suspicion of impending nocturnal hypoventilation and possibly respiratory failure. Physical manifestations of the cardiovascular consequences of significant nocturnal hypoventilation include cor pulmonale with limb oedema, hepatosplenomegaly and elevated jugular venous pressure [4].

Diagnostic Evaluation

Diurnal tests (to predict the presence of SDB), and nocturnal tests (to quantify it and guide its management) are both employed in the evaluation of patients with neuromuscular diseases and suspected sleep dysfunction.

Diurnal Testing

Evaluation of Pulmonary Function and Respiratory Muscle Function

Tests of pulmonary and respiratory muscle function, usually performed in the outpatient setting under the auspices of a pulmonologist, both evaluate the robustness of the ventilatory system in wakefulness and are used to predict nocturnal hypoventilation. Pulmonary function testing using spirometry is a simple, non-invasive and inexpensive method of assessing lung function in patients with intrinsic pulmonary, neurological or musculoskeletal diseases. Lung volumes and capacities are measured and compared with expected normal values. With neuromuscular diseases, there are low lung volumes (specifically a low forced vital capacity [FVC]) and a restrictive pattern characterised by a forced expiratory volume in 1 second to FVC ratio (FEV1/FVC) that is normal or increased, due to preservation of FEV1 in the face of absolute reduction of FVC. Pulmonary function tests (PFTs) are limited by their dependence on patient cooperation and effort.

Respiratory muscle strength can be measured by *maximum (peak) inspiratory pressure* (PImax, or negative inspiratory force, NIF), reflecting inspiratory (mainly diaphragmatic) function, and the *maximum (peak) expiratory pressure* (PEmax), reflecting expiratory muscle function. Normal PImax values in adults (18–65 years old) range from –92 to –121 cm H$_2$O in men and –68 to –79 cm H$_2$O in women; mean PEmax values are 140 cm H$_2$O in men and 95 cm H$_2$O in women. A PImax in the normal range effectively excludes inspiratory muscle weakness. Large ranges of normal values exist for PImax, but it can be used to serially follow respiratory function in a particular patient. Measurement of PImax and PEmax requires the patient to blow into a mouthpiece, requiring both patient cooperation as well as the ability to form a tight lip seal, often difficult for patients with bulbar and facial weakness. Therefore, PImax values below the normal range (usually 50% or less than predicted) need to be interpreted with caution [5].

The exact role of PFTs and respiratory muscle testing in the evaluation of SDB remains unclear. A combination of FVC and PImax measurements appears more sensitive and specific for nocturnal hypoventilation; FVC less than 25% predicted and a PImax less than 4 kPa were determined predictive of nocturnal hypoventilation in both NREM and REM sleep [6,7]. Supine FVC measurements (especially if less than 75% predicted) and differences in FVC readings in the erect and supine positions may predict diaphragmatic weakness with greater reliability [8].

Oesophageal and transdiaphragmatic sniff pressures reflect diaphragmatic function, and may be especially useful in patients with facial weakness (rendering PImax measurement impractical) despite their semi-invasive nature. The non-invasive measurement of *sniff nasal inspiratory pressure* (SNIP) is comparable with oesophageal sniff pressures and may be superior to PImax and FVC in predicting SDB [9]; it has particular usefulness in serially assessing respiratory function in patients with a variety of neuromuscular diseases, and may predict survival in amyotrophic lateral sclerosis (ALS) [10]. Despite being increasingly used however, it is not yet accepted as a standard means to assess for SDB, and many patients find it difficult and unpleasant [11].

In summary, while no single diurnal pulmonary or respiratory muscle function test has been found to be predictive of nocturnal hypoventilation, multiple tests most likely increase diagnostic precision. A combination of PImax and SNIP has been recommended by several authors [12].

Arterial Blood Gases

ABG measurements detect hypoxaemia (a PaO_2 less than 60 mm Hg) and hypercapnia (a $PaCO_2$ greater than 45 mm Hg) resulting from respiratory insufficiency. Early in the course of neuromuscular respiratory dysfunction, ABG abnormalities may be limited to sleep; thus, diurnal ABG abnormalities are insensitive in detecting SDB, although when present, they strongly suggest nocturnal hypoventilation, and may be used to monitor response to nocturnal non-invasive positive pressure ventilation (NIPPV, see below) [13]. While continuous measurement of nocturnal PaO_2 and $PaCO_2$ is too impractical for routine clinical use, comparison of a single nocturnal ABG sample (or a sample drawn immediately upon awakening) with one drawn during the day may demonstrate nocturnal hypoventilation. Per American Academy of Sleep Medicine criteria, hypoventilation is present when the $PaCO_2$ (or a surrogate such as the end tidal carbon dioxide [EtCO2] or transcutaneous carbon dioxide) is greater than 55 mm Hg (or is at least 50 mm Hg and more than 10 mm Hg above the awake supine value) for at least 10 minutes during sleep; in children, it is diagnosed when the $PaCO_2$ or surrogate is greater than 50 mm Hg for more than 25% of the sleep time [1].

Miscellaneous Diurnal Testing

Transdiaphragmatic pressure measurement (comparing oesophageal and gastric pressures through balloon techniques), fluoroscopic chest X-ray evaluation (involving real-time imaging of diaphragm movements during a supine sniff manoeuvre), and intercostal and phrenic nerve conduction studies and diaphragmatic EMG are largely research tools and are not routinely employed clinically [5].

Nocturnal Testing

Surrogate Markers of Blood Gases

In patients with neuromuscular diseases, the presence of significant oxygen desaturation on a screening overnight pulse oximetry suggests SDB. A typical pattern seen, especially early in the course of the illness, is low baseline oxygen saturations with

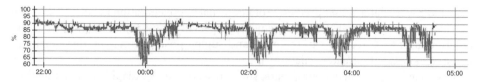

Figure 17.1 Abnormal overnight pulse oximetry tracing from a patient with an underlying neuromuscular disease. Note the low baseline arterial oxygen saturation (SpO2) level consistently below 90% with superimposed cyclical worsening, suggesting sleep hypoxaemia with probable rapid eye movement (REM)-related worsening or significant REM-predominant obstructive sleep apnoea. Full night in-lab polysomnography is necessary to make this distinction. A similar pattern may be seen in patients with pulmonary disorders.

cyclical worsening, suggesting sleep hypoxaemia with either superimposed REM-related worsening or significant REM-predominant OSA (see Figure 17.1). However, a similar pattern may be encountered in patients with alveolar or interstitial lung diseases such as chronic obstructive pulmonary disease (COPD), pulmonary fibrosis or obesity hypoventilation syndrome; these are indistinguishable by pulse oximetry alone. While overnight pulse oximetry is insufficiently sensitive to detect nocturnal hypoventilation, nocturnal EtCO2 measurement may be more reliable [1,14]. However, both pulse oximetry and EtCO2, which are surrogate markers of the underlying blood gas status, have significant limitations. For example, in patients with haemoglobinopathies, the SpO2 may be spuriously low. Similarly, in patients with significant pulmonary ventilation-perfusion mismatch or nasal congestion/obstruction, EtCO2 also be reduced and mislead interpretation. These probes are also very easily displaced during a sleep study. The clinician must bear this in mind while interpreting the data.

Polysomnography

While admittedly expensive and labour-intensive, there is no true substitute for the gold standard full night in-laboratory PSG in the evaluation of SDB in patients with neuromuscular diseases. PSG allows for detailed analysis of multiple simultaneously recorded parameters (electroencephalography, electrooculography, chin and leg electromyography (EMG), airflow, effort, electrocardiography, SpO2 and snoring), staging of epochs as wake, NREM sleep or REM sleep, scoring of respiratory events, the identification of SpO2 desaturations, and analysis of abnormal movements in sleep. PSG diagnoses OSA, central sleep apnoea and Cheyne–Stokes breathing, identifies PLMS, and assesses REM sleep for the absence of atonia, which is required to diagnose RBD (for details, see Chapter 2). Elevated EtCO2 measurements suggest nocturnal hypoventilation, and patterns of SpO2 abnormalities in conjunction with other parameters reveal event-related hypoxaemia (as may occur in OSA), sleep hypoxaemia (as may occur with nocturnal hypoventilation), or, as is common in patients with neuromuscular diseases, a combination of both. Portable monitoring studies with limited channels cannot, therefore, substitute for in-laboratory PSG studies in patients with neuromuscular diseases [15].

Sleep Dysfunction in Specific Neuromuscular Diseases

Motor Neurone Diseases

The muscle atonia and diaphragmatic weakness arising from the relentlessly progressive degeneration of motor neurones in ALS results in a propensity to develop SDB (both nocturnal hypoventilation and OSA), the most frequent reason for sleep complaints. Nocturia, sleep fragmentation and nocturnal cramps commonly occur [16]. On PSG, patients with ALS typically have decreased sleep efficiency with fragmented sleep architecture and, in the early stages, a large number of central apnoeas, possibly due to central drive dysfunction or respiratory muscle fatigue even in the absence of demonstrable diurnal diaphragmatic dysfunction [17,18]. Nocturnal NIPPV (described in detail below), the cornerstone of treatment, prolongs survival [19]. SDB is also seen with *spinal muscular atrophies* (SMA) and Kennedy's disease (X-linked spinobulbar neuronal atrophy) [20]; infants and children with SMA types 1 and 2 have more severe OSA and paradoxical breathing than controls [21] and NIPPV is beneficial [22]. Respiratory disturbances and sleep dysfunction occur in the acute and convalescent stages of *bulbar poliomyelitis* [4], and both RLS and PLMS occur in *post-polio syndrome* [23]. The traditional pharmacological management of RLS symptoms (see below) is generally effective. PSGs in post-polio syndrome patients show poor sleep efficiency with prolonged sleep latencies and high arousal indices [24], and patients frequently have disabling fatigue [25], but it is unclear whether they have a higher likelihood of SDB [26,27].

Myopathies and Neuromuscular Junction Disorders

In general, myopathies present with respiratory involvement and SDB only late in the disease (although with *acid maltase deficiency,* diaphragmatic involvement causing nocturnal hypoventilation may occur even before limb weakness becomes evident [28]). Even in the absence of diaphragmatic dysfunction and nocturnal hypoventilation, however, upper airway dilator muscle weakness may result in OSA, and REM-related hypopnoeas, apnoeas and paradoxical breathing may occur fairly early (Figure 17.2). *Congenital myopathies* (e.g. nemaline rod myopathy, centrotubular and central core disease, merosin myopathies and congenital muscular dystrophies) generally present in childhood (although rare cases of delayed presentation in adulthood with respiratory failure have been described), and sleep complaints, respiratory insufficiency and SDB may occur [29]. Patients with *Duchenne's muscular dystrophy* exhibit a combination of upper airway resistance and hypoventilation occurring in all stages of sleep due to decreased upper airway resistance, respiratory muscle weakness and scoliosis, causing a restrictive pulmonary deficit and severe nocturnal blood gas derangement [5]. Though nocturnal NIPPV is often prescribed, its long-term benefits are still being investigated [30].

Sleep disorders are prime symptoms in myotonic dystrophy types 1 and 2 and are discussed in detail in Chapter 16. Research into sleep dysfunction in patients with neuromuscular junction disorders has been sparse. Interestingly, while it is controversial

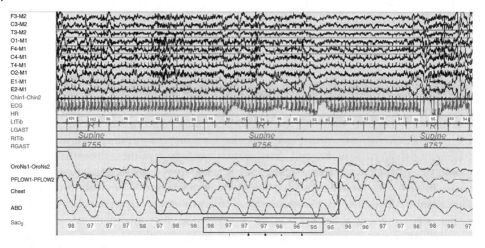

Figure 17.2 A 90-second epoch of rapid eye movement (REM) sleep from the overnight polysomnogram of an 18-year-old woman with limb girdle muscular dystrophy, complaining of orthopnoea, insomnia, frequent awakenings, excessive daytime sleepiness and cognitive concerns. The recording showed mild obstructive sleep apnoea, with an Apnoea–Hypopnoea Index of 10.3/ hour, and an arterial oxygen saturation (SaO2) nadir of 93%. Note paradoxical breathing (upper box) in REM sleep, with alternating movements of the chest and abdominal effort belts, accompanied by a SaO2 desaturation of 3% (lower box).

whether OSA is more common in patients with *myasthenia gravis* than in controls [31,32], anecdotal reports suggest that treating OSA with continuous positive airway pressure (CPAP) in patients with myasthenia gravis improves morning weakness and fatigue [33,34], suggesting that untreated OSA may have a deleterious effect on optimal control of myasthenic symptoms.

Neuropathies

Respiratory involvement, and therefore SDB, is rare in neuropathies. However, OSA is more prevalent with Charcot–Marie–Tooth (CMT) disease than in controls [35], and the 2C subtype, associated with upper airway dysfunction and diaphragmatic weakness, and may in particular predispose to SDB. Patients with CMT report poor sleep quality, daytime sleepiness and fatigue, and RLS [36]. In the first week of illness, most patients with acquired inflammatory demyelinating polyneuropathy (AIDP) have increased sleep latencies, sleep fragmentation, reduced sleep periods [37] and, interestingly, narcoleptic-type symptoms (sleep onset in REM sleep periods, REM sleep without atonia, hypnagogic hallucinations) [38]. The low cerebrospinal fluid hypocretin levels found in the acute phase of AIDP suggest that central demyelination may be partly responsible for sleep dysfunction [39]. As with CMT, patients with chronic inflammatory demyelinating polyneuropathy have a high prevalence of RLS [40].

Management of Sleep Dysfunction in Neuromuscular Disorders

Table 17.2 lists available treatment modalities for sleep dysfunction in neuromuscular diseases. Note that conservative measures and lifestyle modification, such as weight loss, avoiding supine sleep, and minimising agents such as alcohol, narcotic pain medications and benzodiazepines that worsen muscle tone and depress respiration are also important.

Upper Airway Pressurisation

Improving nocturnal gas exchange by reducing upper airway resistance and supporting the ventilatory muscles is the mainstay of treatment of SDB in neuromuscular diseases. Maintenance of adequate alveolar ventilation improves sleep continuity, prevents the long-term cardiovascular effects of chronic hypoxaemia, and improves daytime symptoms such as fatigue, sleepiness, headaches and cognitive dysfunction.

Upper airway pressurisation with a CPAP device is first-line therapy for patients with OSA. CPAP eliminates obstructive events, normalises oxygen saturation and improves sleep continuity. In patients with nocturnal hypoventilation with or without concomitant OSA, bi-level devices are often required to provide pressure support for NIPPV. In patients with ALS, nocturnal NIPPV improves survival, retards pulmonary function decline, enhances quality of life, and improves survival when used for more than four hours a night [41], with sustained long-term benefits [42]. Table 17.3 presents the latest recommendations for the initiation of nocturnal NIPPV in neuromuscular diseases, although they have yet to be universally agreed upon [43,44]. When both OSA and nocturnal hypoventilation coexist, NIPPV may be titrated during in-laboratory PSG, with inspiratory and expiratory positive airway pressures adjusted to eliminate

Table 17.2 Management options for sleep dysfunction in neuromuscular diseases (for details, see text).

Management of SDB

- Upper airway pressurisation
  - Continuous positive airway pressurisation
  - Nocturnal non-invasive positive pressure ventilation
- Supplemental oxygen therapy
- Surgical treatment
  - Tracheostomy
  - Diaphragm pacing
  - Hypoglossal nerve stimulation for OSA
  - OSA-specific surgeries (palatal/nasal/skeletal)
- Dental devices for OSA

Pharmacotherapy for non-SDB sleep dysfunction

- Excessive daytime sleepiness
  - Wakefulness-promoting agents (including modafinil and amphetamine-derivatives)
- Restless legs syndrome
  - Dopaminergics, iron supplemention

OSA, obstructive sleep apnoea; SDB, sleep-disordered breathing.

Table 17.3 Suggested criteria guiding the initiation of nocturnal non-invasive positive pressure ventilation in neuromuscular disorders.

Appropriate clinical symptoms and signs plus at least one of the following:

- $PaCO_2 \geq 45$ mm Hg
- Maximum inspiratory pressure <60 cm H_2O
- Forced vital capacity >50% predicted (in cases of progressive disease)
- Nocturnal $SpO_2 \leq 88\%$ for five consecutive minutes by finger oximetry, or <90% for >1 minute cumulative; with a sniff nasal inspiratory pressure <40 cm H_2O in the presence of orthopnoea

---

Source: Ref. [5]. Reproduced with permission of Elsevier.

respiratory events, and the pressure support adjusted to ensure acceptable EtCO2 and SpO2 levels as well as to maintain desired tidal volumes, with or without supplemental oxygen [45].

Patients with neuromuscular diseases often have considerable weakness of facial, bulbar and intrinsic hand muscles, making the application and tolerance of masks challenging. Careful selection of optimal interfaces and regular follow up with clinicians may improve compliance.

Supplemental Oxygen

Supplemental oxygen therapy alone is not used to treat OSA (upper airway pressurisation, described above, is the recommended therapy), and its role in nocturnal hypoventilation is unclear, with studies suggesting that in patients with neuromuscular disease, there may be worsening of underlying carbon dioxide retention [46]. However, supplemental oxygen is often used to treat residual hypoxia while titrating a patient with bi-level devices.

Miscellaneous Treatment Modalities

New and emerging therapies, while still not in widespread use, are worth discussing briefly. *Diaphragmatic pacing devices,* now approved by the US Federal Drug Administration for ALS, improve diaphragmatic function [47], but contradictory reports on their effect on survival [48] cloud their role in the specific treatment of SDB. *Tracheostomy,* a definitive but invasive method of treating SDB, needs to be carefully considered on a case-by-case basis, but may unfortunately become necessary in patients unable to tolerate treatment with PAP devices.

Patients with neuromuscular disorders and pure OSA (without nocturnal hypoventilation) may be candidates for a variety of *dental devices* (mandibular advancement devices), *hypoglossal nerve stimulators* [49], and *surgeries* (nasal, palatal, tongue-based and skeletal), just as other patients with OSA [50]. Such interventions would, however, be ineffective for patients with nocturnal hypoventilation, who require upper airway pressurisation.

Pharmacological agents have no utility in the treatment of SDB itself, but wakefulness-promoting agents such as modafanil and armodafinil, as well as traditional stimulants such as methylphenidate and amphetamines may be used for residual daytime sleepiness despite optimal compliance with PAP devices. In addition, RLS seen in many neuromuscular disorders, is treated with dopaminergic agents, antiepileptics (gabapentin and pregabalin, especially in patients with coexistent neuropathy) and iron supplementation (in patients with serum ferritin levels lower than 50 ng/ml). The optimal treatment of incidental PLMS that does not disrupt the patient's sleep, without complaints of daytime RLS, is controversial.

Key Points

- Sleep complaints in patients with neuromuscular diseases are common but often overlooked. Familiarity with typical signs and symptoms is important.
- Sleep disordered breathing (SDB), the most common sleep disorder in neuromuscular diseases, may initially be limited to REM sleep, but may also become manifest in NREM sleep as the disease progresses.
- SDB may present as nocturnal hypoventilation from respiratory muscle weakness, and/or OSA from increased upper airway resistance secondary to pharyngeal dilator muscle atonia. Severe nocturnal hypoxia and hypercapnia may result.
- In-laboratory PSG is the recommended diagnostic tool for SDB in patients with neuromuscular diseases. While a variety of diurnal tests are available to predict nocturnal hypoventilation, none have been found to be sufficiently sensitive and specific in isolation, although a combination of maximal inspiratory pressure and nasal sniff pressure testing is generally recommended.
- Optimal management of SDB requires nocturnal upper airway pressurisation, usually with a NIPPV device.

References

1 Berry RB, Brooks R, Gamaldo CE, et al. The AASM Manual for the Scoring of Sleep and Associated Events: Rules, Terminology, and Technical Specifications, Version 2.0.3. Darien, IL: American Academy of Sleep Medicine, 2014.

2 Johns MW. A new method for measuring daytime sleepiness: the Epworth Sleepiness Scale. *Sleep* 1991;14(6):540–545.

3 Steier J, Jolley CJ, Seymour J, et al. Screening for sleep-disordered breathing in neuromuscular disease using a questionnaire for symptoms associated with diaphragm paralysis. *Eur Respir J* 2011;37(2):400–5.

4 Chokroverty S. Sleep and breathing in neuromuscular disorders. *Handb Clin Neurol* 2011;99:1087–108.

5 Bhat S, Gupta D, Chokroverty S. Sleep disorders in neuromuscular diseases. *Neurol Clin* 2012;30(4):1359–87.

6 Ragette R, Mellies U, Schwake C, et al. Patterns and predictors of sleep disordered breathing in primary myopathies. *Thorax* 2002;57(8):724–8.

7 Mellies U, Ragette R, Schwake C, et al. Daytime predictors of sleep disordered breathing in children and adolescents with neuromuscular disorders. *Neuromuscul Disord* 2003;13(2):123–8.

8 Lechtzin N, Wiener CM, Shade DM, et al. Spirometry in the supine position improves the detection of diaphragmatic weakness in patients with amyotrophic lateral sclerosis. *Chest* 2002;121(2):436–42.

9 Heritier F, Rahm F, Pasche P, Fitting JW. Sniff nasal inspiratory pressure; A noninvasive assessment of inspiratory muscle strength. *Am J Respir Crit Care Med* 1994;150(6):1678–83.

10 Morgan RK, McNally S, Alexander M, et al. Use of Sniff nasal-inspiratory force to predict survival in amyotrophic lateral sclerosis. *Am J Respir Crit Care Med* 2005;171(3):269–74.

11 Barnes N, Agyapong-Badu S, Walsh B, et al. Reliability and acceptability of measuring sniff nasal inspiratory pressure (SNIP) and peak inspiratory flow (PIF) to assess respiratory muscle strength in older adults: a preliminary study. *Aging Clin Exp Res* 2014;26(2):171–6.

12 Steier J, Kaul S, Seymour J, et al. The value of multiple tests of respiratory muscle strength. *Thorax* 2007;62:975–80.

13 Hukins CA, Hillman DR. Daytime predictors of sleep hypoventilation in Duchenne muscular dystrophy. *Am J Respir Crit Care Med* 2000;161(1):166–70.

14 Bauman KA, Kurili A, Schmidt SL, et al. Home-based overnight transcutaneous capnography/pulse oximetry for diagnosing nocturnal hypoventilation associated with neuromuscular disorders. *Arch Phys Med Rehabil* 2013;94(1):46–52.

15 Collop N, Anderson M, Boehlecke B, et al. Clinical guidelines for the use of unattended portable monitors in the diagnosis of obstructive sleep apnea in adult patients. Portable monitoring task force of the American Academy of Sleep Medicine. *J Clin Sleep Med* 2007;3(7):737–47.

16 Lo Coco D, Mattaliano P, Spataro R, et al. Sleep-wake disturbances in patients with amyotrophic lateral sclerosis. *J Neurol Neurosurg Psychiatry* 2011;82(8):839–42.

17 Atalaia A, De Carvalho M, Evangelista T, Pinto A. Sleep characteristics of amyotrophic lateral sclerosis in patients with preserved diaphragmatic function. *Amyotroph Lateral Scler* 2007;8(2):101–5.

18 David WS, Bundlie SR, Mahdavi Z. Polysomnographic studies in amyotrophic lateral sclerosis. *J Neurol Sci* 1997;152(S1):S29–35.

19 Hannan LM, Dominelli GS, Chen YW, et al. Systematic review of non-invasive positive pressure ventilation for chronic respiratory failure. *Respir Med* 2014;108(2):229–43.

20 Romigi A, Liguori C, Placidi F, et al. Sleep disorders in spinal and bulbar muscular atrophy (Kennedy's disease): a controlled polysomnographic and self-reported questionnaires study. *J Neurol* 2014; 261(5):889–93.

21 Testa MB, Pavone M, Bertini E, et al. Sleep-disordered breathing in spinal muscular atrophy types 1 and 2. *Am J Phys Med Rehabil* 2005;84(9):666–70.

22 Petrone A, Pavone M, Testa MB, et al. Noninvasive ventilation in children with spinal muscular atrophy types 1 and 2. *Am J Phys Med Rehabil* 2007;86(3):216–21.

23 Marin LF, Carvalho LB, Prado LB, et al. Restless legs syndrome in post-polio syndrome: a series of 10 patients with demographic, clinical and laboratorial findings. *Parkinsonism Relat Disord* 2011;17(7):563–4.

24 Silva TM, Moreira GA, Quadros AA, et al. Analysis of sleep characteristics in post-polio syndrome patients. *Arq Neuropsiquiatr* 2010;68(4):535–40.

25 Tersteeg IM, Koopman FS, Stolwijk-Swüste JM, et al.; CARPA Study Group. A 5-year longitudinal study of fatigue in patients with late-onset sequelae of poliomyelitis. *Arch Phys Med Rehabil* 2011;92(6):899–904.

26 Hsu AA, Staats BA.'Postpolio' sequelae and sleep-related disordered breathing. *Mayo Clin Proc* 1998;73(3):216–24.

27 Chasens ER, Umlauf M, Valappil T, Singh KP. Nocturnal problems in postpolio syndrome: sleep apnea symptoms and nocturia. *Rehabil Nurs* 2001;26(2):66–71.

28 Nabatame S, Taniike M, Sakai N, et al. Sleep disordered breathing in childhood-onset acid maltase deficiency. *Brain Dev* 2009;31(3):234–9.

29 Pinard JM, Azabou E, Essid N, et al. Sleep-disordered breathing in children with congenital muscular dystrophies. *Eur J Paediatr Neurol* 2012;16(6):619–24.

30 Raphael J, Chevret S, Chastang C, Bouvet F. Randomised trial of preventive nasal ventilation in Duchenne muscular dystrophy. French Multicentre Cooperative Group on Home Mechanical Ventilation Assistance in Duchenne de Boulogne Muscular Dystrophy. *Lancet* 1994;343(8913):1600–4.

31 Shintani S, Shiozawa Z, Shindo K, et al. [Sleep apnea in well-controlled myasthenia gravis] (in Japanese). *Rinsho Shinkeigaku* 1989;29(5):547–53.

32 Prudlo J, Koenig J, Ermert S, Juhász J. Sleep disordered breathing in medically stable patients with myasthenia gravis. *Eur J Neurol* 2007;14(3):321–6.

33 Ji KH, Bae JS. CPAP therapy reverses weakness of myasthenia gravis: role of obstructive sleep apnea in paradoxical weakness of myasthenia gravis. *J Clin Sleep Med* 2014;10(4):441–2.

34 Naseer S, Kolade VO, Idrees S, et al. Improvement in ocular myasthenia gravis during CPAP therapy for sleep apnea. *Tenn Med* 2012;105(9):33–4.

35 Boentert M, Knop K, Schuhmacher C, et al. Sleep disorders in Charcot–Marie–Tooth disease type 1. *J Neurol Neurosurg Psychiatry* 2014;85(3):319–25.

36 Boentert M, Dziewas R, Heidbreder A, et al. Fatigue, reduced sleep quality and restless legs syndrome in Charcot–Marie–Tooth disease: a web-based survey. *J Neurol* 2010;257(4):646–52.

37 Karkare K, Sinha S, Taly AB, Rao S. Prevalence and profile of sleep disturbances in Guillain–Barré Syndrome: a prospective questionnaire-based study during 10 days of hospitalization. *Acta Neurol Scand* 2013;127(2):116–23.

38 Cochen V, Arnulf I, Demeret S, et al. Vivid dreams, hallucinations, psychosis and REM sleep in Guillain–Barré syndrome. *Brain* 2005;128(Pt 11):2535–45.

39 Nishino S, Kanbayashi T, Fujiki N, et al. CSF hypocretin levels in Guillain–Barré syndrome and other inflammatory neuropathies. *Neurology* 2003;61(6):823–5.

40 Luigetti M, Del Grande A, Testani E, et al. Restless leg syndrome in different types of demyelinating neuropathies: a single-center pilot study. *J Clin Sleep Med* 2013;9(9):945–9.

41 Lo Coco D, Marchese S, Pesco MC, et al. Noninvasive positive-pressure ventilation in ALS: Predictors of tolerance and survival. *Neurology* 2006 67(5):761–5.

42 Lyall RA, Donaldson N, Fleming T, et al. A prospective study of quality of life in ALS patients treated with noninvasive ventilation. *Neurology* 2001;57(1):153–6.

43 Clinical indications for noninvasive positive pressure ventilation in chronic respiratory failure due to restrictive lung disease, COPD, and nocturnal hypoventilation – a consensus conference report. *Chest* 1999;116(2):521–34.

44 Miller RG, Jackson CE, Kasarskis EJ, et al. Practice Parameter update: The care of the patient with amyotrophic lateral sclerosis: Drug, nutritional, and respiratory therapies (an evidence-based review). Report of the Quality Standards Subcommittee of the American Academy of Neurology. *Neurology* 2009;73(15):1218–26.

45 Berry RB, Chediak A, Brown LK, et al. NPPV titration task force of the American Academy of Sleep Medicine. Best clinical practices for the sleep center adjustment of

noninvasive positive pressure ventilation (NPPV) in stable chronic alveolar hypoventilation syndromes. *J Clin Sleep Med* 2010;6(5):491–509.

46 Gay PC, Edmonds LC. Severe hypercapnia after low-flow oxygen therapy in patients with neuromuscular disease and diaphragmatic dysfunction. *Mayo Clin Proc* 1995;70(4):327–30.

47 Onders RP, Elmo M, Kaplan C, et al. Final analysis of the pilot trial of diaphragm pacing in amyotrophic lateral sclerosis with long-term follow-up: diaphragm pacing positively affects diaphragm respiration. *Am J Surg* 2014;207(3):393–7.

48 Mahajan KR, Bach JR, Saporito L, Perez N. Diaphragm pacing and noninvasive respiratory management of amyotrophic lateral sclerosis/motor neuron disease. *Muscle Nerve* 2012;46(6):851–5.

49 Strollo PJ Jr, Soose RJ, Maurer JT, et al. Upper-airway stimulation for obstructive sleep apnea. *N Engl J Med* 2014;370(2):139–49.

50 Randerath WJ, Verbraecken J, Andreas S, et al. Non CPAP therapies in OSA. *Eur Respir J* 2011;37:1000–28.

18

Headache Disorders

Jeanetta C. Rains[1] and J. Steven Poceta[2]

[1] *Center for Sleep Evaluation at Elliot Hospital, Manchester, USA*
[2] *Scripps Clinic Sleep Center, Division of Neurology, Scripps Clinic, La Jolla, USA*

Introduction

Increasing knowledge of the unequivocal but complex reciprocal relationship between sleep disorders and headache syndromes is likely to facilitate clinical practice. An established example of such a relationship includes the tight timing of certain specific primary headache syndromes to the circadian cycle, particularly hypnic and cluster headaches but also some migraine variants [1]. Furthermore, general disturbance of sleep homeostasis is a well-established acute headache trigger [1]. Available clinical research has also linked the presence of sleep disorders with more frequent and severe headaches. For example, sleep-related variables such as snoring or general sleep disturbance, have been identified among potent risk factors for 'chronification' or progression from episodic migraine to chronic daily episodes [2]. In addition to precipitating and exacerbating existing headache, certain headaches may actually be caused by a sleep disorder. 'Sleep Apnoea Headache' represents the only officially recognised headache diagnosis *secondary* to a defined sleep disorder [3]. Insomnia is by far the most common sleep disorder among headache sufferers, although empirical evidence also links headache with a wide range of sleep disorders such as circadian rhythm disorders, periodic limb movement disorder, as well as the parasomnias. In fact, virtually every sleep disorder examined to date is more prevalent among individuals with headache than those without headache. Irrespective of diagnosis, non-specific headache patterns, especially chronic daily, morning or 'awakening' headaches can sometimes serve as effective general markers for sleep disorders.

The convergence of sleep and headache disorders is believed partly to stem from shared neuroanatomical structures, primarily in the hypothalamus. Adenosine, melatonin, and orexin are all involved in both the regulation of sleep and have been implicated in the pathophysiology of headaches. A recent review explored common neurobiological pathways involved in sleep regulation and generation of certain headache syndromes such as cluster headache and explored potential brain mechanisms that could underlie the effect of sleep on headache [4].

Sleep Disorders in Neurology: A Practical Approach, Second Edition.
Edited by Sebastiaan Overeem and Paul Reading.
© 2018 John Wiley & Sons Ltd. Published 2018 by John Wiley & Sons Ltd.

This chapter highlights headaches empirically shown to be influenced by sleep and describes the classification of sleep-related headache [3,5,6]. It is suggested that those practitioners managing headaches should have low thresholds for screening and recognising sleep disorders. An algorithm for diagnosis and management is suggested which includes focused headache and sleep histories, physical examination, questionnaires or diaries, and objective sleep testing. Though not empirically validated, the algorithm reflects the current literature and accounts for recognised associations of sleep and headache as well as psychiatric co-morbidity.

Epidemiology

Headache is a frequent co-morbid phenomenon with respiratory as well as non-respiratory sleep disorders. These associations tend to be greatest in high frequency headache syndromes and those that specifically emerge from sleep. Chronic daily, morning, or awakening headache patterns occur in 5% of the general population, 18% of insomniacs, 21% of depressed individuals and 18–60% of sleep apnoea subjects across several studies [1].

Sleep-related Breathing Disorders

Headache is more prevalent among habitual snorers and those with obstructive sleep apnoea (OSA) compared with both non-snoring adults and children. Across clinical populations (12 studies), headache prevalence varied widely from 18 to 60% of subjects with OSA [1]. Snoring has also been implicated in the so-called 'chronification' of migraine. A case-control study in the United States, aimed at identifying risk factors for chronic daily headache [7], revealed that daily snoring was more common among 206 chronic daily headache sufferers compared with a large group (507) with episodic headache with an odds ratio (OR) of 2. The OR increased after adjusting for OSA risk factors such as age, gender, body mass index (BMI), alcohol intake, hypertension (adjusted odds ratio, AOR=2.9), and was not accounted for by other potential factors such as caffeine and depression.

Although classified under metabolic headaches [3], the implied pathogenetic mechanisms of hypoxaemia and/or hypercapnoea do not consistently account for OSA headache. Initial data that supported the role of oxygen levels in headache generation came from the Cleveland Family Study of genetics in OSA (n=634) which showed that intermittent nocturnal hypoxemia correlated with morning headache (AOR=1.4), headache disturbing sleep (1.3) as well as chest pain in bed (1.4). The OR for headache doubled when nadir saturation was decreased from 92 to 75% [8]. Conversely, however, Chen and colleagues [9] found no differences in nadir oxygen saturation or other indices of sleep apnoea severity, although morning headache was more common in OSA (27%) compared with primary snorers (16%) from 268 consecutive snorers undergoing polysomnography. Notably, the OR (adjusted for age, gender, smoking habits, and BMI) for sleep apnoea (AOR=2.6) was actually less than other predictors including migraine (6.5), insomnia (4.2), and psychological distress (3.9).

Two clinical subgroups, cluster and chronic headache refractory to standard treatment, appear at significant risk for having underlying OSA. A study of 37 cluster headache patients who underwent polysomnography identified a four-fold increase in the prevalence of OSA relative to age and gender matched controls (58% versus 14% respectively) and this risk strikingly increased over 24-fold amongst patients with a high BMI of >25 kg/m^2 [10]. Another uncontrolled study of 31 cluster headache patients who underwent polysomnography observed OSA in 80% (25/31) of these patients [11]. Likewise, Mitsikostas and colleagues [12] identified OSA in 29% (21/72) of severe headache patients who were refractory to standard treatments and with various diagnoses including medication overuse and cluster headache.

Insomnia

Insomnia is the most prevalent sleep complaint among headache sufferers and reportedly occurs in half to two-thirds of migraineurs in general neurology or specialty practices [1]. Kelman and colleagues [13] reported sleep complaints from a large sample of 1283 migraineurs: 71% reported morning headaches and over half exhibited difficulty initiating or maintaining sleep. As noted above, the study by Chen and colleagues of 268 snorers [9] found higher incidence of insomnia and psychological distress than sleep apnoea. Indeed, 43% of snorers were also diagnosed with insomnia and insomnia was a stronger predictor of morning headache (OR=4.2) than sleep apnoea.

A close dose–response relationship between insomnia and headache frequency has been noted in earlier literature. For example, in a cross-sectional study, Boardman and colleagues [14] identified a clear relationship between headache severity and sleep complaints. Among 2662 respondents, headache frequency was associated with slight [age/gender adjusted OR=2.4 (1.7–3.2)], moderate [OR=3.6 (2.6–5.0)], and severe [OR=7.5 (4.2–13.4)] sleep complaints. The study also identified an association with anxiety. Controlling for anxiety and depression, Vgontzas and colleagues [15] also confirmed the association of sleep problems (trouble falling asleep, inadequate sleep) with migraine. As mentioned previously, insomnia [16] and sleep disturbance [7] have been implicated in headache 'chronification'. Conversely, behavioural sleep interventions have been shown to influence the nature and severity of migraine headaches in an unselected adult headache population [17].

Circadian Rhythm Disorders

Circadian patterns have been identified in migraine [18], cluster [3,11], and hypnic [3,19] headache syndromes. An epidemiological study suggested that 'chronic morning headache' was twice as prevalent in circadian rhythm disorders and that the relationship strengthened when the data were reanalysed in a model that included only 'daily' morning headache [20].

Restless Legs Syndrome

Schürks and colleagues [21] reviewed 24 studies that addressed restless legs syndrome (RLS) and the presence of migraine headache. Across the 18 studies that focused on headache patients, the prevalence of RLS ranged from 9 to 39% in migraine and from 4.6 to 5% in tension-type headache. Across the other six studies describing RLS patients, prevalence of migraine ranged from 15 to 63%. Unfortunately, data could not be easily pooled or compared with control populations due to the heterogeneous nature of the studies.

Parasomnias

Epidemiological studies indicate parasomnias such as nightmares, bruxism and sleep-walking are approximately twice as prevalent in adults with chronic headache [1,20]. Likewise, children with migraine and other headaches exhibited greater incidence of sleepwalking, bruxism, nightsweats, and nocturnal hyperkinesias than in those without headache [22,23].

Other Sleep Disorders

'Exploding head syndrome' may present to either the headache or sleep specialist and is often included in reports of unusual and short-lived headaches. The syndrome is characterised by waking from sleep or the sleep–wake transition with a painless but frightening sense of noise or explosion [5]. This unusual parasomnia is not included in headache classifications such as in the International Classification of Headache Disorders, 3rd edition, beta version (ICHD-3) due to the absence of definite pain.

Classification

Formal diagnosis of sleep-related headaches follows ICHD-3 [3]. Of interest, the recent revision of the International Classification of Sleep Disorders (ICSD-3) [5] has added 'sleep-related headaches' in a five-page appendix describing their diagnosis, clinical features, and course, under the section 'Sleep related medical and neurological disorders'. Although most headache and sleep disorders would be classified by the ICHD-3 and ICSD-3, respectively, familiarity with the Diagnostic and Statistical Manual of Mental Disorders, 5th edition (DSM-5) [6] can also be useful given the close co-morbidity between mental health problems and both headache and sleep disorders. The symptom constellation of sleep–headache–mood disorder is common and frequently poses the most challenging clinical cases. DSM-5 includes diagnoses for 10 major sleep–wake disorders broadly consistent with ICSD-3.

Sleep Apnoea Headache

Sleep apnoea headache is coded under 'Headache attributed to hypoxia or hypercapnia' [3] even though the precise underlying mechanisms and specificity of OSA to headache remain uncertain (Table 18.1). Diagnostic criteria have not yet been fully validated. OSA headache may present as new onset or exacerbation of migraine, tension, cluster or unclassifiable headache with various patterns: bilateral (53%) or unilateral (47%); location frontal (33%), frontotemporal (28%) or temporal (16%); pressing/tightening pain (79%); with intensity mild (47%), moderate (37%), or severe (16%) [24].

Hypnic Headache

Hypnic headache is the quintessential example of a 'pure' sleep-related headache syndrome which tends to occur in the mid to latter portion of the sleep period. It is also referred to as an 'alarm clock' headache due to the tendency to occur at approximately

Table 18.1 International Headache Society diagnostic criteria [3].

Sleep apnoea headache

a) Headache present on awakening after sleep and fulfilling criterion C

b) Sleep apnoea (Apnoea–Hypopnoea Index ≥5) has been diagnosed

c) Evidence of causation demonstrated by at least two of the following:

   1) Headache has developed in temporal relation to the onset of sleep apnoea

   2) Either or both of the following:

     • Headache has worsened in parallel with worsening of sleep apnea

     • Headache has significantly improved or remitted in parallel with improvement in or resolution of sleep apnoea

   3) Headache has at least one of the following three characteristics:

     • Recurs on >15 days per month

     • All of the following:

       (i) bilateral location

       (ii) pressing quality

       (iii) not accompanied by nausea, photophobia or phonophobia

     • Resolves within 4 hours

d) Not better accounted for by another ICHD-3 diagnosis

Hypnic headache

a) Recurrent headache attacks fulfilling criteria B–E

b) Developing only during sleep, and causing wakening

c) Occurring on ≥10 days per month for >3 months

d) Lasting ≥15 minutes and for up to 4 hours after waking

e) No cranial autonomic symptoms or restlessness

f) Not better accounted for by another ICHD-3 diagnosis

Cluster headache

a) At least five attacks fulfilling criteria B–D

b) Severe or very severe unilateral orbital, supraorbital and/or temporal pain lasting 15–180 minutes (untreated)

c) Either or both of the following:

   1) At least one of the following symptoms or signs, ipsilateral to the headache:

     • conjunctival injection and/or lacrimation

     • nasal congestion and/or rhinorrhoea

     • eyelid oedema

     • forehead and facial sweating

     • forehead and facial flushing

     • sensation of fullness in the ear

     • miosis and/or ptosis

   2) A sense of restlessness or agitation

d) Attacks have a frequency between one every other day and eight per day for more than half of the time when the disorder is active

e) Not better accounted for by another ICHD-3 diagnosis

or even precisely the same time each night. A recent review pooled data from all published reports of hypnic headache (250 cases) from 1988 to the present [19]. Hypnic headache is rare and reflects <0.1% of all headaches and 1.4% of geriatric headaches with a female preponderance (65%). Mean age of onset was 61 years although very young patients including five children were noted. Average attack duration was 162±74 minutes, frequency of 21±10 days per month, 68% were bilateral, 94% were moderate or severe, and one-third of cases also had migraine. Two of the included studies assessed and reported very high incidence of OSA (73% and 83%).

Cluster Headache

Cluster headache syndrome is most often seen in men and can have a distinct circadian pattern with 75% of episodes reportedly occurring between the hours of 9:00 p.m. and 10:00 a.m. Headache 'clusters' also have a circannual pattern, lasting for several weeks or months separated by remissions of several months or even years [3,10,11]. These patients, in particular, should be actively screened for OSA since cluster headache patients exhibited 8.4-fold incidence of OSA relative to age- and gender-matched controls and a 24-fold greater incidence among patients with an associated high BMI of >25 kg/m^2 [10].

Sleep-related Headache Triggers

Among migraine and tension-type headache patients, general sleep disturbance, sleep loss, or even oversleeping are frequently cited as acute 'headache triggers', second only to 'stress'. Sleep triggers of migraine and tension-type headache have been confirmed prospectively in time-series analysis [25]. Both short and long sleep patterns have also been associated with chronic migraine. The Kelman and Rains [13] study described the association of sleep duration and migraine severity in 1283 patients; 398 short (<6 hours/night) sleepers exhibited greater headache frequency than 573 normal (6–8 hours) sleepers (17.6 versus 15.1 days/month). Headache frequency for a small group of 73 long sleepers (>8 hours/night) was 17.5 headache days/month, similar to short sleepers, although the trend was not statistically significant.

Diagnostic Procedures

Ideally, diagnosis begins with a thorough and directed headache history, examining the headache onset, chronology, severity, prodromal and associated symptoms, triggers and past treatments to yield an ICHD-3 [3] diagnosis. Headache patterns should be examined in relation to the sleep–wake cycle and screening may be helped by a focused questionnaire (Table 18.2). Positive responses may be followed by more quantitative data, prospective sleep diaries, and possibly sleep studies including polysomnography.

Sleep history

The 24-hour sleep–wake history includes: pre-sleep routine, sleep period (sleep latency, sleep efficiency or total sleep time/time in bed, mid-cycle and early morning awakenings), nocturnal symptoms (respiratory, movement, abnormal behaviours), awakening

Table 18.2 Headache practitioner's brief sleep questionnaire.

Name: _____

Today's date: _____ Your age: _____ Your gender (M/F): _____

(a) My ideal amount of sleep is _____ hours (number of hours sleep you need each night in order to feel and function your best)

1 During the weekdays I usually:			2 During the weekends I:		
Go to bed at _____ a.m. or p.m. (time)			Go to bed at _____ a.m. or p.m. (time)		
Get up at _____ a.m. or p.m. (time)			Get up at _____ a.m. or p.m. (time)		
Sleep _____ (total hours)			Sleep _____ (total hours)		
(b) I awaken from sleep with headache:	daily____	sometimes____	rarely____		never____
(c) Sleep helps my headache:	daily____	sometimes____	rarely____		never____
(d) Oversleeping produces headache:	daily____	sometimes____	rarely____		never____
(e) I snore:	nightly____	sometimes____	rarely____		never____
(f) After a typical night's sleep, I feel:	refreshed____	fairly rested____	somewhat tired____		very drowsy____

Source: Reproduced with permission of author (JSP).

headache features (if reported), daytime function (napping, sleepiness, mood), and use of behavioural measures or substances to promote sleep or wake. Useful information may be obtained not only from the patient, but also from the spouse or other observers.

Predictive Equations

OSA risk may be assessed by history and tools described elsewhere [1]. The Berlin Sleep Questionnaire identified high versus low risk patients for OSA in the primary care environment (sensitivity 86%, specificity 77%, positive predictive value 89%, likelihood ratio 3.79) based on patient's neck circumference, habitual snoring or witnessed apnoea, and hypertension. The STOP-Bang questionnaire was initially developed for screening presurgical patient for sleep apnoea risk, but more recently validated in the general medical population and includes Snoring, Tiredness/sleepiness, Observed apnoea, blood Pressure, BMI, Age, Neck circumference, and Gender. Questionnaires are available for the full range of sleep disorder conditions such as insomnia, restless legs, daytime sleepiness, headache and sleep quality.

Sleep Diary

Diaries track the regularity, duration, and quality of sleep. Combined sleep/headache diaries are available to record sleep patterns and other common headache triggers (https://www.apa.org/pubs/videos/4310731-diary.pdf). The prospective diary helps confirm the sleep history when diagnosing insomnia and circadian rhythm disorders and also may identify headache triggers.

Sleep Studies

Home oximetry and/or polysomnography is needed to confirm sleep-related breathing disorders, hypersomnia and potentially injurious parasomnias. In uncomplicated cases in which there is high pre-test suspicion without confounding co-morbidities, unattended and abbreviated portable monitoring may be sufficient to confirm OSA.

Management

Clinicians are encouraged to diagnose headache according to accepted ICHD-3 criteria (Figure 18.1). The threshold for polysomnography should be particularly low in both cluster and hypnic headache syndromes based on degree of risk for sleep apnoea headache in the literature. Cluster, hypnic, chronic migraine, tension-type or any 'awakening headache' usually warrants further investigation.

Chronic headache patients treated for sleep apnoea with continuous positive airway pressure (CPAP) have improved or resolved headache in one-third to one-half of cases [1,12] although concurrent headache interventions are usually necessary. At this point, variables that predict responders are unknown, so empirical trials in individual patients are justified. Treatment of headache that persists after resolution of sleep apnoea and other sleep disorders depends on the precise headache diagnosis and standard headache therapy recommendations should apply. It is prudent to avoid sedation with hypnotics

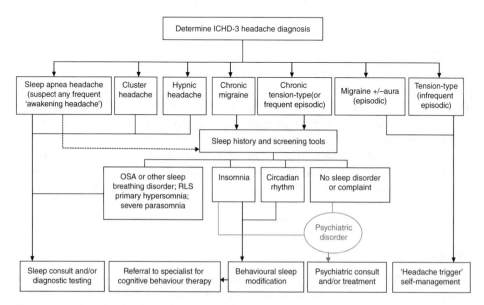

Figure 18.1 Algorithm for sleep-related headache.

or opiates until any sleep-related breathing disorder is treated adequately. After adequate OSA treatment, sedating medications can be usefully considered.

Patients with chronic migraine and chronic or frequent tension-type headache are at increased risk for insomnia and psychiatric disorders. Episodic headache patients should also be screened when history indicates a specific sleep-related headache trigger or sleep complaint. Even when sleep complaints are not volunteered, episodic cases may benefit from sleep education regarding headache triggers.

Behavioural Sleep Modification

Behavioural sleep regulation has been shown to improve chronic migraine and is frequently recommended for chronic headache whether migraine or tension-type. Calhoun and Ford [17] randomised 43 women with transformed migraine to behavioural sleep treatment versus sham control group while both groups received 'usual headache care'. By the sixth week of treatment, 35% of the treatment group reverted from chronic to episodic headache, compared with none of the controls. Following intervention, the treatment group significantly improved over the control group in headache frequency (39% versus 12%) and headache index (28% versus −3%). This relatively brief behavioural sleep intervention was delivered in the headache practice setting. Patients with irregular sleep schedules, poor sleep habits, and those spending less than 6.5 or more than 8.5 hours in bed should be actively counselled in sleep hygiene and provided with more intensive insomnia interventions as needed.

Insomnia Treatment

Although insomnia is the most common sleep complaint in headache, cognitive behavioural therapy (CBT) for insomnia has only rarely been applied to headache patients. One pilot study has been published comparing CBT to sham control for insomnia in chronic migraine [26]. CBT significantly increased total sleep time. A trend for decreased headache frequency did not reach statistical significance. Evidence from parallel literature in chronic pain has demonstrated insomnia improves with CBT. Referral for CBT for insomnia should be considered on a case-by-case basis. Behaviour patterns interfering with sleep may warrant referral for behavioural and/or pharmacological treatment. Antidepressants with sedative properties such as tricyclic antidepressants or anticonvulsants may provide benefit from headache as well as sleep enhancement although response rates are unpredictable in individual cases. The use of benzodiazepine and non-benzodiazepine hypnotics needs to be balanced against the risks, including dependency and tolerance, risk of falls, cognitive problems, and other known adverse effects. Some hypnotic agents may be more appropriate for chronic use than others, but intermittent dosing (two to five times per week) is usually desirable.

Psychiatric Referral or Treatment

Mood and anxiety disorders are co-morbid with insomnia as well as headache. Sleep disturbance and daytime sleepiness are symptoms of a number of psychiatric disorders and occur in the majority of patients with depression, anxiety, and chemical dependencies [6]. There is little research to direct specific treatment. However, recognition of insomnia with depression or anxiety may guide headache prophylaxis toward sedating antidepressants or anticonvulsants, while hypersomnia would call for neutral or more alerting medications.

Conclusions

At this juncture, there is no formal evidence that sleep evaluation or treatment should supersede standard headache care. However, the evidence that sleep and headache mutually influence each other is based on considerable clinical observations, epidemiological data, case-control studies, and proposed common neuro-anatomic pathways. Unfortunately, there are few controlled trials assessing headache outcomes following intervention and management of sleep-related problems. The best data relate to CPAP therapy for sleep apnoea headache syndrome although there are no placebo-controlled or long-term trials. There is preliminary evidence for behavioural sleep regulation as an effective option for all patients with chronic migraine. In advance of evidence-based algorithms, the recommendations are preliminary and unvalidated. As such, identification and management of sleep-related headache should be considered complementary to standard pharmacological and behavioural headache treatments.

Key Points

- Sleep apnoea headache may emerge de novo or may present as an exacerbation of cluster, migraine, tension-type, or other headache. Patients with cluster and hypnic headache are at increased risk for sleep apnoea headache.
- Snoring and sleep disturbance are independent risk factors for progression from episodic to chronic headache.
- Insomnia is the most prevalent sleep disorder in chronic migraine and tension-type headache.
- Sleep disturbance including sleep loss, oversleeping, and shifts in schedule are frequently reported as acute 'headache triggers' for migraine and tension-type headache.
- Besides standard management of headache syndromes, treatment of associated sleep problems may be a useful adjunct. The best data relate to CPAP therapy for sleep apnoea headache and behavioural sleep regulation for chronic migraine.

References

1 Rains JC, Poceta JS. Sleep-related headaches. *Neurol Clin* 2012;30(4):1285–1298.
2 Bigal ME, Lipton RB. Migraine chronification. *Curr Neurol Neurosci Rep* 2011;11(2):139–148.
3 Headache Classification Committee of the International Headache Society (IHS). The International Classification of Headache Disorders, 3rd edn (beta version). *Cephalalgia* 2013;33(9):629–808.
4 Evers S. Sleep and headache: the biological basis. *Headache* 2010;50(7):1246–1251.
5 American Academy of Sleep Medicine. International Classification of Sleep Disorders, 3rd edn. Darien, IL: American Academy of Sleep Medicine, 2014.
6 American Psychiatric Association. Diagnostic and Statistical Manual of Mental Disorders, 5th edn. Arlington, VA: American Psychiatric Association, 2013.
7 Scher AI, Lipton RB, Stewart WF. Habitual snoring as a risk factor for chronic daily headache. *Neurology* 2003;60(8):1366–1368.

8 Doufas AG, Tian L, Davies MF, Warby SC. Nocturnal intermittent hypoxia is independently associated with pain in subjects suffering from sleep-disordered breathing. *Anesthesiology* 2013;119(5):1149–1162.

9 Chen PK, Fuh JL, Lane HY, et al. Morning headache in habitual snorers: frequency, characteristics, predictors and impacts. *Cephalalgia* 2011;31(7):829–836.

10 Nobre ME, Leal AJ, Filho PM. Investigation into sleep disturbance of patients suffering from cluster headache. *Cephalalgia* 2005;25(7):488–492.

11 Graff-Radford SB, Newman A. Obstructive sleep apnea and cluster headache. *Headache* 2004;44(6):607–610.

12 Mitsikostas DD, Vikelis M, Viskos A. Refractory chronic headache associated with obstructive sleep apnoea syndrome. *Cephalalgia* 2008;28(2):139–143.

13 Kelman L, Rains JC. Headache and sleep: examination of sleep patterns and complaints in a large clinical sample of migraineurs. *Headache* 2005;45(7):904–910.

14 Boardman HF, Thomas E, Millson DS, Croft PR. Psychological, sleep, lifestyle, and comorbid associations with headache. *Headache* 2005;45(6):657–669.

15 Vgontzas A, Lihong C, Merikangas KR. Are sleep difficulties associated with migraine attributable to anxiety and depression? *Headache* 2008;48(10):1451–1459.

16 Sancisi E, Cevoli S, Vignatelli L, et al. Increased prevalence of sleep disorders in chronic headache: a case-control study. *Headache* 2010;50(9):1464–1472.

17 Calhoun AH, Ford S. Behavioral sleep modification may revert transformed migraine to episodic migraine. *Headache* 2007;47(8):1178–1183.

18 Alstadhaug K, Salvesen R, Bekkelund S. Insomnia and circadian variation of attacks in episodic migraine. *Headache* 2007;47(8):1184–1188.

19 Liang JF, Wang SJ. Hypnic headache: A review of clinical features, therapeutic options and outcomes. *Cephalalgia* 2014;18 June (epub ahead of print).

20 Ohayon MM. Prevalence and risk factors of morning headaches in the general population. *Arch Intern Med* 2004;164(1):97–102.

21 Schürks M, Winter AC, Berger K, et al. Migraine and restless leg syndrome: A systematic review. *Cephalalgia* 2014;18 June (epub ahead of print).

22 Isik U, Ersu RH, Ay P, et al. Prevalence of headache and its association with sleep disorders in children. *Pediatr Neurol* 2007;36:146–151.

23 Esposito M, Parisi P, Miano S, Carotenuto M. Migraine and periodic limb movement disorders in sleep in children: a preliminary case-control study. *J Headache Pain* 2013;14:57.

24 Alberti A, Mazzotta G, Gallinella E, Sarchielli P. Headache characteristics in obstructive sleep apnea and insomnia. *Acta Neurol Scand* 2005;111:309–316.

25 Houle TT, Butschek RA, Turner DP, et al. Stress and sleep duration predict headache severity in chronic headache sufferers. *Pain* 2012;153(12):2432–2440.

26 Smitherman TA, Walters AB, Davis RE, et al. Randomized controlled pilot trial of behavioral insomnia treatment for chronic migraine with comorbid insomnia. *Headache* 2016;56:276–291.

19

Sleep Epilepsies

Luigi Ferini-Strambi

Sleep Disorders Center, University Vita-Salute San Raffaele, Milan, Italy

Introduction

The close relationship between sleep and epilepsy has been recognised since the time of Hippocrates and Aristotle. The state of sleep itself or sleep deprivation, in particular, may trigger clinical seizures as well as increasing interictal epileptiform discharges (IEDs) in the absence of observable clinical events. As early as 1947 Gibbs and Gibbs [1] first described the potential importance of the sleep state as a means of enhancing or inducing IED in predisposed subjects. They studied 174 patients with generalised seizures and found that 63% had 'seizure discharges' during sleep compared with 19% during wakefulness. Other studies showed that sleep may activate both focal and generalised IEDs and that the occurrence of seizures in the sleep state is observed in nearly one-third of young epileptic patients [2].

In 1885, Gowers was the first to classify epileptic patients into three groups based on the distribution of 'fits' over the day with diurnal, nocturnal, and diffuse patterns noted. More contemporary studies have also confirmed that seizure occurrence is far from random across the 24-hour period. Specific epilepsy syndromes have a marked tendency to manifest only or predominantly during sleep. This group include nocturnal frontal lobe epilepsy, benign epilepsy of childhood with centrotemporal spikes (BCET), juvenile myoclonic epilepsy, continuous spikes waves during non-rapid eye movement (non-REM) sleep, and Landau–Kleffner syndrome (LKS). The latter two entities describe the clinical epileptic syndromes seen in association with electrical status epilepticus in sleep (ESES).

The Influence of Sleep Stages on Seizures

The precise stage of sleep is known to influence the relative likelihood of IEDs and nocturnal seizures. In general, non-REM sleep is associated with an increased incidence and spread of IEDs as well as clinical manifestations of epileptic activity originating

Sleep Disorders in Neurology: A Practical Approach, Second Edition.
Edited by Sebastiaan Overeem and Paul Reading.

from frontal and temporal lobes [3]. Electro-clinical events are most frequent in stage 2 non-REM, followed, in order, by stage 1 and stage 3. REM sleep is a relatively protective against epilepsy with suppression of IEDs and both localised and spreading clinical seizure activity.

The relative epileptic risk of different sleep stages can simply be understood in terms of the varying tendency for wave-like oscillations between the stages. The main structure responsible for generating sleep oscillations is the thalamo-cortical axis that is modulated by the ascending brainstem and basal forebrain inputs [4]. In non-REM sleep, electroencephalography (EEG) activity is more synchronised, leading to long-lasting oscillations of rhythmical burst-phase firing patterns which, in turn, tend to increase the magnitude and propagation of postsynaptic responses that might include epileptic discharges.

Electro-clinical studies have clearly shown that seizures predominantly occur during unstable states. The cyclic alternating pattern (CAP) is a periodic EEG activity of non-REM sleep, characterised by sequences of transient electro-cortical events that are distinct from the tonic background and recur at up to 1-minute intervals [5]. In the dynamic organization of sleep, CAP reflects a state of relative instability and most likely significantly predisposes to the occurrence of nocturnal seizures [6]. In recent years, the use of intracerebral recording methods, such as stereo-EEG (S-EEG), have confirmed that IEDs often not detectable on routine scalp EEGs are related to increased arousal fluctuations in the context of a higher CAP rate [7].

During REM sleep and alert wakefulness, cortical neurones tend to fire asynchronously. This pattern generates divergent synaptic signals both temporally and spatially, making propagation of epileptic discharges far less likely.

It is also conceivable that the different state-dependency of skeletal muscle tone may contribute to the increased susceptibility to clinical seizure activity during non-REM compared with REM sleep. In particular, the atonia and active inhibition of voluntary muscle tone in REM sleep, in contrast to non-REM sleep, may further reduce the likelihood of observing any clinical seizure activity during REM sleep.

Clinical Epidemiology

Nocturnal Frontal Lobe Epilepsy

Nocturnal frontal lobe epilepsy (NFLE) is usually an idiopathic partial epilepsy characterised by a wide spectrum of stereotyped motor manifestations, mostly occurring during non-REM sleep. NFLE appears to be relatively rare but is probably underdiagnosed since semiological similarities with many parasomnias together with non-specific surface EEG findings can make differential diagnosis difficult [8] (see Chapter 12). NFLE generally starts during infancy or childhood and persists into adulthood. A recent retrospective cohort study estimated the prevalence of NFLE in adults of two areas in Italy, the city of Bologna and the province of Modena. The crude prevalence (per 100 000 residents) was 1.8 in Bologna and 1.9 in Modena [9]. Thus, this epidemiologic study establishes that NFLE fulfils the definition for a rare epileptic syndrome.

Benign Epilepsy of Childhood with Centrotemporal Spikes

BECT is the most common epileptic syndrome in childhood [10]. Its prevalence among early schoolchildren diagnosed with epilepsy is 23–24% with an age at onset ranging between 2 years and 13 years (mean 7 years). BECT is more frequent in male subjects, with a male-to-female ratio of 3:2 [11]. The seizures occur during sleep in approximately 75% of the affected children and are characterised by hemi-facial motor seizures, often preceded by somatosensory symptoms involving the inner cheek, tongue, and lips.

Juvenile Myoclonic Epilepsy

Juvenile myoclonic epilepsy (JME) is a common idiopathic generalised and age-related epileptic syndrome. The estimated prevalence in large cohorts is 5–10% of all epilepsies and 18% of idiopathic generalised epilepsies [12]. JME usually starts in puberty or late infancy and is initially characterised by myoclonic limb jerks, mainly on awakening. Early reports suggesting a male predominance have been superseded by recent studies implying the opposite [13].

A diagnosis of JME can be overlooked relatively easily and between 25% and 90% of patients referred to neurology or epilepsy clinics are initially misdiagnosed. Contributory factors include failure to elicit a history of myoclonic jerks; misinterpretation of myoclonic jerks as simple partial seizures or a non-specific movement disorder such as a tic, especially if unilateral; and general lack of familiarity with the syndrome by non-specialists.

Continuous Spikes and Waves During Non-REM Sleep and Landau–Kleffner Syndrome

The exact prevalence or incidence of continuous spikes and waves during non-REM sleep (CSWS) and LKS is unknown [14]. These epilepsies appear to be rare but, again, are probably under-recognised conditions. The medical literature is confined to small series and case reports. Approximately 200 cases of LKS were described between 1968 and 1992. Of interest, in a review of 1497 overnight video-EEG monitoring studies conducted in children over a 5-year interval, Van Hirtum-Das and colleagues [15] found 18 (1.2%) cases which met the criteria for LKS.

Clinical Features

Nocturnal Frontal Lobe Epilepsy

NFLE is characterised by repetitive episodes of predominantly motor phenomena which usually recur through the night and occur several nights per week. Events are highly stereotyped, most often starting in childhood with persistence into young adulthood [8]. Since 1985, a familial clustering of NFLE was apparent from several reports. In 1994 and 1995, Scheffer and colleagues [16] reported five families with NFLE inherited as an autosomal dominant trait and introduced the term 'autosomal dominant nocturnal frontal lobe epilepsy' (ADNFLE). Overall, a family history of possible nocturnal frontal lobe seizures is found in about 25% of all NFLE cases while 40% of NFLE patients also present a family history of nocturnal episodes that would meet the diagnostic criteria for non-REM parasomnias.

Since familial, idiopathic, sporadic, cryptogenetic and symptomatic forms have been recognised, NFLE cannot be considered a homogeneous disorder [8,17]. Moreover, a genetic heterogeneity has been shown even within the familial type [18,19]. However, NFLE and ADNFLE exhibit similar clinical and EEG findings including young onset, high nocturnal frequency of events and decreased frequency during adulthood [8,17]. Seizures during wakefulness have been rarely reported [20].

Different subtypes of sleep-related motor events may be observed in NFLE/ADNFLE [8,17,20–22]:

- Very short-lasting (2–4 seconds) stereotyped movements involving the limbs, the axial musculature, and/or the head.
- Paroxysmal arousals with short (5–10 seconds) sudden 'motor attacks' or behaviours.
- Episodes with complex dystonic-dyskinetic components, formerly known as nocturnal paroxysmal dystonia, lasting 20–30 seconds.
- Episodic complex motor attacks consisting of agitation, violent 'somnambulism', and epileptic nocturnal wanderings, lasting 1–3 minutes.

Paroxysmal arousals consist of brief, sudden and very frequent arousals associated with minimal or minor stereotyped motor activity that might include apparently purposeful or semi-purposeful behaviour. Examples include abrupt elevation of head, neck and sometimes trunk from the bed, screaming, moaning or looking around with a fearful expression. Stereotypy and dystonic arm or leg movements are frequent, as well as facial grimacing and chewing.

Nocturnal paroxysmal dystonia episodes sometimes start as paroxysmal arousals, but usually include more complex motor behaviours with prominent dystonic-dyskinetic components; asymmetric posturing; cycling and kicking of the legs; repetitive and rhythmic limb or arm movement; pelvis or body rocking accompanied by guttural sounds or unspecified words and frightened expression of the face. Subjects tend to have their individual repetitive pattern of epsiodes that do not vary.

Epileptic nocturnal wanderings are considerably rarer than the previous two subtypes: the prolonged episodes are characterised by agitation, sudden standing, and ambulation and may easily mimic sleepwalking episodes.

Interestingly but perhaps not surprisingly, NFLE/ADNFLE patients may complain of non-restorative sleep and of daytime sleepiness [8,17,20].

Neurologic examination is normal and affected individuals are typically of normal intelligence. However, rare families with ADNFLE and intellectual disability and/or psychiatric disorders such as depression, personality disorder, and paranoid schizophrenia have been reported. This suggests that a neuropsychological evaluation may need to be included in the clinical assessment of patients with ADNFLE [23].

Benign Epilepsy of Childhood with Centrotemporal Spikes

BECT is an idiopathic age-specific epileptic syndrome with a high genetic predisposition and a benign course. In BECT, seizures are typically unilateral focal motor (clonic) attacks involving the face, arm, and rarely the leg. The affected side can alternate. The seizures may have a sensory component and may provoke speech impairment, a feeling of dysphagia and suffocation, and audible noise when pharyngeal and laryngeal muscles are involved. They usually appear after children have fallen sleep or close to the time they awaken with a tendency to clusters and prolonged seizure-free intervals [24]. Secondarily generalized seizures have been reported in as many as 20–50% of the patients, with about 15% having only secondarily generalized seizures. These seizures are seen more often in children younger than 5 years of age and remain usually nocturnal.

BECT is considered a benign form of epilepsy, but several studies have demonstrated neuropsychological impairments in patients, involving visuomotor coordination, executive functions, attention, language and poor memory [25,26]. It has been hypothesized that BECT in children produces IEDs in non-REM sleep that interfere with the dialogue between the temporal and frontal cortex, causing declarative memory deficit [26]. A recent neuroimaging study [27] showed that BECT children had alterations in the microstructure of white matter, undetectable with conventional magnetic resonance imaging, predominating in the regions displaying chronic IED. The observed association between neuroimaging changes, duration of epilepsy and cognitive performances suggests that IEDs may alter brain maturation, which could in turn lead to cognitive dysfunction [27]. However, in a prospective population-based cohort of childhood-onset epilepsy [28], the adult social outcome for BECT patients was remarkably better than for those with other major epilepsies.

Juvenile Myoclonic Epilepsy

JME is often not confined to early morning jerks and generalised tonic clonic seizures are very common with absences occurring in about one-third of cases [13]. About 20% of patients experience all three types of seizures, while 75% of patients suffer both myoclonic jerks and generalised tonic clonic seizures [29]. In rare cases, an early onset with typical absences followed many years later by myoclonic jerks may be observed and this may cause diagnostic delay.

JME is generally associated with normal intelligence and clinical neurological examination. However, it has been reported that some patients with JME have subtle executive dysfunction and impulsive traits, especially in treatment-refractory cases [30]. Moreover, a recent neuroimaging study found a widespread thinning of the cortical thickness, as well as smaller cerebellar white matter volume, in JME patients with absences compared with controls or JME patients without absences [31]. These findings support the hypothesis that JME is a heterogeneous syndrome.

Continuous Spikes and Waves During Non-REM Sleep

The age of CSWS onset is variable, ranging from 1 to 14 years (mean between 4 years and 8 years). In 80% of patients with CSWS, seizures are the presenting symptom and most children experience multiple seizures per day. The seizure types include the full range of generalised tonic-clonic, typical absence, atypical absence, simple and complex partial seizures.

Children with CSWS often exhibit global regression. Specifically, a loss of language and temporospatial skills, short-term memory deficits, poor reasoning, hyperactivity, and aggressiveness may all be observed [14]. Concerning the language impairment, an expressive aphasia has been reported, while comprehension is generally spared. There are also motor deficits, resulting in ataxia, dystonia, and dyspraxia, which are sometimes unilateral.

CSWS duration and the localisation of IEDs seem to play an important role in influencing the type and severity of cognitive impairment. This implies that epileptic EEG discharges can interfere with local slow wave activity and adversely affect neuroplasticity processes involved in higher cortical functions occurring during sleep [32].

Long-term outcome of CSWS is variable and strictly related to treatment response, disease duration, and underlying aetiology [33].

Landau–Kleffner Syndrome

The age of onset of LKS ranges from 2 to 8 years with a peak at 5 years and boys are affected twice as frequently as girls [34]. The primary clinical manifestation is language regression. In particular, an acquired auditory agnosia with failure to give a semantic significance to differing sounds may progress over weeks to months. The loss of receptive language in turn leads to an expressive aphasia. Other possible clinical symptoms are hyperkinesia, irritability, attention-deficit disorder, and autistic-like behaviours. By convention, LKS is not related to pre-existing organic brain lesions such that before the onset of LKS, language and behaviour in the majority of children are normal or unremarkable.

Perhaps surprisingly, clinical seizures in LKS are usually infrequent and include generalised clonic, partial clonic, and atypical absence seizures. Actual seizures never occur in 20–30% of patients and when present, they are easy to control. The prognosis of LKS patients in terms of seizure outcome is therefore good but the effects on language and other cognitive functions are variable [34].

There is an overlap between CSWS and LKS but children with CSWS present with a more global regression and have more problematic epilepsy. Future genetic studies are likely to help dissecting these syndromes into different types of epileptic encephalopathies.

Diagnostic Procedures

Nocturnal Frontal Lobe Epilepsy

In NFLE, nocturnal video-polysomnography (video-PSG) is considered the gold standard for diagnosis. Most of the seizures appear during non-REM sleep with preponderance in stage N2 (>60%). Rarely, they emerge from REM sleep. In some cases, the motor attacks (especially paroxysmal arousals) show a clear periodicity (every 20 seconds to 2 minutes). However, a video-PSG study has showed that the inter-observer reliability when diagnosing NFLE, based on videotaped observation of sleep motor phenomena, may not be completely satisfactory [35]. In some cases, especially when nocturnal episodes are infrequent, home video recording for multiple nights may be a useful adjunct [17].

EEG monitoring during attacks is uninformative in almost half of cases due to muscle artifact. However, rhythmic theta or delta waves; sharp waves predominantly in the frontal regions; attenuation of the background activity; and, in a minority of cases, classic spike-and-wave activity or small amplitude fast activity may be recorded during ictal or interictal EEG. A burst of delta activity may frequently precede or be simultaneous with the episode [8,21]. Arousal fluctuations, expressed with periodic delta bursts, are commonly related to the occurrence of both epileptic episodes and parasomnia events such as confusional arousals, sleep terrors or sleepwalking [36]. PSG without video recording may therefore be misleading (Figure 19.1).

It has been postulated that the complexity of the motor behaviour in NFLE reflects the precise pattern of propagation of the epileptic discharge within the frontal lobe. S-EEG studies have shown that the seizure onset in NFLE patients with asymmetric tonic or dystonic posturing was generally localised in the posterior portion of the frontal cingulate gyrus and in the posterior mesial frontal cortex with involvement of the supplementary motor area [37]. In patients with seizures characterised by the association of fear and epileptic nocturnal wandering, a cerebral network including the anterior cingulate, orbito-polar, and temporal regions seems to be involved. According to some authors [38], several of these clinical manifestations may be considered as a seizure-induced release or disinhibition of innate behavioural automatisms and survival behaviours programmed in cortical/subcortical 'central pattern generators'.

Neuroimaging studies are indicated to exclude rare symptomatic forms of NFLE but the majority of subjects have no lesions on routine imaging. Some sophisticated techniques have been used for evaluating NFLE/ADNFLE patients but their clinical applications are very limited.

Mutations in three genes that encode the alpha 2, alpha 4 and beta 2 subunits of the neural nicotinic acetylcholine receptor (nAChR) have been found in a minority of ADNFLE patients [18]. A positron emission tomography (PET) study in patients with

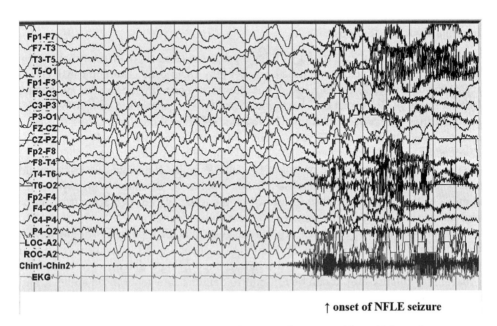

↑ **onset of NFLE seizure**

Figure 19.1 A 20-second EEG epoch, showing the onset of a nocturnal frontal lobe epilepsy (NFLE) seizure.

ADNFLE showed a reduction of the nicotinic receptors in the prefrontal cortex and an increase of these receptors in the brainstem [39]. Interestingly, the nAChRs are extensively distributed in the brain and are known to exert a modulating effect on sleep and arousal oscillations at both cortical and subcortical levels. Experimental studies have shown that a nAChR mutation can facilitate the occurrence of unbalanced excitation/inhibition patterns of activity within the GABAergic reticular thalamic neurons, potentially generating seizures through the synchronising effect of spontaneous oscillations in thalamocortical connections [40]. ADNFLE is not only related to mutations in the cholinergic system as shown by recent studies implicating the corticotropin-releasing hormone and DEPDC5 genes [19,41].

Given the potential difficulty in diagnosing NFLE and the limited availability of resources, a useful tool has been developed, the Frontal Lobe Epilepsy and Parasomnia (FLEP) scale, developed to distinguish NFLE from parasomnias, especially non-REM arousal parasomnias [42,43] (see Chapter 12 for more details). More recently, a structured interview for NFLE (SINFLE) has been proposed [44].

Benign Epilepsy of Childhood with Centrotemporal Spikes

A unique ictal EEG pattern in BECT does not exist. Epileptiform foci are seen in the presence of a normal background activity with activation of epileptic discharges particularly during non-REM sleep. Their morphology reflects a biphasic or triphasic sharp wave of relatively high amplitude, localised to the centrotemporal regions. The electrical field may also include the contralateral homologue zone. The precise morphology of the ictal discharges varies greatly in different patients and sometimes in the same patient [45].

Juvenile Myoclonic Epilepsy

Recently, international experts on JME have proposed two sets of criteria that can be helpful for both clinical and scientific purposes [46]. Diagnostic criteria for JME class I are: (1) myoclonic jerks without loss of consciousness occurring on or after awakening (within 2 hours); (2) normal EEG background and typical generalised epileptiform EEG abnormalities with concomitant myoclonic jerks; (3) normal intelligence; and (4) age at onset between 10 years and 25 years. Diagnostic criteria for JME class II are: (1) myoclonic jerks predominantly occurring on awakening; (2) myoclonic jerks facilitated by sleep deprivation or stress and provoked by visual stimuli; (3) normal EEG background and at least once interictal generalised spike or polyspike discharge with asymmetry allowed in the presence or absence of myoclonic jerks; (4) no mental retardation or regression; and (5) age at onset between 6 years and 25 years.

A simplified summary of both criteria suggests that JME patients should have a clear history of myoclonic jerks predominantly occurring after awakening and an EEG with generalised epileptiform discharges supporting a diagnosis of idiopathic generalised epilepsy [46]. It can be difficult to demonstrate generalised epilepsy and even serial EEGs do not always reveal the suggestive abnormalities in 21–54% of patients [29]. In patients with normal EEGs or with focal/lateralised epileptiform discharges, video-EEG monitoring for 1 or 2 days may be required to make a correct diagnosis of JME [29].

Electrical Status Epilepticus in Sleep

An EEG during sleep is clearly required to make a diagnosis of ESES. In non-REM sleep, the epileptiform discharges are highly activated and become continuous or nearly so. Overall, the sleep structure appears normal, but the presence of almost continuous spike and wave discharges makes the recognition of normal sleep EEG elements, such as K-complexes, spindles, or vertex sharp transients, quite difficult. Although the epileptiform discharges have been described as generalised, they arise focally and are then rapidly propagated within and between hemispheres.

Maximal spike location varies between CSWS and LKS. In CSWS, the wake EEG shows focal, multifocal, or diffuse discharges, often with frontotemporal or frontocentral predominance [14]. In LKS, the EEG during wakefulness is variable and may show focal, multifocal, or generalised epileptic abnormalities or even be normal. The focal epileptiform activity in LKS is usually posterotemporal. This epileptiform activity likely is responsible for the early auditory agnosia that later develops into bilateral EEG abnormalities.

A subgroup of children with ESES may have significantly less activation of epileptiform discharges in stages 1 and 2 non-REM compared with slow wave sleep and a full overnight recording should be considered in some cases.

Neuropsychological tests in ESES patients are important to determine the type and extent of cognitive impairment. Some centres advocate PET and single-photon emission computed tomography (SPECT) studies to correlate neuropsychological dysfunction with altered metabolism in frontotemporal or posterotemporal areas.

Magnetic resonance imaging should be considered in children with CSWS as abnormalities including cortical dysplasia, congenital stroke, diffuse atrophy, white-matter changes, and abnormal or delayed myelination have been described. Patients with LKS, by contrast, generally have normal imaging.

Management

Nocturnal Frontal Lobe Epilepsy

NFLE is considered a relatively benign clinical entity because seizures occur during sleep and most cases respond positively to anti-epileptic drugs. Controlled drug trials are lacking but published data suggest about two-thirds of NFLE patients respond well to carbamazepine at low doses (200–600 mg at bedtime), with greatly reduced seizure frequency and complexity. One study [47] reported a reduction or complete control of nocturnal seizures in three ADNFLE patients with acetazolamide, 500 mg at night, as add-on therapy to carbamazepine.

Of the newer drugs for epilepsy, there is evidence that topiramate (dose range 50–300 mg at bedtime) can be effective in NFLE. The agent was evaluated in 24 patients with a mean age of 29 years. Seizure freedom was achieved in 25% and seizure reduction by 50% in 62.5%. Weight loss was observed in six cases and speech dysfunction in two [48]. Oxcarbazepine (dose range 15–45 mg/kg/day) in eight children aged between 4 years and 16 years was reportedly extremely effective in all cases with mild side effects of transient diplopia in one case and somnolence in another [49]. One case report has tried a transdermal nicotine patch with success [50]. A later study reported a beneficial effect of nicotine on seizure frequency in 9 out of 22 patients from two Norwegian ADNFLE pedigrees with CHRNA4 mutations [51]. These findings support the role of a nicotine defect in the arousal pathway in NFLE/ADNFLE patients.

About 30% of NFLE cases with more frequent and complex attacks in larger samples are resistant to anti-epileptic drugs. Surgical treatment may have an indication in these non-responders who also usually have significant sleep fragmentation, non-restorative sleep, and troublesome daytime sleepiness. An accurate presurgical evaluation, including invasive EEG recording, is mandatory before resective surgery in drug-resistant NFLE is considered.

Benign Epilepsy of Childhood with Centrotemporal Spikes

Overall, prognosis in BECT is excellent with a satisfactory response usually observed with most standard anti-epileptic drugs. However, the evidence base for treatment choice in BECT is acknowledged to be poor, with a few studies suggesting that carbamazepine and sodium valproate are 'possibly' effective, and levetiracetam, oxcarbamazepine, gabapentin and sulthiame 'potentially' effective as initial monotherapy [52].

Subsequent remission of symptoms before age 16 should be anticipated in the majority of the patients once anti-epileptic drugs are discontinued. A minority (6–18%), unfortunately, have numerous events despite therapeutic trials with several drugs. A poor clinical course with frequent seizures is associated with early onset, often before the age of 3 years.

A worsening of BECT has also been observed as a direct side effect of certain anti-epileptic drugs [53]. Indeed, some patients show seizure exacerbation following carbamazepine or oxcarbazepine treatment with progression to atypical absences, neuropsychological disturbances, and even CSWS. Seizure worsening and CSWS have been also reported in a few BECT patients treated with valproate or phenobarbital.

Juvenile Myoclonic Epilepsy

In JME, many studies have reported that 70–90% of patients show a good response to a variety of standard anti-epileptic drugs such as valproate, lamotrigine, topiramate, and levetiracetam. However, carbamazepine and phenytoin may exacerbate seizures [46]. Spontaneous remission is uncommon and lifelong medical treatment with modification of lifestyle issues is often considered appropriate. In JME, epilepsy starts in the vulnerable period of adolescence and avoidance of binge alcohol drinking and sleep deprivation must be strongly recommended.

Electrical Status Epilepticus in Sleep

In ESES, the goal of treatment is not only to control the seizures but also to improve neuropsychological function. With regard to the latter, this provides an incentive to try and normalise EEG abnormalities even if clinical seizures are controlled [14]. Phenytoin, carbamazepine, and barbiturates may reduce the seizures but are probably contraindicated in ESES because they can potentially worsen both the neuropsychological outcome and the neurophysiological abnormalities. Valproate, ethosuximide, levetiracetam, or diazepam have been reported to be beneficial in some small case series. As a rule, polypharmacy should be avoided in ESES. Indeed, one study showed that the reduction of polytherapy coincided with an improvement in the syndrome.

Sinclair and Snyder [54] reported improved speech abnormalities and normalisation of the EEG in all of the three children with LKS treated with corticosteroids. They suggested that steroids should be given in high doses as soon as the diagnosis is established, followed by maintenance doses for several months to years. Other studies have showed that the earlier steroids are started, the shorter the duration required and the better the outcome. Early tapering of steroid doses may be associated with relapse of ESES and neuropsychological deterioration, ultimately necessitating a longer treatment duration.

In the absence of clear evidence, other therapies include intravenous gamma-globulin (2 g/kg over 4 days), ketogenic diets, vagal nerve stimulation, and surgical therapy with multiple subpial transection in drug-resistant cases.

A recent survey conducted in North America on treatment choice for CSWS showed that the preferred first-choice drug was high-dose benzodiazepine (47%), followed by valproate (26%), and corticosteroids (15%) [55].

Although the epileptic seizures resolve with time in most cases, many children are left with significant cognitive or language impairment. Not surprisingly, longer duration of ESES appears to be the major predictor of poor outcome.

Key Points

- An intimate relation between epilepsy and sleep has long been recognised.
- Specific epilepsy syndromes have a marked tendency to manifest only or predominantly during sleep, particularly non-REM stages.
- Some seizure syndromes manifest predominantly at sleep–wake transitions.
- Many generalised epilepsies are sensitive to sleep deprivation, a fact sometimes helpful in diagnostic procedures.
- Diagnosis of nocturnal seizures may be difficult, and generally requires a combination of careful history, nocturnal video recordings and nocturnal EEG recordings.
- Clinical systematic assessment (such as the FLEP scale) and home-made videos may increase diagnostic confidence, reducing the need for video-PSG in a laboratory setting.
- Management depends on the specific syndrome diagnosed although controlled evidence-based information is limited.

References

1 Gibbs EL, Gibbs FA. Diagnostic and localizing value of electroencephalographic studies during sleep. *Res Publ Assoc Nerv Ment Dis* 1947;26:366–376.
2 Kotagal P, Yardi N. The relationship between sleep and epilepsy. *Semin Pediatr Neurol* 2008;15:42–49.
3 Bazil CW, Walczak TS. Effects of sleep and sleep stage on epileptic and nonepileptic seizures. *Epilepsia* 1997;38:56–62.
4 Steriade M, McCarley RW. Brainstem Control of Wakefulness and Sleep. New York: Plenum Press, 1990.

5 Parrino L, Ferri R, Bruni O, Terzano MG. Cyclic alternating pattern (CAP): the marker of instability. *Sleep Med Rev* 2012;16: 27–45.

6 Halasz P. How sleep activates epileptic networks? *Epilepsy Res Treat* 2013;2013:425697.

7 Gibbs A, Proserpio P, Terzaghi M, et al. Sleep-related epileptic behaviors and non-REM related parasomnias: Insights from stereo-EEG. Sleep Med Rev 2015; doi: htpp://dx.doi.org/10.1016/j.smrv.2015.05.002.

8 Zucconi M, Ferini Strambi L. REM parasomnias: arousal disorders and differentiation from nocturnal lobe epilepsy. *Clin Neurophysiol* 2000;111(S2):129–135.

9 Vignatelli L, Bisulli F, Giovannini G, et al. Prevalence of nocturnal frontal lobe epilepsy in the adult population of Bologna and Modena, Emilia-Romagna Region, *Italy. Sleep* 2015;38(3):479–485.

10 Bauma PA, Bovenkerk AC, Westendorp RG, Brouwer O. The course of benign partial epilepsy of childhood with centrotemporal spikes: a meta-analysis. *Neurology* 1997;48:430–437.

11 Tovia E, Goldberg-Stern H, Zeev B, et al. The prevalence of atypical presentations and comorbidities of benign childhood epilepsy with centrotemporal spikes. *Epilepsia* 2011;52(8): 1483–1488.

12 Jallo P, Latour P. Epidemiology of idiopathic generalized epilepsies. *Epilepsia* 2005;46(Suppl. 9):10–14.

13 Camfield CS, Striano P, Camfield PR. Epidemiology of juvenile myoclonic epilepsy. *Epilepsy Behav* 2013;28(Suppl. 1):S15–S17.

14 Nickels K, Wirrell E. Electrical status epilepticus in sleep. *Semin Pediatr Neurol* 2008;15:50–60.

15 Van Hirtum-Das H, Licht EA, Koh S, et al. Children with ESES: variability in the syndrome. *Epilepsy Res* 2006;70S:S248–S258.

16 Scheffer IE, Bhatia KP, Lopes-Cendes I, et al. Autosomal dominant nocturnal frontal lobe epilepsy. A distinctive clinical disorder. *Brain* 1995; 118:61–73.

17 Nobili L, Proserpio P, Combi R, et al. Nocturnal frontal lobe epilepsy. *Curr Neurol Neurosci Rep* 2014; 14: 424–435.

18 Ferini-Strambi L, Sansoni V, Combi R. Nocturnal frontal lobe epilepsy and the acetylcholine receptor. *Neurologist* 2012;18 (6):343–349.

19 Picard F, Makrythanasis P, Navarro V, et al. DEPDC5 mutations in families presenting as autosomal dominant nocturnal frontal lobe epilepsy. *Neurology* 2014;82:2101–2106.

20 Provini F, Plazzi G, Tinuper P, et al. Nocturnal frontal lobe epilepsy: a clinical and polygraphic overview of 100 consecutive cases. *Brain* 1999;122:1017–1031.

21 Oldani A, Zucconi M, Asselta R, et al. Autosomal nocturnal frontal lobe epilepsy. A video-polysomnographic and genetic appraisal of 40 patients and delineation of the epileptic syndrome. *Brain* 1998;121:205–223.

22 Terzaghi M, Sartori I, Mai R, et al. Coupling of minor motor events and epileptiform discharges with arousal fluctuations in NFLE. *Epilepsia* 2008;49(4):670–676.

23 Steinlein OK, Hoda JC, Bertrand S, Bertrand D. Mutations in familial nocturnal frontal lobe epilepsy might be associated with distinct neurological phenotypes. *Seizure* 2012;21:118–123.

24 Kramer U. Atypical presentation of benign childhood epilepsy with centrotemporal spikes: a review. *J Child Neurol* 2008;7:785–790.

25 Piccinelli P, Borgatti R, Aldini A. Academic performance in children with rolandic epilepsy. *Develop Med Child Neurol* 2008;50(5): 353–356.

26 Verrotti A, Filippini M, Matricardi S, et al. Memory impairment and Benign Epilesy with centrotemporal spike (BECTS): A growing suspicion. *Brain Cogn* 2014;84:123–131.

27 Ciumas C, Saignavongs M, Ilski F, et al. White matter development in children with benign childhood epilepsy with centrotemporal spikes. *Brain* 2014;137:1095–1106.

28 Camfield CS, Camfield PR. Rolandic epilepsy has little effect on adult life 30 years later. *Neurology* 2014;82:1162–1166.

29 Park K, Lee SK, Chu K, et al. The value of video-EEG monitoring to diagnose juvenile myoclonic epilepsy. *Seizure* 2009;18(2):94–99.

30 Valente KD, Rzezak P, Moschetta SP, et al. Delineating behavioral and cognitive phenotypes in juvenile myoclonic epilepsy: are we missing the forest for the trees? *Epilepsy Behav* 2015;54:95–99.

31 Park KM, Kim TH, Han YH, et al. Brain morphology in juvenile myoclonic epilepsy and absence seizures. Acta Neurol Scand 2015; doi:10.1111/ane.12436.

32 Tassinari CA, Cantalupo G, Rios-Pohl L, et al. Encephalopathy with status epilepticus during slow sleep: 'The Penelope syndrome'. *Epilepsia* 2009;50(Suppl. 7):4–8.

33 Pera MC, Brazzo D, Altieri N, et al. Long-term evolution of neuropsychological competences in encephalopathy with status epilepticus during sleep: A variable prognosis. *Epilepsia* 2013;54(Suppl. 7):77–85.

34 Caraballo RH, Cejas N, Chamorro N, et al. Landau-Kleffner syndrome: A study of 29 patients. *Seizure* 2014;23:98–104.

35 Vignatelli L, Bisulli F, Provini F, et al. Interobserver reliability of video recording in the diagnosis of nocturnal frontal lobe seizures. *Epilepsia* 2007;48:1506–1511.

36 Parrino L, Halasz P, Tassinari CA, Terzano MG. CAP, epilepsy and motor events during sleep: the unifying role of arousal. *Sleep Med Rev* 2006;10:267–285.

37 Nobili L, Francione S, Mai R, et al. Surgical treatment of drug-resistant nocturnal frontal lobe epilepsy. *Brain* 2007;130:561–573.

38 Tassinari CA, Rubboli G, Gardella E, et al. Central pattern generators for a common semiology in fronto-limbic seizures and in parasomnias. A neuroethologic approach. *Neurol Sci* 2005;26(Suppl. 3): 225–232.

39 Picard F, Bruel D, Servent D, et al. Alteration of the in vivo nicotinic receptor density in ADNFLE patients: a PET study. *Brain* 2006;129:2047–2060.

40 Klaassen A, Glykys J, Maguire J, et al. Seizures and enhanced cortical GABAergic inhibition in two mouse models of human autosomal dominant nocturnal frontal lobe epilepsy. *Proc Natl Acad Sci USA* 2006;103:19152–19157.

41 Combi R, Dalpra L, Ferini-Strambi L, Tenchini ML. Frontal lobe epilepsy and mutations of the corticotropin-releasing hormone gene. *Ann Neurol* 2005;58:899–904.

42 Derry CP, Dvey M, Johns M, et al. Distinguishing sleep disorders from seizure: diagnosing bumps in the night. *Arch Neurol* 2006;63:705–709.

43 Manni R, Terzaghi M, Repetto A. The FLEP scale in diagnosing nocturnal frontal lobe, NREM and REM parasomnias: data from a tertiary sleep and epilepsy unit. *Epilepsia* 2008;49:1581–1585.

44 Bisulli F, Vignatelli L, Naldi I, et al. Diagnostic accuracy of a structured interview for nocturnal frontal lobe epilepsy (SINFLE): a proposal for developing diagnostic criteria. *Sleep Med* 2012;13:81–87.

45 Capovilla G, Beccarla F, Bianchi A, et al. Ictal EEG patterns in epilepsy with centro-temporal spikes. *Brain Develop* 2011;33(4):301–319.

46 Kasteleijn-Nolst Trenitè D, Schmitz B, Janz D, et al. Consensus on diagnosis and management of JME: From founder's observations to current trends. *Epilepsy Behav* 2013;28:S87–S90.

47 Varadkar S, Duncan JS, Cross JH. Acetazolamide and autosomal dominant nocturnal frontal lobe epilepsy. *Epilepsia* 2003;44:986–987.

48 Oldani A, Manconi M, Zucconi M, Ferini-Strambi L. Topiramate treatment for nocturnal frontal lobe epilepsy. *Seizure* 2006;15:649–652.

49 Raju P, Sarco D, Poduri A, et al. Oxcarbazepine in children with nocturnal frontal lobe epilepsy. *Pediatr Neurol* 2007;37:345–349.

50 Willoughby JO, Pope KJ, Eaton V. Nicotine as an antiepileptic agent in ADNFLE: an N-of-one study. *Epilepsia* 2003;44:1238–1240.

51 Brodtkorb E, Picard F. Tobacco habit modulate autosomal dominant nocturnal frontal lobe epilepsy. *Epilepsy Behav* 2006;9:515–520.

52 Glauser T, Ben-Menachem E, Bourgeois B, et al. Updated ILAE evidence review of antiepileptic drug efficacy and effectiveness as initial monotherapy foe epileptic seizures and syndromes. *Epilepsia* 2013;54:551–563.

53 Grosso S, Balestri M, Di Bartolo RM, et al. Oxcarbazepine and atypical evolution of benign idiopathic focal epilepsy of childhood. *Eur J Neurol* 2006;13:1142–1145.

54 Sinclair DB, Snyder TJ. Corticosteroids for the treatment of Landau-Kleffner syndrome and continuous spike-wave discharge during sleep. *Paediatr Neurol* 2005;32:300–306.

55 Sanchez-Fernandez I, Chapman K, Peters JM, et al. Treatment for continuous spikes and waves during sleep (CSWS): survey on treatment choices in North America. *Epilepsia* 2014;55:1099–1108.

20

Sleep–Wake Disorders Following Traumatic Brain Injury

Christian R. Baumann

Department of Neurology, University Hospital Zurich, Zurich, Switzerland

Introduction

Traumatic brain injuries caused by a physical trauma such as a blow to the head or a penetrating head injury are clinically classified as mild, moderate or severe, depending on the duration of loss of consciousness and associated amnesia. In the literature, the annual incidence rates for traumatic brain injury range widely between 7.3 per 100 000 and 300 per 100 000 [1–3]. In the United States, for example, an estimated 1.6 million people sustain traumatic brain injury each year, accounting for 52 000 deaths and 80 000 patients suffering from irreversible neurological impairment [1,2]. Persisting deficits after traumatic brain injury commonly include neuropsychological and psychiatric symptoms, as well as sleep–wake disturbances [3]. This chapter will address the most important sleep–wake consequences of head injury with diagnostic and therapeutic suggestions for each problem.

Clinical Epidemiology

Clearly, traumatic brain injuries are highly heterogeneous with respect to the type, localisation, and severity of trauma. This poses significant restrictions on epidemiological clinical studies and any meaningful conclusions as does the retrospective nature of most of the published studies on post-traumatic sleep–wake disturbances to date. The first systematic and prospective studies on post-traumatic sleep–wake disturbances have been published only very recently. In 65 consecutive patients, sleep–wake disturbances were systematically recorded by means of interviews, questionnaires and electrophysiological sleep laboratory examinations 6 months after the traumatic brain injury [4]. In 47 patients (72% of the population), trauma-related sleep–wake disturbances were identified which were not present prior to the accident (Figure 20.1). Sleep–wake disturbances appeared to arise irrespective of the precise localisation or the severity of the trauma. The most prevalent sleep–wake disturbance following traumatic

Sleep Disorders in Neurology: A Practical Approach, Second Edition.
Edited by Sebastiaan Overeem and Paul Reading.

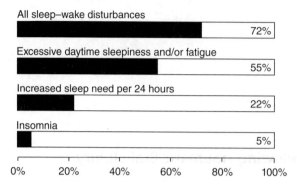

Figure 20.1 Frequency of traumatic brain injury-related sleep–wake disturbances in the first prospective study in 65 consecutive traumatic brain injury patients. Sleep–wake disturbances were assessed and characterised by interviews, questionnaires, sleep laboratory examinations including polysomnography, Multiple Sleep Latency Test and actigraphy.

brain injury was impaired daytime vigilance (excessive daytime sleepiness [EDS] and fatigue in 55%). An increased sleep need over a 24-hour period (≥2 hours more than before traumatic brain injury) was also common (observed in 22%). On the other hand, insomnia was found in only 5% of patients with traumatic brain injury. Another prospective clinical and sleep laboratory study in 87 patients at least 3 months after traumatic brain injury found sleep–wake disturbances in 46% of the examined population, with EDS as the most common finding (25%) [5]. The long-term outcome of sleep–wake disturbances after traumatic brain injury has not been systematically examined yet.

Excessive Daytime Sleepiness

Clinical Features

With regard to impaired daytime vigilance or alertness, there seem to be two potentially separable problems that can occur after traumatic brain injury. On the one hand, there is true EDS, characterised by recurrent lapses into sleep during the daytime, which are often of relatively short duration. On the other hand, some patients develop an increased total amount of sleep over 24 hours, with abnormally long nocturnal sleep time and prolonged subsequent daytime naps. In this chapter, we have used the term 'pleiosomnia' to refer to the latter type [6].

As early as 1983, Guilleminault and colleagues [7] highlighted the potential importance of recognising EDS as a residual symptom after traumatic brain injury. In their study, they found undiagnosed sleep apnoea in a significant portion of their sleepy traumatic brain injury patients. More recent prospective data, however, have shown that in a majority of patients with traumatic brain injury, post-traumatic EDS cannot easily be explained by underlying sleep–wake, neurological, or other disorders [4]. In fact, Castriotta and colleagues [8] have shown that successful treatment of sleep apnoea in brain-injured patients does not relieve symptoms of sleepiness. Rather, it appears that post-traumatic EDS may be directly related to the neuronal injury itself. The precise underlying pathophysiology, however, is not known. A clear or simple association between traumatic brain injury characteristics (such as severity or localisation of the trauma) and post-traumatic EDS has not been identified [4,5]. Early studies revealed that hypothalamus and brainstem – both important regions in the regulation of sleep and wakefulness – are often damaged after traumatic brain injury [9,10]. The preliminary findings of mildly decreased cerebrospinal fluid levels of the wake-promoting hypothalamic neuropeptide hypocretin in sleepy traumatic brain injury patients, and of decreased numbers of hypocretin-producing cells in the hypothalamus of deceased traumatic brain injury patients, suggest that traumatic lesions to wake-promoting neuronal systems may contribute to post-traumatic EDS [4,11].

Although the recent hypocretin findings in traumatic brain injury suggest a relation with narcolepsy, the existence of 'true' post-traumatic narcolepsy remains controversial. Despite previous studies suggesting that narcolepsy might be common after traumatic brain injury [5,12], narcolepsy with typical, unequivocal cataplexy is an exceedingly rare consequence. However, a proportion of head injured subjects may fulfil the criteria for narcolepsy without cataplexy (now termed narcolepsy type 2) based on results from a Multiple Sleep Latency Test. Given the suboptimal specificity of this test [13], whether such patients have true narcolepsy remains a matter of debate.

Diagnosis and Management

EDS can be identified during the clinical interview (Table 20.1; see also Chapter 8) or with questionnaires such as the Epworth Sleepiness Scale or the Karolinska Sleepiness Scale. The Multiple Sleep Latency Test remains the most important objective laboratory technique to detect the presence of EDS [4,5,14]. However, it is important to acknowledge the wide range of normative sleep latency values in control populations. Also, it is always important to consider and rule out other etiologies, especially nocturnal sleep disturbances such as sleep-disordered breathing or periodic limb movements during sleep. Furthermore, other disorders (e.g. hypothyroidism) should be ruled out by appropriate tests.

EDS impairs daytime functioning and quality of life of patients with traumatic brain injury [4,15] and, although treatment is often warranted, no specific therapy for post-traumatic EDS has been rigorously tested or approved. Modafinil is widely used to treat EDS in a variety of disorders. There is one single albeit small prospective, double-blind, randomised, placebo-controlled pilot study in 20 patients with traumatic brain injury providing Class I evidence that modafinil (100–200 mg daily) improves post-traumatic EDS compared with placebo [15]. The use of other psychostimulants such as methylphenidate or of activating antidepressants has not been systematically studied, but would be worthwhile given the prevalence and consequences of post-traumatic EDS. Alternatively, further studies to delineate other treatment strategies for sleepy traumatic brain injury patients are urgently needed.

Pleiosomnia

Clinical Features

Pleiosomnia is defined by increased sleep need per 24 hours, and must be distinguished from EDS (increased daytime sleep propensity with difficulties fighting sleep during waking hours). To prevent confusion, the term hypersomnia should probably be avoided

Table 20.1 Useful 'probes' for sleep–wake disturbances after traumatic brain injury.

Excessive daytime sleepiness

Since the trauma:

- Do you fall asleep unintentionally during the day?
- Do you have difficulties performing activities because of lapses into sleep, including driving a car?
- Do you have an increased need to take daytime naps? If yes, how long do these last?
- Do you perform frequent automatic behaviours, as if on 'autopilot'?

Hypersomnia

Since the trauma:

- How many hours do you sleep per 24 hours (including daytime naps)?
- Has this amount changed compared with before the trauma?
- Do you have difficulties waking up in the morning?

Fatigue

Since the trauma:

- Do you often feel a lack of energy, or physical and mental tiredness?
- Are you easily exhausted?

Insomnia

Since the trauma:

- Do you have difficulties initiating or maintaining sleep at night?
- Do you feel your nocturnal sleep to be 'unrestorative' or poor in quality despite adequate opportunity and circumstances for sleep?

Circadian rhythm sleep disorder

Since the trauma:

- Has your sleep–wake rhythm changed?
- Do you perceive a tendency to go to sleep much earlier or later than before the trauma?
- Do you perceive a tendency to awaken in the morning much earlier or later than before the trauma?

---

in this context, because it is commonly used for both sleepiness and increased sleep need. In the context of traumatic brain injury, a reasonable definition of pleiosomnia could be an increased sleep need of more than 2 hours compared with the situation before the traumatic brain injury [4].

Studies on post-traumatic pleiosomnia are sparse. In a prospective study in 65 patients with traumatic brain injury, most patients with post-traumatic sleep–wake disturbances suffered either from pleiosomnia or from EDS and fatigue [4]. A retrospective case-control study of patients with pleiosomnia revealed that these patients sleep considerable more than matched controls (10.8 compared with 7.3 hours per day) [6]. Furthermore, a positive association between severity of traumatic brain injury and the presence of pleiosomnia was found [4].

In the light of these findings, one may hypothesise that pleiosomnia, rather than EDS per se, is the primary sleep–wake disorder after traumatic brain injury. In other words, patients whose psychosocial environment allows extended sleeping times per 24 hours may avoid increased sleep propensity during daytime, whereas in patients who cannot compensate the increased sleep need, EDS may occur. This hypothesis is supported by the finding of increased EDS in patients between the ages of 30 and 50, whose social environment tends not to allow for longer sleeping times due to tight work schedules or families with young children, compared with pleiosomnia seen in younger or older subjects [4]. The same was found in the case-control study, with Multiple Sleep Latency Tests revealing excessive sleepiness in 15 of 36 patients, 10 of whom had signs of chronic sleep deprivation based upon actigraphy recordings [6].

Diagnosis and Management

Post-traumatic pleiosomnia can be diagnosed using the clinical interview (Table 20.1). A sleep log completed by the patient over 1–2 weeks can also be very helpful. An objective method to estimate total sleep time is wrist actigraphy. Actigraphy measures motor activity continuously over a defined period of usually 1–2 weeks. Patterns of sustained activity or absence of activity correlate well with wake and sleep periods, respectively. There is some evidence that traumatic brain injury patients underestimate sleep need when using sleep logs, thus actigraphy recordings might be preferred [6].

Post-traumatic pleiosomnia can be very difficult to treat. Psychostimulants such as modafinil, possibly in combination with methylphenidate or similar agents may be attempted, but, in practice, efficacy is often disappointing.

Fatigue

Clinical Features

Fatigue is a subjective experience that may encompass such symptoms as persisting lack of energy, exhaustion, physical and mental tiredness, or even apathy [16]. Although often quoted as an important symptom, definite conclusions regarding fatigue after traumatic brain injury cannot easily be drawn due to the inconsistent definitions of fatigue. Furthermore, a multitude of assessment scales have not been validated properly in the few available studies and there is no objective test.

Notwithstanding these difficulties, fatigue as assessed by the Fatigue Impact Scale and the Fatigue Severity Scale was found to be common in patients with traumatic brain injury [17]. Similarly, a recent study used the Global Fatigue Index and observed that fatigue is more common and pronounced in patients with traumatic brain injury compared with healthy controls [18]. The authors found associations with other symptoms such as pain, depression, and sleep–wake disturbances, but not with specific traumatic brain injury characteristics.

Diagnosis and Management

The pathophysiology of fatigue in general and of post-traumatic fatigue, in particular, is not known. Consequently, there are no laboratory tests to diagnose or assess fatigue. Besides structured interviews, there is a multitude of different fatigue assessment scales to diagnose and quantify fatigue. However, only a few of them have been validated, mostly in small studies and for specific disorders. The Fatigue Severity Scale is one of the most commonly used self-report questionnaires to measure fatigue, and has recently been validated in a large sample [19]. A specific therapy of post-traumatic fatigue is not available although treatment of concomitant depression, pain, or sleep–wake disturbances might help alleviate fatigue in some patients with traumatic brain injury. Modafinil has been shown not to be helpful to treat fatigue after traumatic brain injury [15]. In chronic fatigue syndrome, positive effects of specifically developed cognitive behavioural therapies have been reported several times, but data on post-traumatic fatigue is lacking.

Insomnia

Clinical Features

Insomnia is defined as a chronic inability to fall asleep or remain asleep for an adequate length of time at night with adverse consequences for daytime functioning. Previous studies have yielded contradictory results on the prevalence of insomnia in patients with traumatic brain injury. A prospective study based on sleep questionnaires observed a high prevalence (30%) of insomnia symptoms in 50 patients after traumatic brain injury [20]. Furthermore, in a retrospective study comprising a population of 184 somnolent subjects who suffered a traumatic brain injury or head–neck trauma (whiplash injury), almost half of the patients reported additional disturbed sleep at night, mostly due to nocturnal pain [14]. Another study examined sleep–wake diaries of 63 patients with traumatic brain injury and 63 healthy controls. The major finding was an increased number of night-time awakenings and higher latencies from wakefulness to sleep in patients with traumatic brain injury, particularly in those with mild injuries, anxiety, and depression [21]. In a questionnaire study, more than 50% of 452 patients with traumatic brain injury reported insomnia symptoms [22]. Zeitzer and colleagues [23] summarised the evidence on insomnia in the context of traumatic brain injury and concluded that the reported prevalence of post-traumatic insomnia ranged widely from 5 to more than 80%. Risk factors associated with insomnia in these studies were milder injuries, higher levels of fatigue, depression, and pain.

In an intriguing study, 14 patients with traumatic brain injury were compared with 14 healthy good sleepers by the same group, and all subjective measures of sleep as assessed by questionnaires revealed significant sleep disturbances in the traumatic brain injury group [24]. The authors found, however, that traumatic brain injury patients with insomnia have a tendency to overestimate their sleep disturbance compared with objective (polysomnographic) measures of sleep. Of note, a prospective study including objective sleep laboratory tests has found evidence for insomnia in only 5% of patients [4]. Together, these studies suggest that insomnia may be relatively common, but also overestimated after traumatic brain injury.

Diagnosis and Management

Post-traumatic insomnia appears often to be related to depression and anxiety [20–24]. Screening for and subsequent treatment of psychiatric co-morbidities should, therefore, always be performed in patients that complain of post-traumatic insomnia (Table 20.1). Conventional hypnotic medications remain the most frequently used treatment for insomnia in clinical practice although issues remain over long-term use and with tolerance or side effects. A recent study suggested that psychological interventions including cognitive behavioural therapies for insomnia are a promising therapeutic strategy for traumatic brain injury patients [25].

Circadian Sleep–Wake Disorders

Clinical Features

Relevant information on potential circadian sleep–wake disorders following traumatic brain injury is scarce and rather inconclusive. Anecdotal reports suggesting a post-traumatic delayed sleep phase syndrome have been published, but a study of 10 patients using questionnaires, sleep diaries, polysomnography, and saliva melatonin measurements failed to provide evidence of a true shift in circadian timing of sleep subsequent to traumatic brain injury [26,27]. However, a recent study in 42 patients with minor traumatic brain injury and complaints of insomnia were examined by actigraphy, saliva melatonin, and oral temperature measurements [28]. The authors found circadian sleep–wake disorders in 36% of these patients. Two varieties were observed: delayed sleep phase syndrome and irregular sleep–wake pattern. The observation of frequent circadian sleep–wake disorders following traumatic brain injury supports the assumption that post-traumatic insomnia might be overestimated and in fact be an expression of a circadian rhythm disturbance. Furthermore, another study found reduced evening melatonin production in patients with traumatic brain injury, and concluded that this may indicate disruption to circadian regulation of melatonin synthesis [29].

The clinical diagnosis of circadian sleep–wake disturbances is based on a detailed interview (Table 20.1), as well as on sleep diaries and actigraphy studies. Treatments with melatonin or bright light, aiming to synchronise the sleep–wake cycle with the environmental dark–light cycle, are appropriate therapeutic strategies for these patients [28,29] (see also Chapter 11).

Key Points

- Sleep–wake disturbances are common after traumatic brain injury, and may take on a variety of forms.
- Correlating either the severity or site of injury with subsequent sleep–wake symptoms is rarely possible.
- It is probably important to distinguish excessive daytime sleepiness with relatively short-lasting lapses into sleep during waking hours from post-traumatic pleiosomnia (an increased total sleep duration over 24 hours of >2 hours).
- Hypocretin levels may dip severely after head injuries but usually recover. The relation to sleep–wake disturbance needs clarification.
- Treatment strategies are limited. Evidence from clinical practice or the few available trials suggests that agents such as modafinil or conventional psychostimulants are worth trying but effects often disappoint.
- Insomnia appears not as common after traumatic brain injury as previously thought. It is typically associated either with pain or mood and anxiety disorders.

References

1 Sosin DM, Sniezek JE, Thurman DJ. Incidence of mild and moderate brain injury in the United States, 1991. *Brain Inj* 1996;10:47–54.

2 Bruns J Jr, Hauser WA. The epidemiology of traumatic brain injury: a review. *Epilepsia* 2003;44:2–10.

3 Maegele M, Engel D, Bouillon B, et al. Incidence and outcome of traumatic brain injury in an urban area in Western Europe over 10 years. *Eur Surg Res* 2007;39:372–379.

4 Baumann CR, Werth E, Stocker R, et al. Sleep-wake disturbances 6 months after traumatic brain injury: a prospective study. *Brain* 2007;130:1873–1883.

5 Castriotta RJ, Wilde MC, Lai JM, et al. Prevalence and consequences of sleep disorders in traumatic brain injury. *J Clin Sleep Med* 2007;3:349–356.

6 Sommerauer M, Valko PO, Werth E, Baumann CR. Excessive sleep need following traumatic brain injury: a case-control study of 36 patients. *J Sleep Res* 2013;22: 634–9.

7 Guilleminault C, Faull KF, Miles L, van den Hoed J. Posttraumatic excessive daytime sleepiness: a review of 20 patients. *Neurology* 1983;33:1584–1589.

8 Castriotta RJ, Atanasov S, Wilde MC, et al. Treatment of sleep disorders after traumatic brain injury. *J Clin Sleep Med* 2009;5:137–144.

9 Crompton MR. Hypothalamic lesions following closed head injury. *Brain* 1971;94:165–172.

10 Crompton MR. Brainstem lesions due to closed head injury. *Lancet* 1971;1:669–673.

11 Baumann CR, Bassetti CL, Valko PO, et al. Loss of hypocretin (orexin) neurons with traumatic brain injury. *Ann Neurol* 2009;66: 555–559.

12 Verma A, Anand V, Verma NP. Sleep disorders in chronic traumatic brain injury. *J Clin Sleep Med* 2007;3:357–362.

13 Mignot E, Lin L, Finn L, et al. Correlates of sleep-onset REM periods during the Multiple Sleep Latency Test in community adults. *Brain* 2006;129:1609–1623.

14 Guilleminault C, Yuen KM, Gulevich MG, et al. Hypersomnia after head-neck trauma: a medicolegal dilemma. *Neurology* 2000;54:653–659.

15 Kaiser PR, Valko PO, Werth E, et al. Modafinil ameliorates excessive daytime sleepiness after traumatic brain injury. *Neurology* 2010;75:1780–1785.

16 Chaudhuri A, Behan PO. Fatigue in neurological disorders. *Lancet* 2004;363:978–988.

17 LaChapelle DL, Finlayson MA. An evaluation of subjective and objective measures of fatigue in patients with brain injury and healthy controls. *Brain Inj* 1998;12:649–659.

18 Cantor JB, Ashman T, Gordon W, et al. Fatigue after traumatic brain injury and its impact on participation and quality of life. *J Head Trauma Rehabil* 2008;23:41–51.

19 Valko PO, Bassetti CL, Bloch KE, et al. Validation of the Fatigue Severity Scale in a large Swiss cohort. *Sleep* 2008;31(11):1601–1607.

20 Fichtenberg NL, Zafonte RD, Putnam S, et al. Insomnia in a post-acute brain injury sample. *Brain Inj* 2002;16:197–206.

21 Parcell DL, Ponsford JL, Rajaratnam SM, Redman JR. Self-reported changes to nighttime sleep after traumatic brain injury. *Arch Phys Med Rehabil* 2006;87:278–285.

22 Ouellet MC, Beaulieu-Bonneau S, Morin CM. Insomnia in patients with traumatic brain injury: frequency, characteristics, and risk factors. *J Head Trauma Rehabil* 2006;21:199–212.

23 Zeitzer JM, Friedman L, O'Hara R. Insomnia in the context of traumatic brain injury. *J Rehabil Res Dev* 2009;46: 827–836.

24 Ouellet MC, Morin CM. Subjective and objective measures of insomnia in the context of traumatic brain injury: a preliminary study. *Sleep Med* 2006;7:486–497.

25 Ouellet MC, Morin CM. Efficacy of cognitive-behavioral therapy for insomnia associated with traumatic brain injury: a single-case experimental design. *Arch Phys Med Rehabil* 2007;88:1581–1592.

26 Quinto C, Gellido C, Chokroverty S, Masdeu J. Posttraumatic delayed sleep phase syndrome. *Neurology* 2000;54:250–252.

27 Steele DL, Rajaratnam SM, Redman JR, Ponsford JL. The effect of traumatic brain injury on the timing of sleep. *Chronobiol Int* 2005;22:89–105.

28 Ayalon L, Borodkin K, Dishon L, et al. Circadian rhythm sleep disorders following mild traumatic brain injury. *Neurology* 2007;68:1136–1140.

29 Shekleton JA, Parcell DL, Redman JR, et al. Sleep disturbance and melatonin levels following traumatic brain injury. *Neurology* 2010;74: 1732–1738.

21

Sleep Disorders Associated with Stroke

Dirk M. Hermann[1], Markus H. Schmidt[2] and Claudio L. Bassetti[2]

[1] Department of Neurology, University Hospital Essen, Essen, Germany
[2] Department of Neurology, Bern University Hospital, Bern, Switzerland

Introduction

Despite their prevalence and significance, sleep-disordered breathing (SDB) and sleep–wake disturbances (SWDs) following stroke are often either not recognised or poorly managed. Indeed, both SDB [1–4] and SWDs [5,6] are highly frequent, each being found in up to 50% of patients, and recent data suggest that they both negatively affect short- and long-term functional outcomes, length of hospitalisation, and stroke recurrence risk [6–10]. As such, it is reasonable to postulate that diagnosis and therapy of post-stroke SDB and SWDs may have a favourable effect on stroke clinical outcome. This chapter outlines the present knowledge about the role of SDB and SWDs in ischaemic stroke, in addition to analysing their presentation, prevalence and clinical consequences. Despite a paucity of controlled evidence, recommendations for management are also addressed.

Clinical Presentation and Pathophysiological Relevance

Sleep-disordered Breathing

Clinical Presentation

Night-time symptoms of SDB include sleep onset insomnia, excess respiratory noises, irregular breathing, agitated sleep, shortness of breath, palpitations and nocturia [2]. In patients with severe hypoventilation, arousal responses can be suppressed by increasing sleep debt and may, in conjunction with cardiac arrhythmias, even lead to sleep-related death. Daytime symptoms of SDB are headaches, fatigue, sleepiness, and deficits in concentration and memory [2]. Risk factors such as increased age, gender, central obesity and neck circumference may be sufficient, with or without a history of snoring, to reliably predict the presence of SDB [11]. In the general population, as well as in stroke

Sleep Disorders in Neurology: A Practical Approach, Second Edition.
Edited by Sebastiaan Overeem and Paul Reading.

patients, it is important to note that the absence of daytime sleepiness is not uncommon and by no means excludes the presence of significant SDB [2,11].

Approximately 50–70% of acute stroke patients exhibit SDB, defined by an apnoea–hypopnoea index (AHI) ≥10/hour, and about 1/3 of stroke patients exhibit severe SDB which is relevant as an independent predictor of cardiovascular morbidity and mortality (Table 21.1) [1–4,12–28].

Until recently, no convincing link has been found between SDB and stroke severity, topography or presumed etiology [2,3,22,24]. However, newer studies have begun to shed light on some of these interactions. For example, population-based [29] and clinical [30] cohorts have identified a particular association of SDB with brainstem stroke, potentially implicating lower cranial nerve dysfunction in the generation of SDB. One possible aetiology relates to the fact that SDB may provoke paradoxical embolism and 'wake-up' strokes when accompanied by cardiac right-to-left shunts, as was demonstrated in a cross-sectional study on 335 acute stroke or transient ischaemic attack (TIA) patients [31].

The most common form of SDB in stroke patients is obstructive sleep apnoea (OSA), caused by a cessation of nasal flow due to upper airway collapse [1–4]. It is not unusual for patients to present with mixed breathing disturbances involving both OSA and central sleep apnoea (CSA), sometimes resembling Cheyne–Stokes breathing (CSB) [1,4,32–34]. A predominance of CSA/CSB was first described in patients with bilateral strokes associated with disturbed levels of consciousness or heart failure [35]. Nocturnal fluid shifts in heart failure patients from the lower extremities to the upper torso may be relevant in some. Increases in neck circumference may predispose either to upper airway collapse and obstructive events or to pulmonary congestion and central breathing events, respectively [36]. More recently, CSB presenting only during sleep has also been found in patients with unilateral strokes and preserved consciousness in the absence of overt cardiorespiratory dysfunction. Damage to areas involved in autonomic control such as the insula and paramedian thalamus is thought relevant [32,34].

The frequency of SDB was found to be similar in patients with TIA and stroke [1,4,21,37], suggesting that SDB may be not only a consequence of brain injury but a pre-existing condition. However, it seems that SDB may be exacerbated by stroke given the finding that SDB tends to improve from the acute to the subacute stroke phase. Nonetheless, around 50% of patients still exhibit an AHI ≥10/hour after 3 months [2,4,22,38].

Pathophysiological Relevance

SDB may increase predisposition to vascular disease, as has been previously emphasised in a statement paper of the American Heart Association [39]. That SDB elevates the risk for stroke and death, in addition to that of myocardial infarcts and heart failure, was suggested in cohort studies [9,40–42], population-based studies [10,43,44], and meta-analyses [45] in which increased odds ratios were noted even when data were corrected for more established vascular risk factors.

Elevated cardiovascular risk is thought to result from intrathoracic pressure changes and sympathetic activation, which produce acute cerebral blood flow fluctuations, during and after apnoea episodes [7,46]. In the long term, inflammatory responses in the vasculature contribute to endothelial dysfunction, atherosclerosis, arterial hypertension, platelet activation and prothrombotic coagulation changes [7,46]. SDB is also associated with myocardial ischaemia, left ventricular failure and cardiac rhythm abnormalities, all of which contribute to stroke risk [7,46]. Continuous positive airway

Table 21.1 Effect of continuous positive airway pressure after stroke.

Study	Type	Patients	Age (yr)	Body mass index (kg/m^2)	Findings
Sandberg et al. [12]	Randomised single-blind study	63 ischaemic stroke patients with respiratory disturbance index ≥15/h recruited in a rehabilitation unit at 2–4 weeks post stroke; randomisation to CPAP or no CPAP over 28 days	77 ± 8 (no CPAP), 78 ± 6 (CPAP)	25 ± 5 (no CPAP), 24 ± 4 (CPAP	CPAP was used by 31 out of 33 patients for 4 weeks; mean CPAP use was 4.1 ± 3.6 h/night; CPAP treatment improved depressive symptoms, but did not significantly change MMSE score or Barthel index; low cognitive level (MMSE score) predicted poor CPAP use
Hsu et al. [13]	Randomised single-blind study (blind assessment of outcomes)	30 stroke patients with AHI ≥30/h recruited at 21–25 days post stroke; randomisation to CPAP or no CPAP over 8 weeks	Median 73 (Q1, Q3:73, 81) (no CPAP), 74 (Q1, Q3: 65, 77) (CPAP)	Median 25 (Q1, Q3: 21, 29) (no CPAP), 27 (Q1, Q3: 22, 33) (CPAP)	Mean CPAP use was poor (1.4 h/night); the study was prematurely stopped due to poor recruitment; CPAP treatment did not influence neurologic outcome, anxiety, depression, or quality of life; no significant difference in 24-h daytime and nighttime systolic, diastolic, and mean arterial blood pressure between groups; 7 of 15 patients (47%) kept using the CPAP device over >4 weeks; treatment discontinued in 8 patients because of problems with mask or machine, stroke-related confusional states, or upper airway symptoms; CPAP use positively correlated with good Barthel index and good language capabilities
Bravata et al. [14]	Randomised single-blind study	70 TIA patients randomised within 72 h post TIA; patients with AHI ≥5/h received CPAP or no CPAP over 90 days; 12 patients (no CPAP) vs. 30 patients (CPAP) completed study	67 ± 13 (no CPAP), 66 ± 12 (CPAP)	28 ± 7 (no CPAP), 29 ± 4 (CPAP)	Forty per cent of SDB patients had acceptable (≥4 h/night) and 60% some (<4 h/night) CPAP use; 3 CPAP patients and 1 control patient had recurrent vascular events; there was a nonsignificant tendency towards a lower event rate in patients with acceptable (0%) compared with some (6%) CPAP use (p = 0.08)

(Continued)

Table 21.1 (Continued)

Study	Type	Patients	Age (yr)	Body mass index (kg/m²)	Findings
Svatikova et al. [15]	Randomised single-blind cross-over study	In first study phase, 18 ischaemic stroke patients with AHI > 5/h randomised to positional therapy (therapeutic pillow) or no positional therapy (regular pillow) within 14 days post stroke; treatment administered during two consecutive nights in crossover design; in second study phase, the same 18 patients were randomised to positional therapy or no positional therapy for 3 months	Median 58 (Q1, Q3: 54, 68)	Median 29 (Q1, Q3: 28, 33)	In within-participant comparison (first phase), positional therapy reduced AHI from median 39/h (21/h, 54/h) to 27/h (22/h, 47/h); therapeutic pillow reduced time supine from median 142 (31, 295) to 30 (3, 66) min; median and minimum oxygen saturation remained unchanged; in second phase (between-participant comparison), self- reported adherence was 3 (33%) all nights, 1 (11%) most nights, 2 (22%) some nights, and 3 (33%) no nights in participants randomised to positional therapy; of those randomised to the therapeutic pillow, 7 (78%) had a good outcome, while 6 (67%) of those not randomised to the pillow had a good outcome
Ryan et al. [16]	Randomised single-blind study (blind assessment of outcomes)	44 stroke patients with AHI > 15/h recruited within 3 weeks post stroke; randomisation to CPAP or no CPAP over 4 weeks	61 ± 10 (no CPAP), 63 ± 13 (CPAP)	29 ± 5 (no CPAP), 27 ± 6 (CPAP)	Mean CPAP use was 5.0 ± 2.3 h/night; regarding primary outcomes, CPAP treatment improved neurologic deficits evaluated by Canadian Neurologic Scale, but not 6-min walk distance, sustained attention response, and digit and visual spatial span; regarding secondary outcomes, CPAP improved sleepiness evaluated by Epworth Sleepiness Scale, motor component of the functional independence measure, Chedoke–McMaster lower leg function, and affective component of depression
Bravata et al. [17]	Randomised single-blind study	55 ischaemic stroke patients randomised within 72h post stroke; patients with AHI≥5/h received CPAP or no CPAP over 30 days; 15 patients (no CPAP) vs. 16 patients (CPAP) completed study	72 ± 13 (no CPAP), 71 ± 9 (CPAP)	29 ± 7 (no CPAP), 27 ± 4 (CPAP)	A total of 62.5% of SDB patients had acceptable (≥4 h/ night) and 37.5% some (<4 h/night) CPAP use; NIH Stroke Scale improved more in CPAP (−3.0) than control (−1.0) patients (p = 0.03); 1 CPAP patient and 3 control patients had recurrent vascular events; event rate did not differ between groups

Study	Design	Population	Age	AHI	Findings
Parra et al. [18]	Randomised single-blind study	140 ischaemic stroke patients with AHI ≥ 20/h recruited within 3–6 days post stroke; randomisation to CPAP or no CPAP over 5 years	66 ± 9 (no CPAP), 64 ± 9 (CPAP)	29 ± 4 (no CPAP), 30 ± 5 (CPAP)	Of 71 patients randomised to CPAP, 14 refused participation after 1–3 nights and 6 additional patients refused continuation after a mean of 10 months; in the others, mean CPAP use was 5.3 ± 1.9 h/night; percentage of patients exhibiting improvement in Canadian Neurologic Scale and Rankin scale 1 month after stroke was significantly higher in patients receiving CPAP than controls; mean values in Canadian Neurologic Scale and Rankin scale did not differ between groups at any time point; in log rank tests, CPAP increased cardiovascular survival (100% vs. 89.9%; p = 0.02); there was a nonsignificant tendency towards increased cardiovascular event-free survival in CPAP compared with control patients (89.5% vs. 75.4%; p = 0.06)
Minnerup et al. [19]	Randomised single-blind study (blind assessment of outcomes)	50 ischemic stroke patients with AHI > 10/h recruited within 1st night post stroke; randomisation to CPAP or no CPAP over 7 days	63 ± 11 (no CPAP), 69 ± 10 (CPAP)	27 ± 3 (no CPAP), 28 ± 3 (CPAP)	Forty per cent of SDB patients had acceptable (≥4 h/night), 56% some (<4 h/night), and 4% no CPAP use; patients receiving CPAP revealed a nonsignificant tendency towards a better NIH Stroke Scale improvement (−2.0) compared with control patients (−1.4; p = 0.09)
Brown et al. [20]	Randomised double-blind study	32 ischaemic stroke patients with AHI ≥ 5/h recruited within 7 days post stroke; randomisation to CPAP or sham CPAP over 90 days	Median 74 (Q1, Q3: 55, 81) (sham CPAP), 61 (46, 76) (CPAP)	Median 29 (Q1, Q3: 28, 32) (sham CPAP), 28 (23, 31) (CPAP)	Of 15 patients who commenced active CPAP titration, 11 (73%) took the device home and 8 (53%) completed the 90-day follow-up; of 17 participants who commenced sham titration, 11 (65%) took the sham device home and completed the 90-day follow-up; cumulative usage was poor (mean 0.8 h/night for sham CPAP; 0.6 h/night for CPAP); average usage on days used was 3.5 (1.8, 4.1) h/night for sham CPAP, 4.5 (2.6, 5.5) h/night for CPAP; 50% of patients receiving CPAP and 0% of patients receiving sham CPAP felt more awake during the day; stroke outcome evaluated by Barthel index, Rankin scale, and NIH Stroke Scale remained unchanged

AHI, Apnoea–Hypopnoea Index; CPAP, continuous positive airway pressure; MMSE, Mini-Mental State Examination; SDB, sleep-disordered breathing; TIA, transient ischaemic attack.
Source: Adapted from Ref. [8].

pressure (CPAP) therapy reverses the pathophysiological consequences of SDB, improving arterial hypertension and helping to attenuate vascular risk [7,46].

Several studies indicate that SDB negatively affects early neurological worsening [33], hospitalisation duration [47], and short-term [33] and long-term [48] neurological outcomes. In a series of 120 patients, the presence of SDB predicted a worse Barthel index and higher mortality at 6 months after stroke [48]. This finding was reproduced in other studies in patients with first-ever stroke or TIA, in which SDB increased the patients' mortality over several years [2,4]. Stroke recurrence has also been linked with the presence of SDB [49]. The presence of recurrent nocturnal hypoxia is associated with a poor rehabilitation outcome [50]. The detrimental effect of SDB appears to be more pronounced for OSA than for CSA.

A recent systematic review on SDB and stroke outcome, including death or recurrent vascular events, analysed 10 studies involving a total of 1203 stroke and TIA patients [51]. All studies reviewed reported elevated risks for SDB on stroke outcomes. Two studies powered for multivariate regression analyses found that OSA (as defined by an $AHI \geq 15$/hour or $AHI \geq 20$/hour) independently predicted death (hazard ratio 1.76;1.05–2.95) or nonfatal cardiovascular events such as recurrent stroke (hazard ratio 1.76;1.12–2.68), in addition to other variables such as age, sex, vascular risk factors, and Barthel index.

Several reasons have been discussed for the poorer recovery of SDB patients. For example, stroke patients with moderate to severe sleep apnoea ($AHI > 30$/hour) exhibit higher daytime and night-time blood pressure in the early recovery phase, as compared with patients without sleep apnoea ($AHI < 10$/h) [24]. The elevated blood pressure levels, together with recurrent hypoxias and cerebral hypoperfusion, may contribute to the less favourable prognosis. Recent data also implicate the negative impact of sleep disruption on neuroplasticity which is normally upregulated during normal sleep (see below).

Arousal Disorders

Clinical Presentation

The clinical spectrum of altered levels of arousal following stroke is wide. It includes hypersomnia, defined as an abnormal sleep propensity with increased sleep over the 24-hour period; excessive daytime sleepiness (EDS), an increased tendency to fall asleep during the daytime hours; and fatigue, a loosely defined phenomenon, occasionally synonymous with physical exhaustion, reduced energy, or simple tiredness.

Severe post-stroke hypersomnia is most often recognised after striatal, thalamo-mesencephalic, upper pontine and medial ponto-medullary strokes. In a systematic study of 285 consecutive patients at 21 ± 18 months after stroke, a high frequency of reduced arousal levels was observed [52]. Hypersomnia (defined as a sleep need of ≥10hours/day) was seen in 27%, EDS (Epworth Sleepiness Score ≥10) in 28%, and fatigue (fatigue severity scale ≥3) in 46%. Although hypersomnia usually improves during the first months, fatigue often persists, even in the chronic phase [52]. At 6 months after stroke, fatigue is more prevalent after minor stroke than TIA (56 vs. 29%), indicating that fatigue may reflect organic brain damage.

The most dramatic form of post-stroke hypersomnia is noted after paramedian thalamic stroke [53–55]. Indeed, patients typically present with sudden onset of state resembling coma. After awakening, patients exhibit severe hypersomnia and sleep-like behaviour up to 20 hours/day associated with attention, cognitive, and memory deficits [55]. Hypersomnia gradually improves within months, whereas cognitive deficits often persist, particularly after left-sided and bilateral strokes [55]. Those with bilateral strokes may report increased sleep need for several years.

In addition to thalamic infarcts, hypersomnia may be observed in the context of a number of characteristic syndromes linked to vascular diencephalic brain lesions, namely symptomatic Kleine–Levin syndrome (hypersomnia with hyperphagia) [56] and symptomatic narcolepsy (hypersomnia with cataplexy-like episodes, hallucinations, sleep paralysis and low cerebrospinal fluid hypocretin-1 levels) [57,58].

Pathophysiological Relevance

EDS and fatigue are intimately associated with neuropsychiatric and cognitive disturbances including depression, anxiety and reduced attention with negative impacts on rehabilitation, daily functioning and quality of life [6]. Such sleep-related disturbances might, therefore, be expected to influence stroke recovery adversely. That post-stroke fatigue is indeed an independent predictor of independence and death was shown in a cohort of 8194 stroke patients [59]. In a questionnaire, 39.2% of patients reported fatigue 2 years after their stroke. Notably, patients with fatigue were more likely to be institutionalised and had an increased mortality rate in the subsequent year [8,59].

Insomnia

Clinical Presentation

Insomnia is loosely defined as difficulty initiating or maintaining sleep, early awakenings, and insufficient sleep quality causing adverse daytime consequences such as fatigue. Often post-stroke insomnia is directly linked either to the complications of the stroke or to the environment. In particular, factors, including noise, light and intensive care monitoring may play a role together with co-morbidities such as cardiac failure, SDB and infections.

Similarly to hypersomnia, when directly assessed, post-stroke insomnia is not rare. In a systematic study of 277 consecutive patients, insomnia was found in the first months after stroke in 57% of patients [6]. In 18%, insomnia appeared de novo after the stroke [6]. In view of the known consequences of impaired nocturnal sleep, including daytime fatigue, attention and cognitive problems, insomnia might be expected to hinder or slow stroke recovery. Systematic studies directly supporting this hypothesis, however, are lacking.

Occasionally, insomnia may be related directly to brain damage, mostly in the brainstem. Patients with almost complete loss of sleep electroencephalography (EEG) patterns lasting over several months have been reported after pontine and ponto-mesencephalic strokes [60].

Pathophysiological Relevance

After stroke, insomnia may directly lead to attention and memory problems, which may have an unfavourable influence on stroke clinical outcome. The relevance of this influence is well illustrated by the increased risk of institutionalisation and mortality in stroke patients suffering from fatigue [59]. The importance of adequate and good quality nocturnal sleep should be emphasised in the rehabilitation process.

Recent experimental models have shown that sleep loss or deprivation following stroke increases infarct volume size in rodents [61] and impairs both neuroplasticity and functional recovery [62]. In particular, sleep loss following stroke is associated with a reduction in axonal sprouting and greater impairments in the single pellet-reaching task [62]. In contrast, interventions that increase sleep after stroke in rodents, such as pre-stroke sleep deprivation [63–65] or use of sleep-inducing medications following stroke [66,67], show favourable effects on neuroplasticity and stroke recovery. Of interest, in human subjects following stroke, imitation-based speech therapy increased slow-wave activity during sleep as demonstrated using high density EEG [68]. Increased slow-wave activity in speech areas correlated closely with improvements of aphasia scores. Taken together, these data suggest that improving sleep may have a positive impact on stroke outcome and recovery, consistent with the known role for sleep in neuroplasticity and the promotion of learning and memory (see Ref. [69] for a review).

Sleep-related Movements Disorders

Clinical Presentation

In a cohort of 137 patients that were examined 1 month after their stroke, Lee et al. [5] reported a high prevalence of 12% for symptoms suggesting restless legs syndrome (RLS). RLS was observed mainly in patients with pontine, thalamic, basal ganglia and corona radiata infarcts. About two thirds of patients had bilateral RLS symptoms whereas one third reported unilateral complaints contralateral to the stroke [5]. RLS appeared within 1 week post-stroke and was frequently accompanied by periodic leg movements during sleep (PLMS).

Pathophysiological Relevance

RLS/PLMS often has a strong influence on quality of life and should therefore be adequately diagnosed in stroke patients. RLS/PLMS may even affect life expectancy, as suggested by a mid-Swedish population-based study following 5102 subjects (aged 30–65 years) over 20 years [70]. In a multivariable analysis adjusted for age, sleep time, lifestyle factors, medical conditions, including diabetes and hypertension, and depression, women with RLS and daytime sleepiness had an excess mortality compared with women without RLS and daytime sleepiness [70]. No influence of RLS on mortality was found in men. Whether this excess mortality is secondary to a negative impact of RLS on patients' cerebrovascular risk profile remains to be shown.

Diagnosis and Treatment

Sleep-disordered Breathing

Diagnosis

SDB is generally best diagnosed by respiratory polygraphy, in which nasal airflow, thoracic and abdominal respiratory movements in addition to capillary oxygen saturation (oximetry) are monitored. Polysomnography, in contrast, offers additional information on sleep architecture, but is more expensive and may be less commonly available in general medical settings. It should therefore be reserved for complex or diagnostically unclear situations. Based on nasal airflow, respiratory movements, and oxygen desaturation recordings, various forms of SDB can be defined, including OSA, CSA or CSB. The AHI and the number and severity of desaturations are considered approximate indicators of SDB severity although do not always correlate with clinical markers.

Treatment

SDB treatment in stroke patients often represents a clinical, technical and logistical challenge (Table 21.1). Management strategies should always aim to include prevention and early treatment of secondary complications (e.g. respiratory infections) and the avoidance of sedative-hypnotic drugs, including alcohol, which may negatively affect breathing during sleep (Table 21.2). Positioning patients laterally rather than supine overnight in the acute phase may influence oxygen saturation as well (Table 21.2). CPAP is nearly always the treatment of choice for OSA (Table 21.2). Since SDB might be expected to improve in the first weeks, intelligent positive airway pressure (PAP) systems that allow automatic titration of PAP pressure may well be justified. Biphasic positive airway pressure, adaptive servo-ventilation, or supplemental oxygen may be considered in patients with CSA/CSB.

Early studies suggested that patients with stroke and SDB may benefit from active treatment. Wessendorf et al. [71] reported an improvement of subjective well-being and night-time blood pressure values in a group of 41 and 16 patients with stroke and SDB, respectively, who were treated with CPAP over 10 days. Martinez-Garcia et al. [72] studied 51 patients with stroke and an AHI ≥ 20/hour. After 1 month, 29% of patients remained on CPAP. Of these, the large majority continued their treatment over 18 months. This group had a significantly lower incidence of new vascular events.

Eight randomised studies have investigated the effects of CPAP following stroke (Table 21.1) [12–14,16–20], including five studies that initiated therapy within the first week after the initial stroke [14,17–20]. CPAP adherence was ≥4 hours/night in over half of patients [12,14,16–20]. Although study sizes were small, four of the eight studies demonstrated favourable CPAP effects on neurologic recovery, sleepiness, depression and recurrent vascular events.

These and other data have led the American Heart Association to recently change guidelines to include recommendations on diagnosis and treatment of SDB in patients with stroke or TIAs [73]. These suggest that a sleep study might be considered for all patients with an ischaemic stroke or TIA on the basis of the extremely high prevalence of sleep apnoea in this population and that a low threshold for treatment with CPAP might be considered for patients with ischaemic stroke or TIA and sleep apnoea given the emerging evidence in support of improved outcomes (Class IIb; Level of Evidence B recommendations). Although a recent international, multicentre study found that CPAP therapy did not prevent further cardiovascular events in patients with moderate to severe OSA and established cardiovascular disease, adherence with CPAP therapy in this study was low at a mean duration of 3.3 hours per night [74]. However, in patients with coronary artery disease, an adjusted on-treatment analysis has shown a significant cardiovascular risk reduction for patients who use CPAP ≥ 4 hours, a finding not observed for those who used CPAP < 4 hours [75]. Indeed, similar post-hoc analyses from randomised controlled studies confirm cardiovascular benefit in favour of CPAP over the control group for subjects adherent to therapy (Figure 21.1) [77].

Table 21.2 Summary of diagnostics and treatment of sleep–wake disorders following stroke.

Sleep–wake disorder	Diagnostics	Avoid/use with caution	Treatment
Sleep-related breathing disturbances: Obstructive sleep apnoea	Polygraphy (polysomnography)	Alcohol, hypnotics, sedative antidepressants	Continuous positive airway pressure Weight loss, preference of lateral to supine sleeping position
Sleep-related breathing disturbances: Central sleep apnoea/ Cheyne–Stokes-breathing	Polygraphy (polysomnography)	Alcohol, hypnotics, sedative antidepressants	Continuous/biphasic positive airway pressure Adaptive servoventilation Oxygen Tracheotomy/mechanical ventilation in severe central apnoea
Arousal disorders: Hypersomnia/excessive daytime sleepiness/fatigue	Clinical observation/ actigraphy/ polysomnography	Alcohol, hypnotics, sedative antidepressants	Stimulating antidepressants (e.g. venlafaxine 37.5–150 mg/d) Stimulants: modafinil (100–200 mg/d), methylphenidate (5–60 mg/d) Dopaminergic agents (e.g. bromocriptine 20–40 mg or levodopa 100 mg/d)
Insomnia	Clinical observation/ actigraphy/ polysomnography	Alcohol, caffeine, stimulating antidepressants	Zolpidem, sedative antidepressants (amitryptiline 10–100 mg/d; trazodone 50–200 mg/d; mirtazapine 15–30 mg/d) Non-pharmacological sleep hygiene (avoid noises, treat infections, avoid alcohol and caffeine at night)
Sleep-related movement disorders: Restless legs syndrome/ periodic limb movements during sleep	Clinical observation/ leg actigraphy/ polysomnography	Antidepressants, neuroleptics, metoclopramide, lithium	Levodopa (100 mg at night) Dopamine agonists (ropinirole 0.25–1 mg/d, pramipexole 0.125–0.5 mg/d)

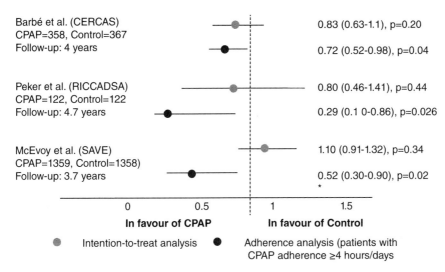

Barbé et al. (CERCAS)
CPAP=358, Control=367
Follow-up: 4 years

0.83 (0.63-1.1), p=0.20

0.72 (0.52-0.98), p=0.04

Peker et al. (RICCADSA)
CPAP=122, Control=122
Follow-up: 4.7 years

0.80 (0.46-1.41), p=0.44

0.29 (0.1 0-0.86), p=0.026

McEvoy et al. (SAVE)
CPAP=1359, Control=1358)
Follow-up: 3.7 years

1.10 (0.91-1.32), p=0.34

0.52 (0.30-0.90), p=0.02
*

0   0.5   1   1.5

In favour of CPAP   **In favour of Control**

Intention-to-treat analysis   Adherence analysis (patients with
CPAP adherence ≥4 hours/days

Figure 21.1 Effect of CPAP treatment on cardiovascular risk. The figure shows the incidence risk for the primary composite endpoints in three randomised controlled trials [74–76] in the CPAP compared with the control group (hazard ratio or incidence density ratio, 95% confidence interval) in the intention-to-treat analysis and in the adherence analysis (patients with CPAP adherence ≥4 hours/day). *In the McEvoy et al. [74] study, the significant cardiovascular improvement in patients who used CPAP ≥ 4 hours/day was only achieved in the risk of a cerebrovascular event, but not in the primary composite outcome. *Source:* Adapted from Javaheri et al. [77]. Reproduced with permission of Elsevier.

In the acute stroke rehabilitation setting, compliance with CPAP therapy may present significant problems. Various groups have reported a wide range of compliance levels although some have achieved up to 70% [2,13,22,72,78,79]. In a randomised trial of stroke patients with severe SDB (AHI ≥ 30/hour) CPAP usage was very low with a mean of 1.4 hours/night (Table 21.1) [13]. In our experience, only ~50% of stroke patients with SDB can be treated in the acute phase, and only half of these patients stay on CPAP in the long-term [2]. Compliance is certainly influenced by any spontaneous improvement of SDB and by the absence of daytime sleepiness in many patients. In addition, compliance can be expected to be a problem in stroke patients with severe facial or bulbar weakness. Clearly, severe peripheral motor deficits may inhibit mask fitting and handling. Confusional states, dementia, aphasia and anosognosia will also hinder treatment protocols in many.

In patients with central apnoea and CSB, improvement can sometimes be achieved with oxygen supplementation or CPAP (Table 21.2) [35] although more sophisticated methods of ventilatory support (e.g. adaptive servo-ventilation) are often needed [80]. Tracheostomy and mechanical ventilation may become necessary in patients with significant central hypoventilation.

Arousal Disorders

Diagnosis
Although most SWDs can be recognised simply on clinical assessment, their presence and severity are often only first fully realised when patients leave hospital. The clinical correlation between post-stroke SWDs and formal sleep investigations, including EEG

parameters, is often poor, particularly when brain damage includes those thalamo-cortical structures involved in wake and EEG generation [53,55].

In patients with post-stroke hypersomnia, sleep EEG may reveal both a reduction and, less commonly, an increase of non-rapid eye movement or rapid eye movement sleep. Particularly in supratentorial strokes, the widely used multiple sleep latency test (MSLT) may be inadequate for assessing post-stroke sleep propensity [55]. Actigraphy may be helpful to estimate changes in sleep–wake rhythms and sleep–rest needs [55], although a differentiating between sleep and inactivity due to apathy or severe motor deficits may be difficult.

Treatment
Treatment of post-stroke hypersomnia is often difficult and the evidence base is minimal (Table 21.2). Case reports of improved apathy and pre-sleep behaviour has been reported following paramedian thalamic stroke treated with 20–40 mg of bromocriptine [54]. A favourable influence on early post-stroke rehabilitation was also reported both after levodopa (100 mg/day) [81] and methylphenidate (5–30 mg/day) [82], an effect that may at least in part be related to improved alertness. A clear-cut improvement of alertness with 200 mg of modafinil was observed in a patient with bilateral paramedian thalamic stroke [60]. Anecdotally, treatment of stroke-associated depression with stimulating antidepressants such as venlafaxine may also improve hypersomnia.

Insomnia

Diagnosis
A directed sleep–wake history will identify significant insomnia. The validity of insomnia rating scales specifically to assess stroke patients remains uncertain.

Treatment
Management of post-stroke insomnia may be helped by placing patients in quiet rooms at night with protection from external stimulation including light while simultaneously increasing light exposure during the day. If hypnotic use is considered unavoidable, temporary use of agents that are relatively free of cognitive and muscle-relaxant effects, such as zolpidem or zopiclone, is preferable (Table 21.2). It should be kept in mind that benzodiazepines may provoke neuropsychological deficits and result in the re-emergence of motor symptoms [83].

Although formal evidence is lacking, sedative antidepressants may improve post-stroke insomnia (Table 21.2). In a study of 51 stroke patients, 60 mg/day of mianserin led to a better improvement of insomnia than placebo, even in patients without depression [84]. If stroke patients with insomnia exhibit clear depressive symptomology, sedative antidepressants should clearly be preferred, especially as management is likely to be for the long term.

Sleep-related Movement Disorders

Diagnosis
RLS is diagnosed using the usual criteria based on history and established rating scales.

Treatment

After treating 17 patients with stroke-related RLS using dopaminergic agonists (ropinirole 0.25–1 mg/day, pramipexole 0.125–0.5 mg/day), Lee et al. [5] reported marked relief in all except two patients who had only mild improvement. All patients had persistent RLS until the end of the study period, indicating that most patients required treatment [5]. Spontaneous improvement was noted in only four out of 17 patients who allowed the authors to terminate the drug prescription [5]. All other patients remained on long-term dopaminergic agonists.

Key Points

- Virtually all types of sleep disorder may increase in prevalence following an ischaemic stroke.
- Most work has focused on SDB, notably OSA, given its proven association with cerebrovascular disease and increasing evidence that early treatment following stroke improves outcome.
- Improving levels of alertness and treating insomnia, when present after a stroke, is likely to help the rehabilitation process and improve quality of life.
- Controlled evidence to guide treatment of sleep disorders following stroke is lacking, but current guidelines on stroke management are increasingly including sleep assessment as an important component.

References

1 Bassetti C, Aldrich MS, Chervin RD, Quint D. Sleep apnea in patients with transient ischemic attack and stroke: a prospective study of 59 patients. *Neurology* 1996;47:1167–73.

2 Bassetti CL, Milanova M, Gugger M. Sleep-disordered breathing and acute ischemic stroke: diagnosis, risk factors, treatment, evolution, and long-term clinical outcome. *Stroke* 2006;37:967–72.

3 Dyken ME, et al. Investigating the relationship between stroke and obstructive sleep apnea. *Stroke* 1996;27:401–7.

4 Parra O, et al. Time course of sleep-related breathing disorders in first-ever stroke or transient ischemic attack. *Am. J. Respir. Crit. Care Med.* 2000;161:375–80.

5 Lee S-J, et al. Poststroke restless legs syndrome and lesion location: anatomical considerations. *Mov Disord* 2009;24:77–84.

6 Leppävuori A, et al. Insomnia in ischemic stroke patients. *Cerebrovasc Dis* 2002;14:90–7.

7 Bassetti CL. Sleep and stroke. *Semin Neurol* 2005;25:19–32.

8 Hermann DM, Bassetti CL. Role of sleep-disordered breathing and sleep-wake disturbances for stroke and stroke recovery. *Neurology* 2016;87:1407–16.

9 Yaggi HK, et al. Obstructive sleep apnea as a risk factor for stroke and death. *N Engl J Med* 2005;353:2034–41.

10 Young T, et al. Sleep disordered breathing and mortality: eighteen-year follow-up of the Wisconsin sleep cohort. *Sleep* 2008;31:1071–78.

11 Marti-Soler H, et al. The NoSAS score for screening of sleep-disordered breathing: a derivation and validation study. *Lancet Respir Med* 2016;4:742–8.

12 Sandberg O, et al. Nasal continuous positive airway pressure in stroke patients with sleep apnoea: a randomized treatment study. *Eur Respir J* 2001;18:630–4.

13 Hsu C-Y, et al. Sleep-disordered breathing after stroke: a randomised controlled trial of continuous positive airway pressure. *J Neurol Neurosurg Psychiatry* 2006;77:1143–9.

14 Bravata DM, et al. Auto-titrating continuous positive airway pressure for patients with acute transient ischemic attack: a randomized feasibility trial. *Stroke* 2010;41: 1464–70.

15 Svatikova A, et al. Positional therapy in ischemic stroke patients with obstructive sleep apnea. *Sleep Med* 2011;12:262–6.

16 Ryan CM, et al. Influence of continuous positive airway pressure on outcomes of rehabilitation in stroke patients with obstructive sleep apnea. *Stroke* 2011;42: 1062–7.

17 Bravata DM, et al. Continuous positive airway pressure: evaluation of a novel therapy for patients with acute ischemic stroke. *Sleep* 2011;34:1271–7.

18 Parra O, et al. Efficacy of continuous positive airway pressure treatment on 5-year survival in patients with ischaemic stroke and obstructive sleep apnea: a randomized controlled trial. *J Sleep Res* 2015;24:47–53.

19 Minnerup J, et al. Continuous positive airway pressure ventilation for acute ischemic stroke: a randomized feasibility study. *Stroke* 2012;43:1137–9.

20 Brown DL, et al. Sleep apnea treatment after stroke (SATS) trial: is it feasible? *J Stroke Cerebrovasc Dis* 2013;22:1216–24.

21 Bassetti C, Aldrich MS. Sleep apnea in acute cerebrovascular diseases: final report on 128 patients. *Sleep* 1999;22:217–23.

22 Hui DSC, et al. Prevalence of sleep-disordered breathing and continuous positive airway pressure compliance: results in Chinese patients with first-ever ischemic stroke. *Chest* 2002;122:852–60.

23 Rola R, et al. Sleep related breathing disorders in patients with ischemic stroke and transient ischemic attacks: respiratory and clinical correlations. *J Physiol Pharmacol* 58(Suppl. 5):575–82.

24 Selic C, Siccoli MM, Hermann DM, Bassetti CL. Blood pressure evolution after acute ischemic stroke in patients with and without sleep apnea. *Stroke* 2005;36:2614–8.

25 Turkington PM, Bamford J, Wanklyn P, Elliott MW. Prevalence and predictors of upper airway obstruction in the first 24 hours after acute stroke. *Stroke* 2002;33:2037–42.

26 Wessendorf TE, et al. Sleep-disordered breathing among patients with first-ever stroke. *J Neurol* 2000;247:41–7.

27 Yan-fang S, Yu-ping W. Sleep-disordered breathing: impact on functional outcome of ischemic stroke patients. *Sleep Med* 2009;10:717–9.

28 Jonas DE, et al. Screening for obstructive sleep apnea in adults: Evidence report and systematic review for the US Preventive Services Task Force. *JAMA* 2017;317:415–33.

29 Brown DL, et al. Brainstem infarction and sleep-disordered breathing in the BASIC sleep apnea study. *Sleep Med* 2014;15:887–91.

30 Manconi M, et al. Longitudinal polysomnographic assessment from acute to subacute phase in infratentorial versus supratentorial stroke. *Cerebrovasc Dis* 2014;37:85–93.

31 Ciccone A, et al. Wake-up stroke and TIA due to paradoxical embolism during long obstructive sleep apnoeas: a cross-sectional study. *Thorax* 2013;68:97–104.

32 Hermann DM, et al. Central periodic breathing during sleep in acute ischemic stroke. *Stroke* 2007;38:1082–4.

33 Iranzo A, et al. Prevalence and clinical importance of sleep apnea in the first night after cerebral infarction. *Neurology* 2002;58:911–6.

34 Siccoli MM, Valko PO, Hermann DM, Bassetti CL. Central periodic breathing during sleep in 74 patients with acute ischemic stroke - neurogenic and cardiogenic factors. *J Neurol* 2008;255:1687–92.

35 Nopmaneejumruslers C, et al. Cheyne-Stokes respiration in stroke: relationship to hypocapnia and occult cardiac dysfunction. *Am J Respir Crit Care Med* 2005;171:1048–52.

36 Yumino D, et al. Nocturnal rostral fluid shift: a unifying concept for the pathogenesis of obstructive and central sleep apnea in men with heart failure. *Circulation* 2010;121:1598–1605.

37 McArdle N, et al. Sleep-disordered breathing as a risk factor for cerebrovascular disease: a case-control study in patients with transient ischemic attacks. *Stroke* 2003;34:2916–21.

38 Harbison J, Ford GA, James OFW, Gibson GJ. Sleep-disordered breathing following acute stroke. *QJM Mon J Assoc Physicians* 2002;95: 741–7.

39 Somers VK, et al. Sleep apnea and cardiovascular disease: an American Heart Association/American College Of Cardiology Foundation Scientific Statement from the American Heart Association Council for High Blood Pressure Research Professional Education Committee, Council on Clinical Cardiology, Stroke Council, and Council On Cardiovascular Nursing. In collaboration with the National Heart, Lung, and Blood Institute National Center on Sleep Disorders Research (National Institutes of Health). *Circulation* 208;118:1080–11.

40 Chang C-C, et al. High incidence of stroke in young women with sleep apnea syndrome. *Sleep Med* 2014;15:410–4.

41 Marin JM, Carrizo SJ, Vicente E, Agusti AGN. Long-term cardiovascular outcomes in men with obstructive sleep apnoea-hypopnoea with or without treatment with continuous positive airway pressure: an observational study. *Lancet* 2005;365:1046–53.

42 Redline S, et al. Obstructive sleep apnea-hypopnea and incident stroke: the sleep heart health study. *Am J Respir Crit Care Med* 2010;182: 269–77.

43 Arzt M, et al. Association of sleep-disordered breathing and the occurrence of stroke. *Am J Respir Crit Care Med* 2005;172: 1447–51.

44 Munoz R, et al. Severe sleep apnea and risk of ischemic stroke in the elderly. *Stroke* 2006;37:2317–21.

45 Loke YK, et al. Association of obstructive sleep apnea with risk of serious cardiovascular events: a systematic review and meta-analysis. *Circ Cardiovasc Qual Outcomes* 2012;5:720–8.

46 Shamsuzzaman ASM, Gersh BJ, Somers VK. Obstructive sleep apnea: implications for cardiac and vascular disease. *JAMA* 2003;290:1906–14.

47 Kaneko Y, et al. Relationship of sleep apnea to functional capacity and length of hospitalization following stroke. *Sleep* 2003;26:293–97.

48 Turkington PM, et al. Effect of upper airway obstruction in acute stroke on functional outcome at 6 months. *Thorax* 2004;59:367–71.

49 Dziewas R, et al. Atherosclerosis and obstructive sleep apnea in patients with ischemic stroke. *Cerebrovasc Dis* 2007;24:122–6.

50 Cherkassky T, Oksenberg A, Froom P, Ring H. Sleep-related breathing disorders and rehabilitation outcome of stroke patients: a prospective study. *Am J Phys Med Rehabil* 2003;82:452–5.

51 Birkbak J, Clark AJ, Rod NH. The effect of sleep disordered breathing on the outcome of stroke and transient ischemic attack: a systematic review. *J Clin Sleep Med* 2014;10:103–8.

52 Winward C, Sackley C, Metha Z, Rothwell PM. A population-based study of the prevalence of fatigue after transient ischemic attack and minor stroke. *Stroke* 2009;40:757–61.

53 Bassetti, et al. Hypersomnia following paramedian thalamic stroke: a report of 12 patients. *Ann Neurol* 1996;39:471–80.

54 Catsman-Berrevoets CE, von Harskamp F. Compulsive pre-sleep behavior and apathy due to bilateral thalamic stroke: response to bromocriptine. *Neurology* 1988;38:647–9.

55 Hermann DM, et al. Evolution of neurological, neuropsychological and sleep-wake disturbances after paramedian thalamic stroke. *Stroke* 2008;39:62–8.

56 Drake ME. Kleine–Levin syndrome after multiple cerebral infarctions. *Psychosomatics* 1987;28:329–30.

57 Rivera VM, et al. Narcolepsy following cerebral hypoxic ischemia. *Ann Neurol* 1986;19:505–8.

58 Scammell TE, Nishino S, Mignot E, Saper CB. Narcolepsy and low CSF orexin (hypocretin) concentration after a diencephalic stroke. *Neurology* 2001;56:1751–3.

59 Glader E-L, Stegmayr B, Asplund K. Poststroke fatigue: a 2-year follow-up study of stroke patients in Sweden. *Stroke* 2002;33:1327–33.

60 Autret A, et al. Sleep and brain lesions: a critical review of the literature and additional new cases. *Neurophysiol Clin Clin Neurophysiol* 2001;31:356–75.

61 Gao B, et al. Sleep disruption aggravates focal cerebral ischemia in the rat. *Sleep* 2010;33:879–87.

62 Zunzunegui C, et al. Sleep disturbance impairs stroke recovery in the rat. *Sleep* 2011;34:1261–9.

63 Cam E, et al. Sleep deprivation before stroke is neuroprotective: a pre-ischemic conditioning related to sleep rebound. *Exp Neurol* 2013;247:673–9.

64 Moldovan M, et al. Sleep deprivation attenuates experimental stroke severity in rats. *Exp. Neurol.* 222, 135–143 (2010).bBravata, D. M. *et al.* Auto-titrating continuous positive airway pressure for patients with acute transient ischemic attack: a randomized feasibility trial. *Stroke* 2010;41:1464–70.

65 Pace M, Adamantidis A, Facchin L, Bassetti C. Role of REM sleep, melanin concentrating hormone and orexin/hypocretin systems in the sleep deprivation pre-ischemia. *PloS ONE* 2017;12:e0168430.

66 Gao B, et al. Gamma-hydroxybutyrate accelerates functional recovery after focal cerebral ischemia. *Cerebrovasc. Dis.* 26, 413–419 (2008).bBrown, D. L. *et al.* Sleep apnea treatment after stroke (SATS) trial: is it feasible? *J Stroke Cerebrovasc Dis Off J Natl Stroke Assoc* 2013;22:1216–24.

67 Hodor A, et al. Baclofen facilitates sleep, neuroplasticity, and recovery after stroke in rats. *Ann Clin Transl Neurol* 2014;1:765–77.

68 Sarasso S, et al. Plastic changes following imitation-based speech and language therapy for aphasia: a high-density sleep EEG study. *Neurorehabil Neural Repair* 2014;28:129–38.

69 Duss SB, et al. The role of sleep in recovery following ischemic stroke: A review of human and animal data. *Neurobiol Sleep Circadian Rhythms* 2017;2:94–105.

70 Mallon L, Broman J-E, Hetta J. Restless legs symptoms with sleepiness in relation to mortality: 20-year follow-up study of a middle-aged Swedish population. *Psychiatry Clin Neurosci* 2008;62:457–63.

71 Wessendorf TE, et al. Treatment of obstructive sleep apnoea with nasal continuous positive airway pressure in stroke. *Eur Respir J* 2001;18:623–9.

72 Martínez-García MA, et al. Continuous positive airway pressure treatment in sleep apnea prevents new vascular events after ischemic stroke. *Chest* 2005;128:2123–9.

73 Kernan WN, et al. Guidelines for the prevention of stroke in patients with stroke and transient ischemic attack: a guideline for healthcare professionals from the American Heart Association/American Stroke Association. *Stroke* 2014;45:2160–236.

74 McEvoy RD, et al. CPAP for prevention of cardiovascular events in obstructive sleep apnea. *N Engl J Med* 2016;375:919–31.

75 Peker Y, et al. Effect of positive airway pressure on cardiovascular outcomes in coronary artery disease patients with nonsleepy obstructive sleep apnea. The RICCADSA randomized controlled trial. *Am J Respir Crit Care Med* 2016;194: 613–20.

76 Barbé F, et al. Effect of continuous positive airway pressure on the incidence of hypertension and cardiovascular events in nonsleepy patients with obstructive sleep apnea: a randomized controlled trial. *JAMA* 2012;307:2161–8.

77 Javaheri S, et al. Sleep apnea: Types, mechanisms, and clinical cardiovascular consequences. *J Am Coll Cardiol* 2017;69:841–58.

78 Palombini L, Guilleminault C. Stroke and treatment with nasal CPAP. *Eur J Neurol* 2006;13:198–200.

79 Scala R, et al. Acceptance, effectiveness and safety of continuous positive airway pressure in acute stroke: a pilot study. *Respir Med* 2009;103:59–66.

80 Brill A-K, et al. Adaptive servo-ventilation as treatment of persistent central sleep apnea in post-acute ischemic stroke patients. *Sleep Med* 2014;15:1309–13.

81 Scheidtmann K, Fries W, Müller F, Koenig E. Effect of levodopa in combination with physiotherapy on functional motor recovery after stroke: a prospective, randomised, double-blind study. *Lancet* 2001;358:787–90.

82 Grade C, et al. Methylphenidate in early poststroke recovery: a double-blind, placebo-controlled study. *Arch Phys Med Rehabil* 1998;79:1047–50.

83 Lazar RM, et al. Reemergence of stroke deficits with midazolam challenge. *Stroke* 2002;33:283–5.

84 Palomäki H, et al. Complaints of poststroke insomnia and its treatment with mianserin. *Cerebrovasc Dis* 2003;15:56–62.

22

Sleep Disorders in Multiple Sclerosis and Related Conditions

Jeroen J.J. van Eijk[1], Thom P.J. Timmerhuis[1], Brigit A. de Jong[2] and Paul Reading[3]

[1] Department of Neurology, Jeroen Bosch Hospital, Den Bosch, The Netherlands
[2] Department of Neurology, VU University Medical Center, Amsterdam, The Netherlands
[3] Department of Neurology, James Cook University Hospital, Middlesbrough, UK

Introduction

Over the last decade there has been an explosion of new treatment options for multiple sclerosis (MS), the commonest cause of nontraumatic neurodisability in younger populations. The vast majority of new drugs are powerful immunomodulatory agents that have striking effects on limiting inflammatory relapses in active disease in the expectation of reducing long-term disability. Despite these therapeutic advances, symptom control in many patients, particularly those with progressive disease, remains unsatisfactory. Only recently has there been particular attention turned to the sleep–wake cycle in MS. It is increasingly appreciated that specific and treatable sleep disorders are common in this population, probably affecting around 50% [1,2], with profound adverse effects on quality of life. Given the nature of MS, its range of physical symptoms, together with the commonly used drug treatments and associated psychological stress, it should come as no surprise that the sleep–wake cycle is rarely spared.

Several reviews have highlighted how sleep issues have been overlooked or overshadowed by more obvious physical symptoms and how sleep problems often correlate well with a poorer prognosis [3]. Moreover, the symptoms of fatigue, almost universally reported in over 90% of severely and mildly affected individuals alike, may actually reflect an abnormal sleep–wake cycle rather than an inevitable and often untreatable aspect of this significant neuro-immune disorder [4].

Fatigue Versus Sleepiness

Elsewhere in this book, the distinctions between fatigue, a self-reported lack of physical and/or mental 'energy' that adversely impacts on daily functioning, and excessive daytime sleepiness (EDS) have been emphasised. However, in the MS population, this

Sleep Disorders in Neurology: A Practical Approach, Second Edition.
Edited by Sebastiaan Overeem and Paul Reading.
© 2018 John Wiley & Sons Ltd. Published 2018 by John Wiley & Sons Ltd.

issue is particularly important, given the high prevalence of sleep and mental health disorders that may masquerade as simple fatigue but have distinct treatment options. Fatigue is clearly difficult to assess quantitatively although specific scales have been developed. The MFIS (Modified Fatigue Impact Scale) is an extended questionnaire developed from the Fatigue Severity Score (FSS) which may have utility in monitoring MS-related fatigue [5]. Of interest, such fatigue scales have better correlations with the prevalence of sleep disorders in MS populations than specific 'sleepiness' measures such as the Epworth score, underscoring the intimate relation between the two phenomena [6]. Anecdotally, a useful question to separate the two might be: 'Would you normally want to sit in a large comfortable armchair when relaxing in the afternoon?' Fatigued patients will often readily choose this option whereas sleepy subjects will want to avoid sitting down through fear of actually falling asleep.

In conclusion, put simply, if a patient is fatigued, specific attention should be directed to identifying a specific problem with the sleep–wake cycle as well as exploring the possibility of significant mood disorder. The bidirectional interactions of sleep problems with many factors such as fatigue, pain and low mood cannot be over-emphasised.

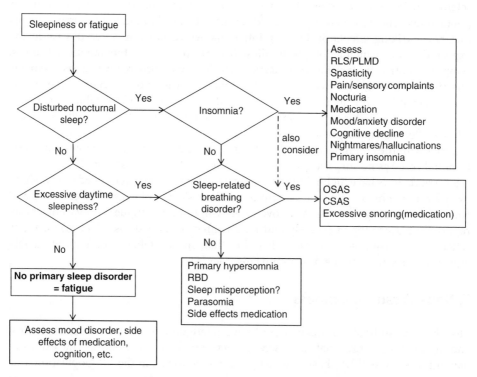

Figure 22.1 A practical stepwise approach to assess sleep disturbances and fatigue in MS.

Clinical Assessment

A practical approach to assess sleep disturbances and fatigue in MS is provided in a stepwise scheme (Figure 22.1). Acknowledging the difficulties sometimes encountered in differentiating fatigue and excessive sleepiness, sleep quality and potential side effects of medication should be evaluated in all subjects and active screening undertaken for the presence of common disorders. If no sleep disorders or significant pharmacological influences are present, fatigue should be treated symptomatically. Often this centres on occupational therapy or improving coping mechanisms by psychological and mindfulness techniques rather than pharmacological interventions.

Specific Sleep Disorders in MS and Management Options

Insomnia

It is not surprising that the majority of patients with significant MS sleep badly given the high prevalence of potential sleep 'toxins' such as nocturia, nocturnal pain, and mental health problems including anxiety or depression. However, a sizeable proportion will also have a primary disorder such as psychophysiological insomnia that may respond to specific treatments, notably cognitive behaviour therapy [7] or potentially (short-acting) hypnotic agents. If pain or spasticity are thought to be contributing to poor sleep, agents such as pregabalin or baclofen sometimes given before bed as surrogate hypnotics may be more acceptable for long-term use than traditional sleep-inducing agents. Identifying primary insomnia necessitates excluding other (co-morbid) causes and may be helped by questionnaires such as the Insomnia Severity Index which can also evaluate treatment effects [8]. Using such scales, a prevalence of over 30% of chronic insomnia disorder has been reported in MS populations [9].

Symptomatic drug treatments for MS, whether over-the-counter preparations or prescribed psycho-active agents, are also commonly overlooked as major factors in promoting poor sleep. Selective serotonin reuptake inhibitors may interfere greatly with sleep quality in a minority of patients [10] and most classes of antidepressants have the potential to worsen restless legs syndrome (RLS) as might antihistamines [11]. Disease-modifying drugs such as interferons are generally associated with insomnia although sedation can also be seen, potentially via a cytokine mechanism. Either way, moving treatment schedules from evening to morning may be beneficial in some [12]. The monoclonal antibody treatments also frequently have adverse but poorly characterised effects on the sleep–wake cycle.

Sleep-related Breathing Disorders

Obstructive sleep apnoea (OSA) and central sleep apnoea (CSA) are clearly both encountered in MS and are frequently worthy of treatment. Depending on the criteria and methodology used, the prevalence of OSA in MS differs from 12 to 70%, with some studies suggesting a higher prevalence compared with control populations [13–15]. Of interest, those MS patients taking disease-modifying therapies were reportedly less prone to OSA, suggesting to some a possible role for inflammatory factors in the genesis of OSA [14]. As a group, however, MS patients seem to have higher Apnoea–Hypopnea Indices (AHIs) and are more symptomatic compared with control subjects with OSA. Positive correlations have also been made between OSA severity and reduced MS quality of life measures as well as impaired cognition [16,17]. A relation between the level of MS plaque lesion load and OSA has been proposed but is debated [14]. Patients with progressive MS generally display worse OSA although this may reflect many confounding factors such as medication (antispasmodic drugs, analgesics, narcotics), increased age and obesity.

Not surprisingly, CSA is seen more commonly in those with prominent brainstem and cervical cord disease involvement with or without concomitant respiratory depressants such as opioids [14].

The usual screening tools, diagnostic strategies and treatment options for OSA subjects in the general population should equally apply to MS patients. Lifestyle changes, weight loss, dental appliances, positional therapy or continuous positive airway pressure therapy are all appropriate although may be tolerated less well in disabled patients. Treating OSA in MS populations is generally rewarding [18]. Regarding CSA, if drug causes, particularly opiates, have been eliminated, it may be difficult to manage effectively and sophisticated masks with so-called 'adaptive servo-ventilation' may be appropriate or even diaphragmatic pacing [19].

Sleep-related Movement Disorders

A number of studies have shown that RLS is approximately four times more prevalent in MS populations when compared with controls [20,21]. In MS patients, despite validated rating scales, RLS can be difficult to distinguish from spasticity, pain or pure sensory complaints that might be largely positional in nature. Examination findings such as spasticity and the timing of symptoms can be helpful in this respect. In particular, painful stiffness due to spasticity is often worsened by movement and commonly more noticeable in the morning in contrast to RLS. Pain and sensory discomfort is also generally exacerbated by movement when secondary to myelopathy ('claudication medullae'). However, given it is also likely that spinal cord pathology accounts for the higher prevalence of RLS in MS, coexistent significant lower limb spasticity and RLS is common. In support of this, cord lesion load has been shown to correlate with RLS severity [22]. There is no evidence that MS patients with RLS are more prone to iron depletion as an explanation for the higher prevalence [20] although serum ferritin levels should be checked.

Despite any specific evidence regarding the treatment of RLS associated with MS, most would suggest that symptomatic therapy should mirror that of the idiopathic syndrome with dopamine agonists or intermittent opioids as the mainstay in moderate or severe cases (see Chapter 13). Nocturnal discomfort with or without likely RLS may also respond well to neuropathic agents, particularly pregabalin. If RLS is present, tricyclics before bed such as amitriptyline are best avoided through fear of worsening leg movements during sleep. Severe spasticity, when coexistent, also merits medical or physiotherapeutic treatment.

As in the general population, it remains controversial whether periodic limb movements (PLMs) during sleep in the absence of RLS are important or worthy of treatment in MS. However, at least 23% of MS patients referred for polysomnography display significant PLMs [23] and treatment would seem appropriate if significant daytime fatigue or frank sleepiness is reported, particularly if the limb movements generate micro-arousals or heart rate rises during sleep [24]. A low dose of a benzodiazepine such as clonazepam (0.5 mg) can be helpful in eliminating excessive leg movement if more specific therapies are unsuccessful.

Although rapid eye movement sleep behaviour disorder is most often closely associated with synucleinopathies, rare cases have been reported in MS, presumed secondary to plaques in the dorsolateral pons that interfere with the generation of normal rapid eye movement (REM) sleep atonia [25]. If present and clinically severe, usual treatment strategies (clonazepam or melatonin) should be considered given the risk of injury.

Secondary Narcolepsy in MS and Neuromyelitis Optica

It has been proposed although unproven that narcolepsy (types 1 and 2) is commoner in MS [26,27]. Potentially, this may relate either to demyelinating plaques in the region of the hypothalamus, causing deficits in the hypocretin system, or result through shared auto-immunological risk factors for the two conditions. Severe sleepiness in MS, not due to more common disorders, especially in the presence of prominent REM sleep-related phenomena, should always raise the possibility of narcolepsy and lead to appropriate management.

Neuromyelitis optica (NMO) can present in a similar fashion to MS but is at least 10 times rarer and predominantly affects certain ethnic groups. It has been recognised as a distinct disorder for some time, largely based on clinical and radiological findings. In particular, NMO may have a different auto-immune pathophysiology and involve different parts of the central nervous system to typical cases of MS with lesions predominantly in the spinal cord and optic nerves. Brain involvement, as seen on magnetic resonance imaging, has traditionally thought to be much less marked than in MS although certain areas such as the hypothalamus might be more preferentially affected. Of interest, a specific auto-antibody has now been established as a pathognomonic marker for NMO, anti-aquaporin 4 (anti-AQP4) [28]. Furthermore, AQP4, a water channel protein, is preferentially expressed in hypothalamic and periaqueductal areas [29] in non-neuronal structures such as astrocytes and ependymocytes.

Several cases are described in the literature in which a syndrome resembling either narcolepsy or idiopathic hypersomnolence has occurred acutely in patients with NMO with corresponding lesions in the hypothalamus and very low cerebrospinal fluid hypocretin levels [30,31]. Interestingly, these cases are often associated with bilateral symmetric hypothalamic lesions. Furthermore, both the EDS and hypocretin deficiency have been seen to resolve after adequate therapeutic interventions.

Key Points

- Sleep-related symptoms are almost certainly very common in conditions such as MS although remain poorly characterised and overlooked.
- Insomnia is probably the commonest consequence and is usually secondary to physical symptoms such as pain, spasms and nocturia.
- RLS may be much commoner in MS populations, especially in those with myelopathy. It is likely to respond to standard RLS treatment strategies although specific evidence is lacking.
- In demyelinating conditions such as MS, fatigue is extremely prevalent. Distinguishing fatigue from excessive somnolence may be particularly difficult.
- Sleep-disordered breathing may be slightly commoner in MS populations and should be actively sought as a treatable condition.
- A form of secondary narcolepsy has been well described in MS and the related condition NMO almost certainly arising from damage to the hypocretin system. In some cases, this appears reversible with immunomodulation.

References

1 Carnicka Z, Kollar B, Siarnik B, et al. Sleep disorders in patients with multiple sclerosis. *J Clin Sleep Med* 2015;11(5):553–557.

2 Bamer AM, Johnson KL, Amtmann D, Kraft GH. Prevalence of sleep problems in individuals with multiple sclerosis. *Multiple Sclerosis* 2008;14(8):1127–1130.

3 Merlino G, Fratticci L, Lenchig C, et al. Prevalence of 'poor sleep' among patients with multiple sclerosis: an independent predictor of mental and physical status. *Sleep Med* 2009;10:26–34.

4 Krupp L. Fatigue is intrinsic to multiple sclerosis (MS) and is the most commonly reported symptom of the disease. *Multiple Sclerosis* 2006;12:367–368.

5 Kos D, Kerckhofs E, Carrea I, et al. Evaluation of the Modified Fatigue Impact Scale in four different European countries. *Multiple Sclerosis* 2005;11(1):76–80.

6 Braley TJ, Chervin RD, Segal BM. Fatigue, tiredness, lack of energy, and sleepiness in multiple sclerosis patients referred for clinical polysomnography. *Multiple Sclerosis Int* 2012;2012:673936.

7 Baron KG, Corden M, Jin L, Mohr DC. Impact of psychotherapy on insomnia patients with depression and multiple sclerosis. *J Behav Med* 2011;34:92–101.

8 Morin CM, Belleville G, Belanger L, Ivers H. The Insomnia Severity Index: psychometric indicators to detect insomnia cases and evaluate treatment response. *Sleep* 2011;34:601–608.

9 Brass SD, Li CS, Auerbach S. The underdiagnosis of sleep disorders in patients with multiple sclerosis. *J Clin Sleep Med* 2014;10:1025–1031.

10 Byerley WF, Reimherr FW, Wood DR, Grosser BI. Fluoxetine, a selective serotonin uptake inhibitor, for the treatment of outpatients with major depression. *J Clin Psychopharmacol* 1988;8:112–115.

11 Bliwise D, Zhang R, Kutner N. Medications associated with restless legs syndrome: a case-control study in the US Renal Data System (USRDS). *Sleep Med* 2014; 15:1241–1245.

12 Nadjar Y, Coutelas E, Prouteau P, et al. Injection of interferon-beta in the morning decresses flu-like syndrome in many patients with multiple sclerosis. *Clin Neurol Neurosurg* 2011; 113:316–322.

13 Kaminska M, Kimoff RJ, Benedetti A, et al. Obstructive sleep apnea is associated with fatigue in multiple sclerosis. *Multiple Sclerosis* 2012;18(8):1159–1169.

14 Braley TJ, Segal BM, Chervin RD. Sleep-disordered breathing in multiple sclerosis. *Neurology* 2012;79(9):929–936.

15 Tachibana N, Howard RS, Hirsch NP, et al. Sleep problems in multiple sclerosis. *Eur Neurol* 1994;34(6):320–323.

16 Trojan D, Kaminska M, Bar-Or A, et al. Polysomnographic measures of disturbed sleep are associated with reduced quality of life in multiple sclerosis. *J Neurol Sci* 2012;316:158–163.

17 Braley TJ, Kratz AL, Kaplish N, Chervin RD. Sleep and cognitive function in multiple sclerosis. *Sleep* 2016;39(8):1525–1533.

18 Cote I, Trojan D, Kaminska M, et al. Impact of sleep disorder treatment on fatigue in multiple sclerosis. *Multiple Sclerosis* 2013;19:480–489.

19 Eckhart D, Jordan A, Merchia P, Malhotra A. Central sleep apnea: pathophysiology and treatment. *Chest* 2007;131:595–607.

20 Italian RSG, Manconi M, Ferini-Strambi L, et al. Multicenter case-control study on restless legs syndrome in multiple sclerosis: the REMS study. *Sleep* 2008;31(7):944–952.

21 Manconi M, Fabbrini M, Bonanni E, et al. High prevalence of restless legs syndrome in multiple sclerosis. *Eur J Neurol* 2007;14:534–539.

22 Manconi M, Rocca M, Ferini-Strambi L, et al. Restless legs syndrome is a common finding in multiple scelrosis and correlates with cervical cord damage. *Multiple Sclerosis* 2008;14:86–93.

23 Veuthier C, Radbruch H, Gaede G, et al. Fatigue in multiple sclerosis is closely related to sleep disorders: a polysomnographic cross-sectional study. *Multiple Sclerosis* 2011;17(5):613–622.

24 Montplaisir J, Boucher S, Poirier G, et al. Clinical, polysomnographic, and genetic characteristics of restless legs syndrome: a study of 133 patients diagnosed with new standard criteria. *Mov Disord* 1997;12;61–65.

25 Plazzi G, Montagna P. Remitting REM sleep behavior disorder as the initial sign of multiple sclerosis. *Sleep Med* 2002;3:437–439.

26 Poirier G, Montplaisir J, Dumont M, et al. Clinical and sleep laboratory study of narcoleptic symptoms in multiple sclerosis. *Neurology* 1987;37(4):693–695.

27 Nishino S, Kanbayashi T. Symptomatic narcolepsy, cataplexy and hypersomnia, and their implications in the hypothalamic hypocretin/orexin system. *Sleep Med Rev* 2005;9(4):269–310.

28 Roemer SF, Parisi JE, Lennon VA, et al. Pattern-specific loss of aquaporin-4 immunoreactivity distinguishes neuromyelitis optica from multiple sclerosis. *Brain* 2007;130(Pt 5):1194–1205.

29 Pittock SJ, Weinshenker BG, Luchinetti CF, et al. Neuromyelitis optica brain lesions localized at sites of high aquaporin 4 expression. *Arch Neurol* 2006;63(7):964–968.

30 Nozaki H, Shimohata T, Kanbayashi T, et al. A patient with anti-aquaporin 4 antibody who presented with recurrent hypersomnia, reduced orexin (hypocretin) level, and symmetrical hypothalamic lesions. *Sleep Med* 2008;10(2):253–255.

31 Carlander B, Vincent T, Le Floch A, et al. Hypocretinergic dysfunction in neuromyelitis optica with coma-like episodes. *J Neurol Neurosurg Psychiatry* 2008;79(3):333–334.

23

Tumours and Paraneoplastic Syndromes

Alex Iranzo[1-3] *and Francesc Graus*[1,2]

[1] *Neurology Service, Hospital Clínic de Barcelona, Barcelona, Spain*
[2] *Institut d'Investigació Biomèdiques August Pi i Sunyer (IDIBAPS), Barcelona, Spain*
[3] *Centro de Investigación Biomédica en Red sobre Enfermedades Neurodegenerativas (CIBERNED), Barcelona, Spain*

Sleep in Patients with Systemic Tumours

Even though they do not directly involve the central nervous system, systemic neoplasms are frequently associated with sleep disturbances. A wide range of symptoms are reported including insomnia, excessive daytime sleepiness (EDS), fatigue, and general disruption of the sleep–wake cycle. Insomnia is particularly common in subjects both with a recent diagnosis of cancer, most likely secondary to anxiety and depression, and in those with advanced disease. Fatigue is particularly associated with chemotherapy but may occur at any stage of the disease [1,2].

As with any severe chronic illness, disturbed or non-restorative sleep in cancer worsens the quality of life in patients, interfering with activities of daily living and ability to face the disease. However, patients with cancer often fail to spontaneously report their sleep disturbances to their oncologists, usually because they feel they are intrinsic problems and therefore unlikely to be easily solved. Compounding the issue, physicians rarely ask specifically about sleep, potentially allowing sleep disturbances to go unrecognised and untreated in oncology patients.

Studies Evaluating Sleep in Patients with Cancer

Over the last 20 years, several studies have assessed the quality of sleep in patients with cancer and its consequence on the quality of life. The majority of published studies are descriptive, evaluating sleep with scales and questionnaires rather than formal polysomnography. Overall, studies have shown that sleep quality is frequently poor among both newly diagnosed and advanced cancer patients. Commonly identified factors include poor health-related quality of life, anxiety, depression, pain, nausea and vomiting, difficulty in turning in bed and the effect of powerful medications including chemotherapy and opioids for pain relief. However, during the course of the disease, patients may develop specific or

Sleep Disorders in Neurology: A Practical Approach, Second Edition.
Edited by Sebastiaan Overeem and Paul Reading.
© 2018 John Wiley & Sons Ltd. Published 2018 by John Wiley & Sons Ltd.

primary sleep disorders such as obstructive sleep apnoea due to upper airway obstruction, especially in head and neck cancers, or restless legs syndrome secondary to iron deficiency anaemia in gastrointestinal carcinomas, for example.

A cross-sectional survey in 982 patients examined the prevalence and characteristics of reported sleep problems in patients attending six clinics at a regional cancer centre. Patients attending clinics for breast, gastrointestinal, genitourinary, gynaecologic, lung, and non-melanoma skin cancers were offered a brief sleep questionnaire. The most prevalent sleep-related problems were excessive fatigue (44%), leg restlessness (41%), insomnia (31%), and EDS (28%). The lung cancer clinic had the highest or second-highest prevalence of all problems. The breast clinic also had a high prevalence of insomnia and fatigue. Recent cancer treatment with chemotherapy was associated with excessive fatigue and frank hypersomnolence. When reported, insomnia most commonly involved multiple awakenings and, in 48% of cases, its onset was reported to occur around the time of cancer diagnosis. The most frequently identified contributors to insomnia were ruminations, medical concerns, and pain or discomfort. Insomnia was positively associated with fatigue, increasing age, restless legs, sedative or hypnotic use, low or variable mood, vivid dreams, and recent cancer surgery [3].

A new diagnosis of lung cancer is associated with marked sleep disturbances, combining insomnia and EDS. Similar findings are observed in patients with advanced cancer receiving elective and palliative treatment. Indeed, one study in 82 advanced cancer patients referred to a palliative care unit for control of pain and other symptoms showed that 96% of patients were poor sleepers, as defined by the Pittsburgh Sleep Quality Index. Positive correlations were found between the Pittsburgh Sleep Quality Index and scales of quality of life, depression and hopelessness. Post-traumatic experiences and quality of life were the strongest predictors of sleep quality. Perhaps not surprisingly, desire for death was associated with poor sleep quality, depression and hopelessness [4].

In another study, a consecutive sample of 123 oncology patients admitted to a pain relief and palliative care unit were studied. Thirty per cent reported sleeping less than 5 hours per night with men more affected than women. Anxiety, sleep onset insomnia, frequent awakening, early awakening and nightmares were significantly associated with the reduced sleep time. No differences, however, were found for age, primary tumour, level of information, Karnofsky status, depression, and use of opioids or hypnotics. Patients admitted for pain control and those receiving opioids more frequently had drowsiness. Anxiety created particular difficulties in falling asleep and having less restorative sleep with nightmares. Depression was associated with early awakening, poorly restorative sleep, fatigue and nightmares. The authors concluded that sleep problems are a significant issue for advanced cancer patients and that more attention should be paid to them. Indeed, detailed sleep evaluation should become routine practice in palliative care evaluation [5].

Recent further epidemiological studies of cancer patients have shown that the high prevalence of insomnia at baseline (59%) generally declines over time but remains pervasive even at the end of an 18-month period (36%). Furthermore, the effects of radiotherapy and chemotherapy frequently aggravate insomnia symptoms [6,7].

Few studies have evaluated detailed sleep architecture in patients with systemic cancer. Polysomnography in patients with lung cancer have confirmed long sleep onset latency, low sleep efficiency and high wake time after sleep onset (WASO) when compared with controls. In one study, 114 patients with advanced solid tumours underwent ambulatory polysomnography for 42 hours in their home. Patients had reduced quantity and quality of nocturnal sleep with episodes of sleep scattered throughout the day. Increased daytime sleep was negatively associated with several parameters of nocturnal sleep quantity and quality [8].

Treatment of Sleep Disturbances in Patients with Systemic Cancer

Treatment should always be individualised although advice on sleep hygiene in an attempt to restore an abnormal sleep–wake cycle is mandatory. Maintenance of physical activity with additional psychotherapy is also often recommended. The use of sedating antidepressants such as mirtazapine, trazodone or agomelatine may improve sleep quality as may serotonin selective reuptake inhibitors in patients with depression, although response is often unpredictable. Short-acting benzodiazepines such as lorazepam are often used to improve sleep onset insomnia when anxiety appears prominent. Long-acting opioids such as morphine and transdermal fentanyl might be expected to improve nocturnal pain. Fatigue and sleepiness can be treated empirically with psychostimulants in the absence of a controlled evidence base.

The Influence of Sleep Disorders in Patients with Systemic Cancer

Available epidemiological and experimental data have led to the speculation that the intermittent hypoxia with sleep fragmentation that occurs in obstructive sleep apnoea may adversely affect cancer development and progression [9]. In particular, malignant cell transformation (tumorigenesis), tumour proliferation and even metastatic invasion (tumour progression) may be enhanced [10]. An epidemiological link between circadian rhythmic disruption (shift work) and sleep duration with cancer has also been postulated but no strong data are available.

Sleep in Patients with Brain Tumors

Specific symptoms of patients with neoplasms of the central nervous system will clearly depend on the structures involved. However, other than the direct effects of any space-occupying tumour, surrounding oedema or secondary damage after treatment with surgery or radiotherapy may be equally important factors. Sleep disturbances, particularly EDS, are very frequent in those with brain tumours although the full spectrum of sleep disorders may be seen. The posterior hypothalamus and rostral brainstem are the two most common locations where tumours are particularly associated with severe sleep disorders.

Symptomatic Narcolepsy

EDS combined with other narcoleptic features occurs as a secondary phenomenon in the setting of several neurological conditions [10–21]. So-called 'secondary' or 'symptomatic' narcolepsy is associated with intracranial space-occupying lesions (e.g. tumours, histocytosis, sarcoidosis), neurodegenerative diseases (e.g. Parkinson's disease, myotonic dystrophy) and head trauma [10–16]. Brain tumours are one of the most frequent causes of symptomatic narcolepsy occurring in 29% of reported cases [15]. However, it remains a very rare situation with no more than 50 cases reported in the medical literature. Not surprisingly, tumours causing symptomatic narcolepsy are most frequently seen in the hypothalamus or its adjacent structures including the pituitary gland, suprasellar region, third ventricle and pineal gland. These patients represent 70% of tumour-related narcolepsy cases and frequently have other symptoms related to hypothalamic damage such as obesity, diabetes insipidus, and panhypopituitarism. However, other sites of damage proposed to cause symptomatic narcolepsy include the upper brainstem (9%), multiple brain areas (9%), cerebellum (6%), temporal lobe (3%) and the frontal lobes (3%). The tumour type is very variable with all the following associated: craniopharyngioma, angioma, hemangioblastoma, astrocytoma, glioblastoma, adenoma, ganglioma, choroid plexus carcinoma, primary central nervous system lymphoma, pineal tumor, medulloblastoma, subependymoma and germinoma. Craniopharyngioma, a congenital suprasellar epidermoid cyst that originates from remnants of Rathke's pouch seen more frequently in children, is the most common tumour causing narcoleptic features. Some tumours causing secondary narcolepsy are predominantly in children (e.g. craniopharyngioma, medulloblastoma) while others mainly affect adults (e.g. glioblastoma, lymphoma).

Development of narcolepsy-cataplexy with normal cerebrospinal fluid (CSF) hypocretin-1 levels may occur as a result of significant ischaemic damage to the hypothalamus after resection of a brain tumour in this area [19]. Narcolepsy without cataplexy has been described after removal of a hypothalamic astrocytoma although reduced CSF hypocretin-1 levels were seen [20]. Cranial radiotherapy for a pituitary adenoma has also been implicated in narcolepsy-cataplexy, several weeks after treatment [16].

Although all have EDS to varying degrees, the precise phenotype of tumour-related narcolepsy is often different to idiopathic cases. Sleep paralysis and hypnologic hallucinations may occur in some patients with brain tumours located in the brainstem and hypothalamus [12]. Cataplexy is absent in 45%, the association with HLA DR2 and DQB1*0602 is not high (around 50%), sudden onset rapid eye movement (REM) sleep may not be demonstrated in the Multiple Sleep Latency Test (MSLT), and low levels of hypocretin-1 may not be detected in the CSF [15]. Measurement of hypocretin-1 in the CSF has been evaluated only in a few subjects with brain tumors and symptomatic narcolepsy [15,18,22]. Levels were found to be undetectable, low (<110 pg/ml), intermediate (110–200 pg/ml) or normal (>200 pg/ml). In subjects with reduced hypocretin-1 level in the CSF, severe damage either in the hypocretin-producing neurons in the posterior hypothalamus or in the hypocretin projections are thought to occur. Interestingly, it has been reported that effective treatment of a brain tumour was associated with normalisation of the CSF hypocretin-1 level in a patient with previous undetectable value [18].

The pathophysiology of narcoleptic features in patients with normal CSF hypocretin-1 level remains speculative and it is often not known whether damage to brain areas containing high levels of hypocretin receptors or another neurotransmitter system is largely responsible.

Hypersomnolence associated with brain tumors may respond to central nervous system stimulants [11]. In some cases, effective treatment of the tumour itself may result in improvement of the narcoleptic features in conjunction with other neurological symptoms such as visual field defects. In such cases normalisation of hypocretin-1 levels in the CSF may be seen [18]. In contrast, disabling hypersomnolence in children often persists after effective brain tumour removal [16].

Excessive Daytime Sleepiness Without Narcoleptic Features

Some patients with brain tumours develop subacute EDS lacking cataplexy and with normal levels of hypocretin-1 in the CSF. In these cases, HLA DR2 and DQB1*0602 are usually negative and tumours are located in non-hypothalamic structures involved in sleep–wake cycle regulation such as the thalamus [15]. However, subtle disruption of the hypocretin system may still be responsible in such cases in the absence of grossly altered levels of hypocretin-1 measured in the CSF.

In some tumours involving the hypothalamus, weight gain may lead to obstructive sleep apnoea and associated hypersomnolence. Transient or permanent EDS can occur after several weeks of cranial radiation in patients with brain tumours [16].

Isolated Symptomatic Cataplexy

A few adult cases of symptomatic cataplexy not linked to EDS have been reported in the literature. Interestingly, isolated symptomatic cataplexy is not always associated with tumours located in the hypothalamus [15]. A temporal association between cataplexy onset and meningiomas located in the frontal and parietal lobe was reported in five adults aged 50–68 years [23]. A 6-year-old girl with a pontomedullary pylocitic astrocytoma developed isolated cataplexy [24]. An adult with glioblastoma of the hypothalamus and upper brainstem developed continuous cataplectic attacks and sleep paralysis [25].

Rapid Eye Movement Sleep Behaviour Disorder

Rapid eye movement sleep behaviour disorder (RBD) is a parasomnia characterised by dream enactment, unpleasant dreams and lack of muscle atonia during REM sleep. It is thought that RBD is mediated by dysfunction of the brainstem structures in the dorsolateral pontine tegmentum and medial medulla that regulate muscle tone during REM sleep, and their anatomic connections. In humans, RBD is usually linked to neurodegenerative diseases involving this area, particularly the synucleinopathies [26]. Rare cases have been reported with RBD secondary to a focal lesion in the brainstem and/or limbic system, including the amygdala. The nature of these lesions may be inflammatory, vascular or space-occupying [27]. In fewer than 10 published reports, tumours are located in the brainstem or in the pontocerebellar angle [28,29]. A 59-year-old man with a neurinoma of the left pontocerebellar angle developed deafness of the left side over a period of 6 years and RBD symptoms (dream enactment with associated unpleasant dreams) over a period of 5 years. RBD was confirmed by polysomnography and symptoms were successfully treated with clonazepam. RBD symptoms disappeared after the tumour was surgically removed and clonazepam was discontinued allowing the authors to postulate that the tumour interfered with the brainstem circuitry responsible for REM sleep atonia [28]. In one case series, two cerebello-pontine angle meningiomas and one petroclival meningioma causing brainstem mass effect were reported to occur in three adults with RBD. In one case, resection of the meningiomas led to resolution of RBD symptoms. The authors speculated that the parapontine lesions resulted in compression and/or distortion of those dorsolateral pontine structures involved in REM sleep atonia regulation [29]. In another publication, a 30-year-old man with RBD confirmed by polysomnography had a B-cell lymphoma at the pontomes-encephalic junction. Chemotherapy subsequently diminished the dream-enacting behaviour [30].

Sleep in Paraneoplastic Syndromes

Paraneoplastic neurological syndromes (PNS) such as limbic encephalitis and suba-cute cerebellar syndromes are uncommon disorders related to neoplasms outside the nervous system [31]. PNS are not caused by metastases or direct infiltration but reflect immune-mediated phenomena linked to onconeuronal antibodies against neural antigens expressed both by the tumour and the nervous system. Antibodies react with specific proteins expressed in the cytoplasm, nuclei or surface membrane although in most PNS, the direct pathogenic role of the antibodies is debatable and hard to prove. Autopsy findings reveal neuronal loss, gliosis and inflammatory infil-trates of cytotoxic T lymphocytes. Interestingly, PNS often precede the diagnosis of the underlying systemic malignancy. PNS are common in patients with lung, ovary, breast, testicular cancer and Hodgkin's disease with a clinical course that is usually subacute and progressive. Symptomatology can be severe and involve any area of the nervous system depending on the brain structures where the relevant antigens are prominently expressed. Involvement of dorsal root ganglia, cerebellum, amygdala, hippocampus, brainstem, hypothalamus and thalamus are the sites most commonly involved in PNS [31].

Sleep disorders in patients with PNS have received attention only recently [32] although prospective and well-designed studies are yet to be published. Small series and case reports have described patients with PNS suffering from a range of sleep disturbances such as EDS, RBD and central respiratory abnormalities. In most of the reported cases, sleep studies were not performed and CSF hypocretin-1 was not measured. Sleep disorders tend not to occur in isolation and often coexist with symptoms of limbic lobe dysfunction, brainstem symptomatology and hypothalamic disturbances. Rarely, however, sleep abnormalities are the first or most severe com-plain among patients with PNS. Hypersomnia has frequently described in patients with anti-Ma2 encephalitis, a PNS affecting diencephalic, limbic and brainstem structures in any combination. Central hypoventilation is sometimes seen either with anti-Hu brainstem encephalitis associated with small cell lung cancer or anti-NMDA receptor encephalitis linked to ovarian teratoma. Morvan's syndrome, most often associated with malignant thymoma, results in profound insomnia as the main sleep-related problem although related limbic encephalitis due to voltage-gated potassium channel complex anti-LGI1 may be associated with insomnia, hypersom-nia and RBD (Table 23.1).

By contrast, sleep problems seem to be uncommon in PNS patients with either sensory neuronopathy due to anti-Hu antibodies against the dorsal root ganglia or subacute cerebellar syndrome associated with anti-Yo antibodies against Purkinje cells.

Table 23.1 Sleep disturbances recognised in paraneoplastic syndromes.

Onconeuronal antibody	Associated cancer	Neurologic syndrome	Sleep disorder
Anti Ma1 and Ma2	Germ cell tumour of the testis	Limbic, brainstem and diencephalic encephalitis	Hypersomnia Cataplexy Rapid eye movemnt sleep behaviour disorder
Anti-NMDA receptor	Ovarian teratoma	Encephalitis	Hypersomnia Insomnia Central hypoventilation
Anti LGI1/Caspr2	Thymoma, adenocarcinomas	Morvan's syndrome Limbic encephalitis	Hypersomnia Insomnia Agrypnia excitata Rapid eye movemnt sleep behaviour disorder
Anti Hu (ANNA-1)	Small cell lung cancer	Encephalomyelitis	Central hypoventilation

However, it should be noted that it is possible the frequency and nature of sleep disorders in the setting of any PNS may have been overlooked due to the low profile of sleep disorders and because it is rare for patients and bed partners to spontaneously report them.

Excessive Daytime Sleepiness

The majority of reported PNS cases with severe EDS had anti-Ma2 antibodies linked to lung and testicular cancers, probably because this PNS commonly affects diencephalic structures (Figure 23.1). In a detailed review of 38 cases with anti-Ma2-associated encephalitis published in 2004, the authors noted that 'EDS affected 32% of the patients, sometimes with narcolepsy-cataplexy and low CSF hypocretin' [33]. Of the 13 patients that developed hypothalamic dysfunction characterised by weight gain, hyperthermia, diabetes insipidus, gelastic seizures, 12 had EDS and two of them presented a frank narcoleptic phenotype characterised by cataplexy and hypnagogic hallucinations. Unfortunately, none of these 12 patients underwent sleep studies and hypocretin was not evaluated in the two patients with cataplexy. One of the patients without cataplexy was 'lethargic and napping more than usual' and CSF hypocretin was undetectable while magnetic resonance imaging (MRI) showed abnormalities in the right thalamus, midbrain and mesial temporal lobe but not in the hypothalamus [34]. This review [33] included six patients with anti-Ma2 encephalitis previously published [35] in whom CSF hypocretin was undetectable in four presenting with EDS and normal in two without EDS. None of these six patients underwent sleep studies and the presence of cataplexy could not be determined because the study was retrospective. HLA haplotypes were not determined. Brain MRI did not detect abnormalities in the hypothalamus. This was the first report indicating that hypocretin deficiency can have a definite autoimmune-mediated aetiology [35]. In another case series

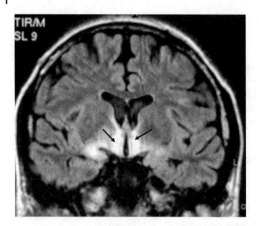

Figure 23.1 Coronal brain MRI showing amygdalar and hypothalamic high signal (see arrows to the hypothalamus) in a FLAIR sequence in a patient with anti-Ma2 encephalitis and testicular germinoma who presented with hypersomnia.

that involved 22 newly diagnosed patients with anti-Ma2 encephalitis, four presented with EDS but sleep studies and hypocretin status were not evaluated [36].

A number of additional case reports have described subjects with EDS and paraneoplastic anti-Ma2 encephalitis. One patient with testicular carcinoma presented with a full-blown limbic encephalitis syndrome with EDS and brief cataplectic episodes triggered by emotions. Nocturnal polysomnography showed reduced sleep efficiency of 44% and a reduced sleep latency onset of 4.5 minutes. A MSLT performed the following day demonstrated a sleep latency of 9 minutes with two episodes of REM sleep onset. HLA DR2 was negative and CSF hypocretin was not measured. MRI revealed bilateral medial temporal lobe damage but no hypothalamic impairment. Cataplexy was controlled with imipramine but EDS did not improve with high doses of modafinil [37]. In another case report, a patient with anti-Ma2 encephalitis presented with subacute onset of severe hypersomnia, memory loss, parkinsonism and gaze palsy. The patient did not experience cataplexy, sleep paralysis or hallucinations. Brain MRI showed bilateral damage in the dorsolateral midbrain, amygdala and paramedian thalami. Video-polysomnography disclosed RBD, a reduced sleep efficiency of 48% and a subsequent MSLT revealed a mean sleep latency of 7 minutes and four sleep-onset REM periods. HLA typing was negative for the DQB1*0602 and DRB1*15 antigens. CSF hypocretin level was pathologically low (49 pg/ml) [21]. A patient with anti-Ma2 encephalitis and lung cancer presented with EDS in the absence of cataplexy or hallucinations but with a low CSF hypocretin level (58 pg/ml). MRI showed prominent high signal intensity in the hypothalamus and hippocampus. However, sleep studies and HLA typing were not done [38]. Hypothalamic damage demonstrated by MRI was documented in another patient with anti-Ma2 encephalitis and breast cancer who presented with severe hypersomnia. Sleep studies, HLA typing and hypocretin measurement were not assessed [39]. Other case reports noted the presence [40,41] or absence of EDS [42–44] in subjects with anti-Ma2-associated encephalitis. A 55-year-old man presented with hypersomnolence, cataplexy, abnormal sleep behaviour, parkinsonism and vertical supranuclear palsy. Polysomnography showed disrupted sleep architecture with RBD and MSLT demonstrated reduced sleep latency and multiple sleep onset REM sleep periods. The patient had positive Ma1 and Ma2 antibodies and a tonsillar squamous cell carcinoma [45]. A 63-year-old man with anti-Ma2 antibodies had diencephalic encephalitis with sleepiness, cataplexy, hypocretin deficiency and RBD demonstrated by polysomnography. Neuropathology demonstrated inflammation induced by cytotoxic CD8+ T lymphocytes and complete loss of hypocretinergic neurons within the hypothalamus [46].

It is difficult to assess which factors cause EDS in patients with anti-Ma2-associated encephalitis due to the small number of published cases and lack of sleep and hypocretin status characterisation (Table 23.2). In some patients, however, detection of low levels of CSF hypocretin indicates that EDS is secondary to deficient hypocretin transmission. Normal appearance of the hypothalamus in MRI probably does not exclude hypocretin dysfunction due to small but critical cell infiltrates and hypocretinergic cell loss [46].

Hypersomnia may be one of the many symptoms occurring in young women with ovarian teratoma and anti-NMDA receptor encephalitis. In one such case, brain MRI showed a suprasellar lesion [47,48]. Inversion of the sleep pattern with insomnia at night and daytime somnolence occurs in 27% of patients with anti-NMDA receptor encephalitis after recovery [48]. Hypersomnia has also been described in subjects with limbic encephalitis associated with voltage-gated potassium channel-complex antibodies against the leucine-rich, glioma inactivated protein (LGI1) that are associated with adenocarcinoma of the colon and prostate, and melanoma [49].

Rapid Eye Movement Sleep Behaviour Disorder

RBD, confirmed by video-polysomnography, was reported in a patient with anti-Ma2 encephalitis who presented with parkinsonism among other symptoms [21]. RBD severity was mild. MRI demonstrated damage of the dorsolateral mesopontine tegmentum and bilateral amygdala. It should be noted that RBD has also been described in other autoimmune disorders such as narcolepsy [50], multiple sclerosis [51], Morvan's syndrome [52] and idiopathic potassium channel antibody-associated limbic encephalitis due to ILGI1 antibodies [53], the latter associated with direct damage of the limbic system and no apparent primary brainstem impairment. It may be speculated that in RBD, limbic system dysfunction contributes to development of the characteristic frightening dreams and brainstem dysfunction to lack of muscle atonia and dream-enacting behaviours during REM sleep. A patient with systemic lymphoma presented with subacute confusional state. The patient's sleep was disturbed by hallucinatory experiences, increased motor activity, violent purposeful movements and vocalisations. Diagnosis of RBD was only presumed because polysomnography was not performed. Brain MRI was normal. The presence of anti-Ma2 and anti-voltage-gated potassium channel antibodies was not evaluated in this case [54].

RBD is also described in subjects with limbic encephalitis associated with voltage-gated potassium channel-complex antibodies against the leucine-rich, glioma inactivated protein (LGI1) that are associated with adenocarcinoma of the colon and prostate, and melanoma [49,55].

Table 23.2 Studies reporting excessive daytime sleepiness in patients with paraneoplastic anti-Ma2 encephalitis.

Author and reference number	EDS (n)	Cataplexy (n)	HLA DR2	PSG	MSLT	MRI hypothalamic lesion	CSF hypocretin (pg/ml)
Overeem et al. [35]	4 of 6	Unknown	ND	ND	ND	No	Low in four with EDS (<100) and normal in two without EDS (218, 237)
Blumenthal et al. [34]	1	NR	ND	ND	ND	No	Undetectable
Dalmau et al. [33]	12 of 38[a]	2	ND	ND	ND	No	Low in five with EDS. Not reported in the remaining seven with EDS[a]
Hoffmann et al. [36]	4 of 22	NR	ND	ND	ND	NR	ND
Landolfi et al. [37]	1	Yes	Neg	SE = 44%	SL = 9 min SOREMP = 2	No	ND
Rojas-Marcos et al. [38]	1	No	ND	ND	ND	Yes	58 (low)
Compta et al. [21]	1	No	Neg	SE = 48%	SL = 7 min SOREMP = 4 RBD	No	49 (low)
Sahashi et al. [39]	1	NR	ND	ND	ND	Yes	ND
Bennet et al. [40]	1 of 2	NR	ND	ND	ND	Yes	ND
Waragai et al. [41]	1	NR	ND	ND	ND	No	ND
Adams et al. [45]	1	Yes	ND	Disrupted sleep architecture RBD	SL = 2 min SOREM = 3	No	ND
Dauvilliers et al. [46]	1	Yes	ND	Reduced SE RBD	SL = 7 min SOREMP = 2	Yes	Undetectable

[a] Dalmau et al. article [33] includes the patient reported by Blumenthal et al. [34] and the six patients reported by Overeem et al. [35].
CSF, cerebrospinal fluid; EDS, excessive daytime sleepiness; MSLT, Multiple Sleep Latency Test; ND, not done; Neg, negative; NR, not reported; PSG, polysomnography; RBD, rapid eye movement sleep behaviour disorder; SE, sleep efficiency; SL, sleep latency; SOREMP, sleep onset rapid eye movement periods.

Sleep-disordered Breathing

Central hypoventilation has been described in patients with anti-Hu [56–59], anti-NMDA receptor encephalitis [47,48], and anti-Ri antibody associated paraneoplastic brainstem syndrome [60].

Of 22 patients with anti-Hu-associated pure brainstem encephalitis, central alveolar hypoventilation occurred in five with isolated medulla involvement who also exhibited other bulbar symptoms such as dysphagia, dysphonia and dysarthria [55–58]. The clinical course was rapidly progressive and required orotracheal intubation with immediate mechanical ventilation for a few days after admission because of subacute respiratory failure. Respiratory failure was the problem that led to admission in all cases. During wakefulness patients exhibited dyspnoea but could breath spontaneously while central apnoeas occurred during sleep due to failure of automatic respiration (Ondine's curse). Underlying malignancies were prostate adenocarcinoma, small cell lung cancer and kidney cancer. Prognosis was usually poor.

Central hypoventilation is a common finding in young women with ovarian teratoma and anti-NMDA receptor encephalitis. In a recent series of 100 patients with anti-NMDA receptor encephalitis, central hypoventilation occurred in 66 [48]. Central hypoventilation is usually severe requiring mechanical support for a few weeks or many months [48,61]. Of interest, knockout animals of the NR1 subunit of the NMDA receptor die of hypoventilation [62]. Patients typically present with hallucinations, delusions, seizures, short-term memory loss, movement disorders, and decreased level of consciousness. Brain MRI is normal or shows abnormalities in the mesial temporal lobes, basal ganglia and brainstem [47]. Autopsies reveal extensive microgliosis, rare T-cell infiltrates and neuronal degeneration in the hippocampus and other regions including the brainstem [47]. Most patients recover after tumour removal and immunotherapy.

Ondine's curse, failure of autonomic respiration when asleep and normal respiration while awake, was described in a 54-year-old woman with breast cancer and anti-Ri antibodies. She had horizontal gaze palsy and recurrent episodes of oxygen desaturation and carbon dioxide retention during sleep needing mechanical ventilation due to persistent respiratory failure episodes during sleep [60].

Insomnia

Insomnia may occur in the acute phase of anti-NMDA receptor encephalitis in association with psychiatric symptoms [48]. However, insomnia is a cardinal characteristic feature of Morvan's syndrome accompanied by encephalopathy, dysautonomia and neuromyotonia. Morvan's syndrome is linked to autoantibodies reactive against the voltage-gated potassium channel complex and malignant thymoma. Polysomnography shows so-called 'agrypnia excitata' that is characterised by the absence of a recognisable sleep pattern or brief fragments of sleep-theta activity and REM sleep without atonia in association with increased motor activity, especially general agitation and complex semi-purposeful activities [55]. This pattern has to be distinguished from a similar phenomenon that occurs in fatal familial insomnia and the Iglon5 syndrome, two non-paraneoplastic conditions [63,64].

Key Points

- When studied systematically, it is clear that cancer patients frequently have severe but potentially reversible sleep-related problems in both early and late disease.
- Evidence is accumulating that improving sleep in cancer patients may have a direct positive effect on cancer prognosis.
- Brain tumours, most commonly in the region of the hypothalamus such as childhood craniopharyngioma, may cause sleep-related symptoms closely resembling narcolepsy, occasionally with hypocretin deficiency and associated cataplexy.
- Profound insomnia may occur in the context of paraneoplastic syndromes, particularly those that involve anti-NMDA and anti-voltage-gated potassium channel antibodies.
- Excessive sleepiness, resembling narcolepsy, is most commonly associated with anti-Ma2 encephalitis, a syndrome usually seen in testicular cancer.
- Severe nocturnal central hypoventilation, resembling Ondine's curse, can be seen in several paraneoplastic syndromes, especially those involving anti-NMDA, anti-Hu and anti-Ri antibodies.

References

1 Sateia MJ. Sleep in patients with cancer and HIV/AIDS. In: Sleep Medicine. Lee-Chiong TL, Satela MJ, Carskadon MA (eds). Hanley and Belfus, Philadelphia, 2002;489–496.

2 Savard J, Savard MH, Anconi-Israel S. Sleep and fatigue in cancer patients. In: Principles and Practice of Sleep Medicine, 6th edn. Kryger MH, Roth T, Dement WC (eds). Elsevier, Philadelphia, 2017;1286–1293.

3 Davidson JR, Maclean AW, Brundage MD, Schulze K. Sleep disturbance in cancer patients. *Soc Sci Med* 2002;54:1309–1321.

4 Mystakodou K, Parapa E, Tsilika E, et al. How is sleep quality affected by the psychological and symptom distress of advanced cancer patients? *Palliat Med* 2009;23:46–53.

5 Mercadante S, Girelli D, Cassucio A. Sleep disorders in advanced cancer patients: prevalence and factors associated. *Support Care Cancer* 2004;12:355–359.

6 Savard J, Ivers-H, Villa J, et al. Natural course of insomnia comorbid with cancer: an 18-month longitudinal study. *J Clin Oncol* 2011;29:3850–3856.

7 Palesh OG, Peppone L, Innominato PF, et al. Prevalence, putative mechanisms. And current management of current problems during chemotherapy for cancer. *Nat Sci Sleep* 2012;4:151–154.

8 Parker KP, Bliwise D, Ribeiro M, et al. Sleep/wake patterns of individuals with advanced cancer measured by ambulatory polysomnography. *J Clin Oncol* 2008;26:2464–2472.

9 Gozal D, Farré R, Nieto FJ. Obstructive sleep apnea and cancer: epidemiologic links and theoretical biological constructs. *Sleep Med Rev* 2016;27:43–55.

10 Aldrich MS, Naylor MW. Narcolepsy associated with lesions of the diencephalon. *Neurology* 1989;39:1505–1508.

11 Autret A, Lucas B, Henry-Lebras F, Toffol B. Symptomatic narcolepsies. *Sleep* 1994;17:S21–S24.

12 Malik S, Boeve BF, Krahn LE, Silber MH. Narcolepsy associated with other central nervous system disorders. *Neurology* 2001;57:539–541.

13 Snow A, Gozal E, Malhotra A, et al. Severe hypersomnolence after pituitary/ hypothalamic surgery in adolescents: clinical characteristics and potential mechanisms. *Pediatrics* 2002;110(6):e74.

14 Marcus CL, Trescher WH, Halbower AC, Lutz J. Secondary narcolepsy in children with brain tumors. *Sleep* 2002;25:435–439.

15 Nishino S, Kanbayashi T. Symptomatic narcolepsy, cataplexy and EDS, and their implications in the hypothalamic hypocretin/orexin system. *Sleep Med Rev* 2005;9:269–310.

16 Rosen G. Sleep and wakefulness in children with brain tumors. In: Sleep Medicine Clinics. Neurological Disorders and Sleep. Silber MH (ed.). Elsevier, New York, 2008;3(3): 455–-468.

17 Malik S, Boeve BF, Krahn LE, Silber MH. Narcolepsy associated with other central nervous system disorders. *Neurology* 2001;57:539–541.

18 Dauvilliers Y, Abril B, Charif M, et al. Reversal of symptomatic tumoral narcolepsy, with normalization of CSF hypocretin level. *Neurology* 2007;69:1300–1301.

19 Scammell TE, Nishino S, Mignot E, Saper CB. Narcolepsy and low CSF orexin (hypocretin) concentration after a diencephalic stroke. *Neurology* 2001;56:1751–1753.

20 Arii J, Kanabayashi T, Tanabe Y, et al. A hypersomnolient girl with decreased CSF hypocretin level after removal of a hypothalamic tumor. *Neurology* 2001;56:1775–1776.

21 Compta Y, Iranzo A, Santamaria J, et al. REM sleep behavior disorder and narcolpetic features in anti-Ma2 encephalitis. *Sleep* 2007;30:767–769.

22 Tachibana N, Taniike M, Okinaga T, et al. Hypersomnolence and increased REM sleep with low cerebrospinal fluid hypocretin level in a patient after removal of craniopharyngioma. *Sleep Med* 2005;6:567–569.

23 Smith T. Cataplexy in association with meningiomas. *Acta Neurol Scand (Suppl.)* 1983;94:45–47.

24 D' Cruz O, Vaughn B, Gold S. Symptomatic cataplexy in pontomedullary lesions. *Neurology* 1994;44:2189–1291.

25 Stahl SM, Layzer RB, Aminoff MJ, et al. Continuous cataplexy in a patient with a midbrain tumor: The limp man syndrome. *Neurology* 1980;30:1115–1118.

26 Boeve BF, Silber MH, Saper CB, et al. Pathophysiology of REM sleep behaviour disorder and relevance to neurodegenerative disease. *Brain* 2007;130:2770–2788.

27 Iranzo A, Aparicio J. A lesson from anatomy: focal brain lesions causing REM sleep behavior disorder. *Sleep Med* 2009;10(1);9–12.

28 Zambelis T, Paparrigopoulos T, Soldatos CR. REM sleep behaviour disorder associated with a neurinoma of the left pontocerebellar angle. *J Neurol Neurosurg Psychiatry* 2002;72:821–822.

29 McCarter SJ, Tippmann-Peikert M, Sadness DJ, et al. Neuroimaging evident lesional pathology associated with REM sleep behavior disorder. *Sleep* 2015;16:1502–1510.

30 Jianhua C, Xiuquin L, Quancai C, et al. Rapid eye movement sleep behavior disorder in a patient with brainstem lymphoma. *Intern Med* 2013;52:617–621.

31 Höftenberfg R, Rosenfeld M, Dalmau J. Update on neurological paraneoplastic syndromes. *Curr Opin Oncol* 2015;27:489–495.

32 Silber MH. Autoimmune sleep disorders. *Handb Clin Neurol* 2016;133:317–326.

33 Dalmau J, Graus F, Villarejo A, et al. Clinical analysis of anti-Ma2-associated encephalitis. *Brain* 2004;127:1831–1844.

34 Blumenthal DT, Salzman KL, Digre KB, et al. Early pathologic findings and long-term improvement in anti-Ma2-associated encephalitis. *Neurology* 2006;67:146–149.

35 Overeem S, Dalmau J, Bataller L, et al. Hypocretin-1 CSF levels in anti-Ma2 associated encephalitis. *Neurology* 2004;62:138–140.

36 Hoffmann LA, Jarious S, Pellkofer HL, et al. Anti-Ma and anti-Ta associated paraneoplastic neurological syndromes: 22 newly diagnosed patients and review of previous cases. *J Neurol Neurosurg Psychiatry* 2008;79:767–773.

37 Landolfi JC, Nadkarni M. Paraneoplastic limbic encephalitis and possible narcolepsy in a patient with testicular cancer: Case study. *Neuro-Oncology* 2003;5:214–216.

38 Rojas-Marcos I, Graus F, Sanz G, et al. Hypersomnia as presenting symptom of anti-Ma2-associated encephalitis: Case study. *Neuro-Oncology* 2007;9:75–77.

39 Sahashi K, Sakai K, Mano K, Hirose G. Anti-Ma2 related paraneoplastic limbic/brain stem encephalitis associated with breast cancer expressing Ma1, Ma2, and Ma3 mRNAs. *J Neurol Neurosurg Psychiatry* 2003;74:1332–1335.

40 Bennet JL, Galetta SL, Frohman LP, et al. Neuro-opthalamic manifestations of a paraneoplastic syndrome and testicular carcinoma. *Neurology* 1999;52:864–867.

41 Waragai M, Chiba A, Uchibori A, et al. Anti-Ma2 associated paarneoplastic neurological syndrome presenting as encephalitis and progressive muscular atrophy. *J Neurol Neurosurg Psychiatry* 2006;77:111–113.

42 Scheid R, Voltz R, Guthke T, et al. Neuropsychiatric findings in anti-Ma2-positive paraneoplastic limbic encephalitis. *Neurology* 2003;61:1159–1160.

43 Sutton I, Winner J, Rowlands D, Dalmau J. Limbic encephalitis and antibodies to Ma2: a paraneoplastic presentation of breast cancer. *J Neurol Neurosurg Psychiatry* 2000;69:266–268.

44 Barnett M, Prosser J, Sutton I, et al. Paraneoplastic brain stem encephalitis in a woman with anti-Ma2 antibody. *J Neurol Neurosurg Psychiatry* 2001;70:222–225.

45 Adams C, McKeon A, Silber MH, Kumar R. Narcolepsy, REM sleep behavior disorder, and supranuclear gaze palsy associated with Ma1 and Ma2 antibodies and tonsillar carcinoma. *Arch Neurol* 2011;68:521–524

46 Dauvilliers Y, Bauer J, Rigau V. Hypothalamic immunopathology in anti-Ma-associated diencephalitis with narcolepsy-cataplexy. Hypothalamic immunopathology in anti-Ma-associated diencephalitis with narcolepsy-cataplexy. *JAMA Neurol* 2013;70:1305–1310.

47 Vitaliani R, Mason W, Ances B, et al. Paraneoplastic encephalitis, psychiatric symptoms and hypoventilation in ovarian teratoma. *Ann Neurol* 2005;58:594–604.

48 Dalmau J, Gleichman AJ, Hughes EG, et al. Anti-NMDA-receptor encephalitis: case series and analysis of the effects of antibodies. *Lancet Neurol* 2008;7:1091–1098.

49 Irani SR, Alexander S, Waters P, et al. Antibodies to Kv1 potassium channel-complex proteins leucine-rich, glioma inactivated 1 protein and contactin-associated protein-2 in limbic encephalitis, Morvan's syndrome and acquired neuromyotonia. *Brain* 2010;133:2734–2748.

50 Schenck CH, Mahowald MW. Motor dyscontrol in narcolepsy: Rapid-eye-movement (REM) sleep without atonia and REM sleep behavior disorder. *Ann Neurol* 1992;32:3–10.

51 Gomez-Choco M, Iranzo A, Blanco Y, et al. Prevalence of restless legs syndrome and REM sleep behavior disorder in multiple sclerosis. *Multiple Sclerosis* 2007; 13:805–808.

52 Josephs KA, Silber MH, Fealey RD, et al. Neurophysiologic studies in Morvan syndrome. *J Clin Neurophysiol* 2004;21:440–445.

53 Iranzo A, Graus F, Clover L, et al. Rapid eye movement sleep behavior disorder and potassium channel antibody–associated limbic encephalitis. *Ann Neurol* 2006;59:178–182.

54 Mocellin R, Velakoulis D, Gonzales M, et al. Weight loss, falls, and neuropsychiatric symptoms in a 56-year-old man. *Lancet Neurol* 2005;4:381–388.

55 Cornellius JR, Pittock SJ, McKeom A, et al. Sleep manifestations of voltage-gated potassium channel complex autoimmunity. *Arch Neurol* 2011;68:733–738.

56 Ball JA, Warner T, Reid P, et al. Central alveolar hypoventilation associated with paraneoplastic brain-stem encephalitis and anti-Hu antibodies. *J Neurol* 1994;241:561–566.

57 Lee KS, Higgins MJ, Patel MB, et al. Paraneoplastic coma and acquired central alveolar hypoventilation as a manifestation of brainstem encephalitis in a patient with ANNA-I antibody and small-cell lung cancer. *Neurocrit Care* 2006;4:137–139.

58 Gómez-Choco MJ, Zarranz JJ, Saiz A, et al. Central hypoventilation as the presenting symptom in Hu associated paraneoplastic encephalomyelitis. *J Neurol Neurosurg Psychiatry* 2007;78:1143–1145.

59 Saiz A, Bruna J, Stourac P, et al. Anti-Hu-associated brainstem encephalitis. *J Neurol Neurosurg Psychiatry* 2009;80:404–407.

60 Kim KJ, Yun JY, Lee JY, et al. Ondine's curse in anti-Ri antibody associated paraneoplastic brainstem syndrome. *Sleep Med* 2013;14:382.

61 Iizuka T, Sakai F, Ide T, et al. Anti-NMDA receptor encephalitis in Japan. Long-term outcome without tumor removal. *Neurology* 2008;70:504–511.

62 Forrest D, Yuzaki M, Soares HD, et al. Targeted disruption of the NMDA receptor 1 gene abolishes NMDA response and results in neuronal death. *Neuron* 1994;13:325–338.

63 Sabater L, Gaig C, Gelpi E, et al. A novel non-rapid-eye movement and rapid-eye-movement parasomnia with sleep breathing disorder associated with antibodies to IgLON5: a case series, characterisation of the antigen, and post-mortem study. *Lancet Neurol* 2014 13:575–586.

64 Högl B, Heidbreder A, Santamaria J, et al. IgLON5 autoimmunity and abnormal behaviours during sleep. *Lancet* 2015;385:1590.

Index

Locators in *italic* refer to figures; those in **bold** to tables

Sleep Disorders in Neurology: A Practical Approach, Second Edition.
Edited by Sebastiaan Overeem and Paul Reading.
© 2018 John Wiley & Sons Ltd. Published 2018 by John Wiley & Sons Ltd.